Getting Pregnant with PCOS

An evidence-based approach to treat the root causes
of polycystic ovary syndrome and boost your fertility

Clare Goodwin
Registered Nutritionist

To all the incredible women who have entrusted me to help them understand their bodies. I'm eternally grateful to you. x

Designed by Kate Barraclough
Printed and bound in Australia by Ovato Print
First published in 2020 through Point Publishing Limited, Auckland

www.the pcosnutritionist.com

978-0-473-53860-6 (paperback)
978-0-473-53861-3 (epub)
978-0-473-53862-0 (Kindle)
978-0-473-54662-5 (audiobook)

Contents

About the author

Clare Goodwin is a Registered Nutritionist, with a first-class honors degree in Exercise Prescription from the University of Otago, New Zealand. She has trained in Functional Medicine (an individualized approach to medicine with a focus on root causes) through the Kresser Institute, and is a certified trained teacher in Natural Fertility Education through Dr. Kerry Hampton, researcher and lecturer at Monash University, Australia.

A competitive multisport athlete, Clare was diagnosed with PCOS and insulin resistance in her mid-twenties, having just retired from international athletics and triathlon competition, and was told she wouldn't be able to have children. Determined not to accept this fate, Clare kept researching, learning, and seeking out specialists to find the lifestyle changes which could help her reverse her symptoms.

After finding what worked for her, Clare started working with other women with PCOS, both one-to-one and in a group program. Clare's *PCOS Protocol*, a 12-week supported online e-learning program for all women with PCOS, has helped over 2,000 women understand what's driving their hormonal imbalance. This is important for understanding all PCOS symptoms, as well as helping women to not just get pregnant but also have a healthy pregnancy and a healthy baby.

Introduction

THE PCOS DIAGNOSIS—A PERSONAL EXPERIENCE

I was diagnosed with polycystic ovary syndrome (PCOS) when I was 25 years old. I'd just finished university and was working for a tech company in my first graduate role. I was still having to deal with acne, even though I thought I would have grown out of it by my mid-twenties. Trying to be taken seriously at meetings with the GM while worrying about whether my makeup really was covering the pimple that had just erupted on my chin wasn't the best recipe for a calm, confident demeanor.

I had the loveliest doctor, who could probably tell from that first meeting that PCOS was the culprit. She ran some blood work, including testosterone and glucose levels, and two days later I got a call to come in to see her again. In New Zealand, where I live, you only get a callback if your blood work is abnormal, so I knew something was up. I sat down and was told I had PCOS. She explained that this was why I was struggling to lose weight, why my periods were irregular, and why I was still getting acne. She then explained the other consequence of PCOS: "You're going to struggle to conceive."

I was devastated. I walked out to my car, put my head on the steering wheel, and wailed. While I didn't want to get pregnant right then, I certainly wanted children in my future. Feeling like that dream had been taken away from me was devastating. My mind raced forward a few years when all my friends would be happily popping babies out, while *I* dealt with infertility.

The next day, I went to the bank and opened up an account to start saving for IVF.

Like many of you will have experienced, this wasn't the first time I'd thought my symptoms weren't typical or visited the doctor. But this was the first time that someone had been able to put it all together for me.

I'd just finished five years at university, doing a joint honors degree in Exercise Prescription (more well known now as exercise physiology) and nutrition. I'd also just retired as a competitive athlete, having spent the previous 10 years racing for New Zealand in athletics (track) and cross-country, and then later triathlon when running injuries got the better of me. Although retired from international racing, I was now aiming to compete in one of the world's longest multisport events, the arduous Coast to Coast Race, involving running, cycling, and kayaking for 151 miles (243 kilometers) from the west coast to the east coast of New Zealand's South Island, over the Southern Alps. While no longer training 17 to 20 hours a week (that wasn't conducive to working 50-plus hours a week in one of the top graduate programs), I was still doing 12 hours every week minimum. So I was no slob.

I had all the hallmarks of PCOS: I hadn't had a period for about three years, my weight was going up and up (but only accumulating around my stomach), and I had acne. I'd visited the student campus doctor many times about these separate issues, but the picture had never been put together from all its separate parts. Instead, I was given a low-grade antibiotic for the acne and told that the missing periods were due to my being a competitive athlete. I was prescribed hormonal birth control to "regulate" my periods and was told to "eat less" and exercise more to control my weight.

The problem was that I knew too much to accept this diagnosis. My honors thesis was on female athletes with eating disorders (how ironic), and the research supported that the main reason why athletes lose their period is due to low bodyweight—which didn't fit my situation because I was gaining about 10 lb (5 kg) per year.

After five years of training in nutrition and exercise science, I was severely disappointed that weight gain or weight loss was merely being put down to calories. It went like this: If you were eating more than you burned (calorie surplus), you would put on weight; if you were eating less (calorie deficit), you'd lose weight. But I knew I wasn't in calorie surplus.

Every weekday I'd get up and swim for an hour of high-intensity interval training (HIIT), followed by lectures and labs, and then either a run or a bike ride for one to two hours in the evening. At the weekend I did a four-hour swim and some bike fun on Saturday, and a three-hour bike ride on Sunday. On average, I was training for 17 hours a week and burning 300 to 400 calories an hour. The average female needs 1,800 calories (kcal) a day to maintain weight, without exercise, and I was burning an extra 800 to 1,500 a day. In theory, I would have needed to eat 3,000 to 3,300 kcal to put on weight. Have you ever tried eating 3,300 kcal a day? It's a LOT! It would be the equivalent of my usual day of food—muesli, apple, and yogurt for breakfast; pumpkin soup and two slices of toast for lunch; roast chicken and vegetables for dinner; two bottles of sports drink, two crackers with cheese mid-morning; and a yogurt and apple in the evening—PLUS five Krispy Creme donuts, a cheeseburger, and two KFC drumsticks. Spoiler alert: I wasn't doing this. I was meticulously tracking everything I ate and burned and should have been in calorie deficit.

I'm talking about weight gain here because this was one of my symptoms with PCOS. But it may not be the same for you. In this book, you'll learn that weight gain is almost irrelevant, and that even if you are "lean," lifestyle changes can be very effective.

Blood sugar and cravings

When I was diagnosed with PCOS, my doctor also tested my blood glucose and diagnosed insulin resistance (i.e. pre-diabetes). I was stunned. I'd just spent five years learning that pre-diabetes and type 2 diabetes could be avoided if you followed a healthy diet and did enough exercise. Here I was, the "healthiest" person I knew, staring down the barrel of chronic disease. It was a cruel blow. If I couldn't ward off type 2 diabetes while doing a huge amount of exercise, what hope did anyone else have?

Although, according to the food pyramid, I was eating "healthily," I was also having severe sugar cravings and "hangry" attacks. For anyone who gets hangry, you know what I mean. It's the kind of hunger that comes on suddenly, approximately two hours after your last meal, and if you don't eat something in the next half-hour you're in danger of biting someone's hand off. I understand now that this wasn't *just me*—it was a red flag that my insulin wasn't working correctly.

My sugar cravings were another red flag. Come 3 p.m., sugar was all I could think about. I even restructured my day to have meetings in the afternoon, to distract me from the intensity of needing sugar; otherwise, I would inevitably end up at the vending machine. The same thing would happen after dinner. I'd be eating my meal, but my mind would be 100 percent on what sugary treat I'd have afterward.

I knew this wasn't good; I hadn't spent five years learning that a chocolate bar a day is healthy. But my craving for sugar was so intense that I couldn't stay away from it. It was mortifying. I knew all this information, and yet I couldn't stop myself. The real kicker happened one day at work—I'd just got back to my desk after a trip to the vending machine, when my colleague Brenda said to me, "For a nutritionist, you sure eat a lot of sugar." She was right, and I knew it. But I didn't know how to stop it.

THE REAL PICTURE—PCOS IN OUR MEDICAL SYSTEM

In the aftermath of my PCOS diagnosis, I had mixed feelings. I was relieved to finally have an answer to my symptoms, but also devastated that there was something "wrong" with me. I felt like a victim with no control over the situation. I didn't really know what PCOS was, but it sounded serious—like I had pre-cancerous growths on my ovaries. I felt completely helpless because I couldn't get in there and get rid of them.

Even though I had a lovely doctor who'd finally been able to piece together the real picture of my health, she didn't have enough knowledge to be able to explain what was really driving my PCOS. I now know that my high insulin levels were actually causing a hormonal imbalance, and this was stopping me from ovulating. No egg equals no baby, so hello fertility issues. But it didn't mean that I'd never ovulated or never would again. I now know that if I could address the root cause (my high insulin and stress hormones), by changing my diet and exercise routine, and by focusing on reducing stress and increasing sleep, then I could improve the hormone imbalance and ovulate again.

What was true for me is also the case for almost all women with PCOS. I've witnessed time and time again that if we can find the root cause and tweak a few lifestyle factors, most women can conceive. The reason that many women with PCOS haven't been offered the information they need to do this is that often their doctor simply doesn't know.

Our medical system is incredible at treating acute and life-threatening conditions. If I got hit by a bus or fell off a cliff while skiing, there isn't anywhere I'd want to be but the hospital. Medics know how to diagnose thousands of conditions from the few vague symptoms we give them; how to work the end of a scalpel like a pro; and all the ins and outs of what medication to use for what symptoms (and have pharmacists to back them up here).

But when it comes to chronic conditions like PCOS, it can all get a bit unstuck. There isn't a surgical procedure or a pill that can simply "fix" it, and the correct tests often don't get carried out. We get pinballed from one medication to the next to alleviate our symptoms, but none of these really address the root cause. Despite extensive research showing that lifestyle interventions are as effective, if not more so, than medication, it's the medication that seems to always be the answer.

The most recent (2018) international evidence-based guidelines for PCOS state that "Lifestyle intervention (preferably multicomponent including diet, exercise, and behavioral strategies) should be recommended in all those with PCOS." [1] But when physicians get little nutrition education in their medical training, how can they be expected to know all of the specifics for PCOS? Not just the different vitamin and mineral requirements, but also the various forms of exercise, sleep, and stress management that help those with PCOS. Asking your doctor how to eat, sleep, and move to improve your PCOS symptoms is like asking your carpenter to install plumbing for your shower. Your carpenter will have an idea how to do it because they work with plumbing contractors all the time. However, plumbers have a training program that's independent of carpentry for a reason: It's specialized work that requires a specific set of skills.

CASE STUDY

As well as suffering from PCOS, Danah is a doctor. I got to know her as she went through my *PCOS Protocol* program. Danah had struggled for years with an ever-expanding waistline, irregular periods, and thinning hair, and then, in her late twenties, she developed acne. She joined me on my podcast to tell her story and explain to other women with PCOS why doctors might not be able to offer them the best advice.

Because of her medical training, Danah had thought that she would be able to figure out what was happening with her body and how to fix it, but she was none the wiser. There was very little education on PCOS in her course, and what she did get taught was just the standard treatment of symptoms: hormonal birth control, lose 5 percent of bodyweight, and take medications like antibiotics for acne, spironolactone, and metformin. The only additional training occurred during her gynecological rotation, where the students would examine women with PCOS. However, there was no training in precisely what lifestyle modifications would work—so she couldn't fix her own symptoms, let alone really help her patients.

Danah felt she had tried everything. She was paying to see a personal trainer a few times a week and was getting zero results. She tried the very, very low-carb keto diet, and only lost an ounce (30 grams) of weight, felt like hot trash, and had brain fog. She tried consulting dieticians and eating low-calorie food, and every exercise that Google said would help her lose belly fat, but with no success. Like me, she also had the most unbearable sugar cravings.

"I knew better than to be eating sugar, but come mid-afternoon I just had to pray I didn't pass a shop or vending machine, as I knew self-control wouldn't be enough to overcome the cravings. I also felt like such a hypocrite—here I was, a doctor, telling my patients to lose weight and reduce sugar intake while I was overweight and eating candy and chocolate every day. Up until this point I felt like PCOS was my fault because the only advice I'd been given was to lose weight, and I thought that I'd gained weight through lack of self-control."

When Danah contacted me, we figured out that her insulin wasn't functioning correctly—even though it was within the "normal" medical reference ranges. The insulin issue came as a surprise to Danah, and while she wasn't trying to conceive, with her irregular periods she would have found this problematic if she was.

"As a doctor, I knew about the connection between PCOS and insulin, and I'd ordered labs (blood tests)—and everything looked in range, including my insulin. I even took my results to my gynecologist, who said 'You're not diabetic, you're not even pre-diabetic. There is nothing to worry about with your insulin.' However, while Danah wasn't pre-diabetic, her insulin certainly wasn't functioning optimally, and (as you'll find out in Chapter 6), this is the important thing—not whether you're clinically pre-diabetic or not.

Once Danah changed her lifestyle to improve her insulin function, everything started to fall into place. Within eight months she'd lost almost 30 lb (14 kg) and 6 inches (15 cm) off her waist. Her blood markers for insulin improved, and she lowered her HbA1c (a measure of blood sugar) to the optimal range. Her acne cleared up, her periods became regular, and her hair loss was a lot less. She also noticed improvements in areas that she didn't think were connected:

"I can see now that I was really just existing, getting through the 24 hours and completely dependent on coffee. I wasn't sleeping well and was unhappy and very irritable. I am much, much happier now!"

Danah's story may strike a chord with many of you: irregular cycles, weight gain, cravings, fatigue, and acne. She was following the standard

PCOS guidelines to just "eat well and exercise," and yet it wasn't helping. In fact, her symptoms were getting worse. This is where the research falls short for any medical professionals wanting to know how to improve PCOS via lifestyle changes. Those same 2018 international evidence-based guidelines I mentioned before state that "General healthy eating principles should be followed for all women with PCOS across the life course, as per general population recommendations." I think that I, you, and Danah would all agree: "general guidelines" don't work. If they did, you wouldn't be reading this book, searching for answers.

So why is there such an incredibly small amount of research on lifestyle treatments for PCOS, even though this is recommended for all women with the syndrome? A major reason is that research studies are expensive to conduct, and when a lifestyle treatment can't be patented, then companies can't make money out of it. It ends up being left up to public funding, which is tiny and has many demands on it, so PCOS research can get only a minuscule amount of it. This is where having many years of experience working with thousands of women with PCOS is helpful. I've been able to use the existing research and an understanding of how our body and hormones work, along with real-life clinical experience to figure out what lifestyle changes are most effective. No single human can know everything about every condition, which is why I work only with PCOS. I'm not trying to be an expert in PCOS, and an expert in sports nutrition working with elite athletes, and an expert in pediatric nutrition—that's just too much information for one person to know. So I encourage you to have on your team both your doctor AND someone else who specializes in a lifestyle approach to PCOS.

ABOUT THE FERTILE INGREDIENTS

When it comes to getting pregnant and staying pregnant, what you need is what I call your "fertile ingredients," because baking a baby is like baking a cake:

- ✓ An egg and sperm of good quality (quality ingredients) . . .
- ✓ that meet in the fallopian tubes (timing).

✓ A uterine lining to act as a safe nest for your fertilized egg, without collapsing (cake mold).

In PCOS we can have issues with each of these steps:

✗ The egg can be exposed to high levels of androgen hormones (testosterone) and insulin, and can therefore be of poor quality (not to mention the quality of your partner's sperm).

✗ You may not be ovulating, or, more likely, you are ovulating at irregular times and you don't know when so can't time sex correctly.

✗ Your hormones, especially progesterone, are not at the right levels to hold your uterine lining in place long enough for your egg to burrow in, or to make it to 12 weeks when the fetus starts producing its own progesterone.

The great news is that nothing here is irreversible. But it does require a professional to find out which parts of the process are not working correctly. They then, crucially, also need to know precisely how you can change your lifestyle to fix it. Then, if you need them, you will have many medical fertility treatments available to you to assist conception.

If you've been trying to conceive without success, I can only imagine how hard this is for you. Most of us love being organized and in control. We love planning for the next step in our career, the next step in our lives. But fertility is the one thing that feels totally out of our control. Every month you wait for those excruciating weeks, only to see a negative pregnancy test or feel the telltale signs of a period on its way. It feels like everyone around you is getting pregnant. This won't be accurate, but it feels like it. It feels exponentially unfair.

Having PCOS and going through fertility challenges makes you feel like your body is broken—like your body is failing, that it doesn't know how to do its job correctly. In turn, this can affect your feelings of self-worth and make you feel less of a woman. But none of this is true.

You aren't broken. Your body isn't failing you. And you're certainly no less of a woman.

The messenger system (your hormones) that tells your body when to ovulate has just gotten a little confused. But when you understand why your hormones become confused, i.e. the root cause, you can fix this and help them to communicate normally again. This is precisely what I want to share with you in this book.

WHAT'S IN THIS BOOK

We'll begin by exploring PCOS and the problems around it:

- What PCOS is, why hormone imbalance can affect all three of your fertile ingredients, and what the most common causes of those are.
- Why just being told to lose weight to improve your fertility is useless advice.
- The current fertility treatments, how they work, and the risks.

Next, we'll cover off my five-step plan to help you conceive:

- How to find out which of your fertile ingredients isn't working for you at the moment. This is what we call the "root cause." Then we'll focus on the most important factors to help you address that root cause, as follows.
- How to optimize your diet for *you*. There is no single PCOS diet, and therefore there isn't a single list of foods you should and should not eat. Optimizing your diet involves understanding your root cause and how different foods affect that.
- How to address stress. Stress can come in many forms, from psychological stress to over-exercising, undersleeping, and just plain doing too much.
- How to chart your cycle. You can only get pregnant about four to six days per cycle. Learn to use your body temperature and cervical fluid to ensure you're catching these precious days.
- How to use nutrients and herbs to improve your root cause.

Finally, we'll do some troubleshooting:

- What to do if you're still not pregnant after six months to a year of doing everything in the five-step plan. This includes issues such as endometriosis, genetics, and the male factor.

- Once you do get pregnant, how to reduce your risk of PCOS-related pregnancy complications.

- And, if you're not looking to conceive right now but want to in the future, or you want to check that everything is working correctly (which is crucial for your health), then massive kudos to you, and I'll show you how to protect your fertility.

I strongly encourage every woman with PCOS to read this book, because being fertile isn't just about getting pregnant—it's also about your health! If your insulin is high so you're not ovulating, then you're also going to be at risk of developing type 2 diabetes. If your eggs aren't forming correctly because your body is chronically inflamed, then your immune system is going to be compromised. If you are so chronically stressed that your uterine lining is collapsing before your body has time to bake that baby properly, then that stress is also going to be breaking down other cells in your body. If you're not ovulating regularly because your hormone levels are too high to allow the egg to be released, then you're more likely to develop osteoporosis later in life, because your body needs to ovulate to maintain bone density.

You'll learn in this book that there is always a reason, a root cause, for why the steps in the process of conceiving aren't working correctly—and how to fix them. So let's go on and improve your health, your PCOS, and your fertility!

UNDERSTANDING PCOS AND HOW IT AFFECTS FERTILITY

Chapter 1
What is PCOS?

PCOS is a syndrome rather than a disease, like irritable bowel syndrome (IBS), chronic fatigue syndrome (CFS), and premenstrual tension syndrome (PMS). Notice anything about those syndromes? Well,

- the names really just describe the symptoms, and
- if you've ever had any of them, you'll know that there's not much your doctor can really do to help.

None of these syndromes has a single medication or surgical procedure that will relieve the symptoms, because for each patient the root cause can be very different. For example, one patient's CFS could be due to a combination of mold toxicity, Lyme disease, subsequent Hashimoto's thyroiditis, and an inadequate intake of vitamins and minerals. Another patient's CFS might be caused by a combination of a parasite infection, adrenal burnout, and poor nutrition.

It is precisely the same for PCOS. Polycystic ovary syndrome is just a name that describes one symptom of PCOS—the "cyst-like appearance" of the ovaries—while other symptoms include irregular periods, and sometimes symptoms of high testosterone or androgens, such as acne, unwanted hair growth, or hair loss. Likewise, the "root cause" of PCOS can be completely different for different patients. For one woman it could be chronically high insulin due to a combination of genetics and not eating food that suits her genetic makeup. For another woman it could be that she's just come off hormonal birth control.

> When you have PCOS, what's on your ovaries isn't actually cysts—it's follicles (baby eggs) that don't "hatch" (ovulate). Instead, they keep growing and form a fluid-filled sac that looks like a cyst. About 25 percent of all women have these cysts on their ovaries (polycystic ovaries), but only 10 percent of women have PCOS (the syndrome).

HOW PCOS IS DIAGNOSED

PCOS is currently diagnosed via the "Rotterdam criteria." You can be diagnosed as having PCOS if you have two out of three of the following:[1]

1. Irregular periods
2. Follicles or "cysts" on your ovaries
3. High levels of androgens (testosterone, androstenedione or DHEA-S) in your blood, or a symptom that would suggest that levels are high such as acne around the chin and jaw, unwanted facial or body hair growth, or hair loss in the "male pattern balding" areas.

I'm not really a fan of these criteria, as their use can lead doctors to over-diagnose PCOS. There are also other conditions (such as hypothalamic amenorrhea or hypothyroidism) that can stop the body ovulating. Both of these conditions can be misdiagnosed as PCOS because they fit two out of the three criteria, but they have different root causes and require different treatments. (There's more information about both hypothalamic amenorrhea and hypothyroidism later in the book.) Conditions such as these are supposed to be ruled out before a diagnosis of PCOS is given,[2] but in my experience this very rarely happens.

Anna and her partner had decided to try for a baby, so she came off hormonal birth control (HBC), aka the pill. Anna wasn't getting her periods and noticed that she had a few chin and nipple hairs. She had a scan that showed she had polycystic ovaries, so because of this and the lack of a period she was diagnosed with PCOS.

However, when I looked at Anna's blood test results I saw that her testosterone was very low—in PCOS it is often high. Plus, her luteinizing hormone (LH) was also low, whereas it is also often high in many cases of PCOS. I suggested to Anna that she get a second opinion from a gynecologist, who diagnosed her with hypothalamic amenorrhea, not PCOS, even though she technically met the diagnostic criteria for PCOS. The new diagnosis completely changed Anna's treatment, and the result was that she had a period and was ovulating within a month of that new treatment.

It's a good idea to check whether you've been correctly diagnosed with PCOS, especially if you've only had a scan. If you don't have many of the other PCOS symptoms, ask for a second opinion to check the diagnosis.

WHAT HAPPENS TO YOUR HORMONES IN PCOS

In PCOS, there is often an increase in the androgen hormones. You've likely heard of testosterone, but few people know that testosterone has two brothers from another mother: DHEA-S (dehydroepiandrosterone sulfate) and androstenedione. These two do the same thing as testosterone but are produced in different areas of the body. DHEA-S is mostly produced in your adrenal (stress) glands, whereas testosterone is produced by your ovaries and also other tissues like fat and skin.[3]

The androgen hormones are often called the "male" hormones because they are higher in men than in women and produce more "male" symptoms. They are converted into a more potent form called dihydrotestosterone (DHT), which gets into the hair follicles on your face and body and turns any soft, light "peach fuzz" into thick, dark hairs. They also get into the oil glands under your skin and cause those to overproduce oil, which then causes acne; and into your scalp and kill the hair follicles, causing hair loss (androgenic alopecia).

Women often tell me "I don't have high testosterone, so this isn't relevant to me." However, if you have PCOS, you're almost always going to have high androgen levels, as this defines the syndrome. Many groups have actually lobbied to change the name of PCOS to something like "hyperandrogenic persistent ovulatory dysfunction syndrome," which is a much more accurate description of what's going on.[4] However, high androgen levels may not show up in blood tests because of the way the levels are measured—the tests only measure the "whole" forms rather than the broken-down (metabolized) forms.

CASE STUDY

Bethany came to see me after failing to conceive. She was confused about whether or not she had PCOS, as her blood androgen levels were low. She also had low libido and other symptoms of low testosterone. We performed a more sensitive test called the DUTCH test, which measures the levels of both "whole" hormones and their metabolites (broken-down forms) in urine and saliva.

What we found was that while Bethany's testosterone ("whole" hormone) was low, the metabolites—especially the very potent form DHT—were high, which was the likely reason for her facial hair and would be contributing to her fertility struggles.

It's therefore important to not just accept blood test levels of androgens as gospel; they are often misleading. If you have PCOS, you're very likely to have some high androgens.

HOW PCOS AFFECTS YOUR PERIODS AND FERTILITY

By now you're probably thinking, okay—that makes sense for my facial hair, but how does this affect my periods and fertility? Well, when it comes to getting pregnant and staying pregnant, we need the three fertility ingredients I outlined in the introduction (see page 16)—quality egg and sperm, meeting at the right time, with a safe nest available. In PCOS there can be issues with any of these ingredients, but *they are all treatable*, if not wholly reversible.

PCOS does not equal infertility. If you are infertile, this means that you can never conceive naturally due to a physical reason, such as missing sexual organs—which only applies to 2 to 4 percent of the population.[5] I prefer to use the term "subfertility," which means that while you may not be ovulating at this moment, or your partner's sperm may not be optimal right now, *it doesn't mean that you will never be able to conceive*. You just need to work on the issues you have, and in most cases these are fixable and/or treatable with medical intervention.[4]

> ## All hope is not lost—you are not infertile. You are just in a state of subfertility, which can be reversed.

HOW YOU GET PREGNANT

Before we dive into restoring you to magnificent health to help you conceive (if that's your goal), let's explore what we should have been taught in school (instead of spending days on genetics and figuring out what color eyes baby rabbits would have): about our periods and how we actually get pregnant.

It all starts with your menstrual cycle, which is like a synchronized orchestra of hormones. None of the hormones that make up your menstrual cycle act alone—they are all perfectly linked to influence each other. So if one hormone is too high or too low, or is released at the wrong time, then it disrupts the whole cycle. This is precisely the way that any team sport works. If one player is off their game or playing out of position, it affects the whole team—whether it's football, basketball, or my favorite (because I'm from the Commonwealth) rugby.

The first part of your cycle starts with **estrogen** rising. This signals the uterine lining (uterine bed) to start developing in readiness for a fertilized egg (called a zygote) to implant in it. Think about estrogen as a mother hen, nesting away. In the team sport analogy, this is like the warm-up. The team is getting everything ready, laying the foundations for a successful game.

As estrogen is rising, another hormone, **follicle-stimulating hormone (FSH)**, starts to increase. FSH does what it says on the tin: It stimulates the follicles (the baby eggs) to grow. (I'm just going to call follicles "eggs" from here onward, to keep things simple and easy to remember.) While hundreds of eggs are developing in your ovaries at all times, only the strongest and largest of them is chosen to go on and be the dominant egg. Your body doesn't want to waste a whole lot of energy developing eggs that are never going to grow to size; it literally wants to put all its eggs into one basket. Once the dominant egg is chosen, it is grown to full size so it can be released.

In the team sport analogy, think about this as the ground play (or the ruck in rugby). This is an essential part of the game where the attacking play is decided on, and who's going to be the main playmaker who gets the ball to where it needs to be to score. The players need to assess the other team's defense and which play they are going to make, and, therefore, who's going to take the ball. They don't just throw it into the air or knock it into space, hoping that one of their teammates will catch it.

As FSH peaks, at the end of the follicular phase, our next hormone comes into play—**luteinizing hormone (LH)**. LH is here for a good time, not a long time. Its job is to lay low for the first part of your cycle, not drawing too much attention to itself and just slowly creeping up; then, when the time is perfect, it shoots up rapidly. This massive spike of LH causes the dominant egg to be projected out of the ovary and into the fallopian tube, so that it's ready to meet any awaiting sperm. This is called ovulation, and is the start of what we call the luteal phase. Think of LH as the wide receiver in football or the wing in rugby. Their job is to hang back from the line, not really getting involved in the midfield play, and then when the time is right, grab the ball and sprint through the defensive line to score the goal or pass the ball to a supporting player to do so.

Progesterone is the last hormone in the mix. Progesterone is virtually non-existent until after ovulation, because it's mainly produced by the sac (corpus luteum) that the egg is encased in before being projected out. If the egg has been fertilized, it will make its way down the fallopian tube and into your uterus, where it burrows into your uterine lining, making a little nest for itself while it grows. Progesterone's job is to keep your uterine lining intact and to protect the fertilized egg, while also increasing your core body temperature to incubate the egg. If the egg hasn't been fertilized and so doesn't implant itself, after a couple of weeks your body detects this and your progesterone comes crashing down. This triggers the uterine lining to shed—and you get your period.

You can think about progesterone as the supporting player, running in behind the wing, ready to take a pass or fend off attackers. If the goal is scored (the egg is released and fertilized), it carries the scorer and winning trophy ball on its shoulders to celebrate the win and protect that trophy. But if the goal isn't scored, it throws the biggest tantrum ever and burns down the entire stadium.

What is different when you have PCOS

In PCOS, it's like our team is just a bit hamstrung by poor timing and injured players. The consequence is that our synchronized hormonal team—estrogen, FSH, LH, and progesterone—gets very unsynchronized.

FSH in PCOS

One of the first hormone functions to suffer in PCOS is that of FSH, because this hormone is often simply too low to stimulate egg production or grow the dominant egg to size. This often occurs because the eggs have been exposed to high levels of androgens and/or insulin over three to six months. Such exposure could mean that their development is hindered, or they are of poor quality, which can result in miscarriage later.[6]

Instead of continuing to try to grow the egg, the body cuts its losses and discards the egg (this is what forms a cyst on the ovary), and a new dominant egg is then chosen to grow. This can happen multiple times before the dominant egg has been exposed to enough FSH to grow to size. One result of this is an irregular cycle—each time a dominant egg doesn't grow big enough you have to produce a new dominant egg, and this takes about a week each time. The length of your cycle is determined by how many times your body has tried to ovulate.

Back to the sporting analogy: it's like a play is selected, but the main player chosen to pass the ball to the receiver isn't in position, so the whole play is mucked up. Instead of continuing with that play, the team cuts their losses, and chooses a new play and playmaker. This can go on and on until they get it right, and the playmaker gets the ball.

LH in PCOS

Unlike FSH, in PCOS the levels of LH are often too high. To be able to release the egg into the fallopian tube to meet the sperm, LH needs to be in the right ratio with FSH (2:1 or less).[7] In PCOS this ratio is often 3:1, and I've seen it up to 10:1. The high LH level also increases testosterone, which not only affects the quality of the egg but also worsens other symptoms (acne, hair growth, hair loss, etc.).[6] Even if the dominant egg is the right size, it won't be released if LH is too high. However, you will continue to try to release that egg again and again until finally your LH and FSH are in the right ratio. This is another reason why you might have long cycles.

In the sports analogy, if the main player (FSH) isn't in position, then the wing or the wide receiver will run forward but the ball won't be passed at the right time; they'll end up overshooting the mark. They'll reset that play and keep trying until they get the timing right and a goal is scored.

Progesterone in PCOS

The other hormone that is disrupted in PCOS is progesterone. Progesterone levels are very sensitive and are easily disturbed by imbalances in LH and FSH. The result is that progesterone is too low, and does not stay high enough for long enough in your luteal phase for the fertilized egg to burrow into the uterine lining and signal to your brain that you're pregnant and so need to keep the uterine lining in place. Consequently, the lining sheds, and you get your period. Or, in another scenario, it stays high for long enough for the egg to burrow into the lining, but there isn't enough to maintain the lining before the fetus produces its own progesterone (after 12 weeks), and you miscarry.

In the sporting analogy, progesterone is the supporting player that helps keep the ball-carrier safe until they can score. But in PCOS, that player is injured and can't keep up, so can't provide any support. Consequently, the goal isn't scored and an epic tantrum follows.

The lesson to take away

As with any team, the raw talent is there to enable us to succeed; we just need a few tweaks to fire correctly in the next game. Your body wants to reproduce; it's the next most basic human desire after survival. You just need to give it the right environment to do so, and this means understanding which of your three fertility ingredients (an egg and sperm of good quality; that meet in the fallopian tubes; and a uterine lining to act as a safe nest for your fertilized egg, without collapsing) is— or are—not working correctly.

CASE STUDY

Destynne is a triathlete who was preparing for a half ironman, as well as working as a recruiter and being mom to a two-year-old boy. Talk about having a bit on!

She struggled for three years to conceive before becoming pregnant with her son, and after her first pregnancy, things didn't get any easier. Destynne's periods were irregular, and she gained weight even though she was working out for 90 minutes a day. Her weight had increased so much that she was now clinically obese even though she ate more healthily than most of her friends and ran six days a week.

Together, we identified that Destynne's insulin wasn't working normally, and the stress she was placing on her body through endurance training, working, and parenting wasn't helping either— not to mention the sugary gels and sports drinks she was using to fuel her training. Destynne changed her diet, decided to give her body a bit of a break from all the endurance exercise, prioritized her sleep, and increased her intake of vitamins and minerals. Within two months of implementing these changes she ovulated and got pregnant naturally with a beautiful baby girl.

Unfortunately, many medical professionals (even fertility specialists) don't always have the time to do a thorough analysis of what's going wrong, and they may not know which lifestyle tweaks will fix a particular problem. In Destynne's case, they may even have told her to eat less and exercise more—not realizing that, in fact, this was part of the problem. Many women are prescribed medications to force ovulation or are recommended to go down the IVF route. These medical interventions— while incredible if you need them—often aren't necessary. Not only that, but, coupled with not fixing the root cause, some can have long-term effects on your body and your baby's health, which I explain in more detail in Chapter 4.

Chapter 2
Hormonal imbalance and PCOS

One morning I was running one of our live Q&A sessions in the *PCOS Protocol* program, and one of the women participating had her mother join us on the call so that she too could learn a bit more about PCOS. When I started talking about the "root cause," the mom said, "What do you mean about this 'root cause?' I thought PCOS *was* the root cause?"

This is a common misconception. PCOS is not a root cause in itself; it is actually a result of our genes not playing nicely with our environment. While we can't change our genes, we *can* change our environment and therefore the root cause.

PCOS has been around for thousands of years—it was first described by Hippocrates (460–377 BC).[1] You might think that a condition that affects fertility would have been bred out through natural selection years ago, but PCOS was likely much less prevalent and not as severe when we moved a lot and didn't have an abundance of food available to us.[2] That is the way we have lived for most of human existence; it has only been in the past 60 or so years that most of us have had an abundance of food and led very sedentary lives. Alternatively, other researchers suggest that PCOS may have provided a physiological advantage during the Paleolithic or hunter-gatherer era, 2,000,000 BC to 20,000 BC. The theory is that we needed to be able to survive prolonged periods of famine, and therefore the ability to store and use body fat very efficiently (by making our body less sensitive to insulin and possibly reducing thyroid hormone too) was a massive advantage. So was not carrying 13 children on your back while running from a lion, or ovulating and getting pregnant during a famine or while under threat from another tribe or animals.[1] Therefore, having more time between pregnancies was favorable. The genes that conferred these characteristics (known as the "thrifty genes")[1] were passed from generation to generation because it's very possible to get pregnant with PCOS (they just probably had fewer children).

But genes don't account for everything when it comes to PCOS. Identical twins have the same genetic makeup, so if PCOS were purely genetic we would see that 100 percent of identical twins would both develop PCOS. This isn't the case at all.[3] What accounts for this difference is our environment.

THE ENVIRONMENT FACTOR

The typical environment in today's Western world is not what it was back in the hunter-gatherer era. Most of us now have an abundance of food, particularly manufactured food, rather than a scarcity. This change happened very rapidly, mostly just over the past 60 years. A study in Sweden between 1960 and 2010 found that the consumption of processed food products increased by 116 percent, and that of ultra-processed products increased by 142 percent. Among the ultra-processed products, there were particularly large increases in soda/soft drinks (315 percent) and snack foods such as chips and candy (367 percent).[4] This is how much our *environment* has changed in 50 years—it takes a lot longer for our genes to catch up and for us to adapt and evolve. New research estimates that we only gain 30 to 50 new DNA changes (or mutations) each generation every 20 to 40 years. This might sound a lot, but when you put it into context you can see that it took 7 million years for us to evolve from apes to humans.[5]

And it's not all about food. We also live in a hyper-stressful world, which has become worse for women over the past 60 years as we've cemented our place in the paid workforce. While getting to work outside the home has been an incredible achievement, we haven't been able to share the workload equally at home, especially the "mental load"—your total sum of responsibilities and "the remembering of things." The Office for National Statistics in the UK found that women do 60 percent more unpaid work than men.[6] In the US, the OECD found that in 2018, women spend almost twice the amount of time doing unpaid work each day compared with men.[7] In 2020 this had improved (only very slightly), with men doing 145 minutes unpaid work per day compared with 241 minutes for women.[8] And this doesn't mean doing the gratifying work of helping underprivileged families or a church community. It's the unpaid work of remembering and organizing things for the household.

We are also no longer living in family communities where we share the burden of childcare, cooking, cleaning, and food sourcing. We get far less sleep than our hunter-gatherer ancestors, and consequently our stress levels skyrocket. We move much less, and we sit a whole lot more.

While the stakes aren't often as high as life and death, our brain doesn't see it this way. It still produces high levels of stress hormones and detects that we are in danger. We don't want to bring a baby into a dangerous world, so our body stops ovulation, which is why stress can be a significant factor in PCOS and fertility. Like with food, our genes can't keep up with this change, and so we are not well adapted to our current environment.

The combination of all the factors I've mentioned here is likely why the prevalence of PCOS has increased noticeably over the past few decades to about 10 percent of the female population.[9]

WHAT WE CAN AND CAN'T CHANGE

We can't change our genes, but
we can improve our environment
to work with our genes.

This statement is what I mean when I talk about treating the root cause. It's not that we caused our PCOS through doing things "wrong," but that we've got to work *with* our genes rather than against them. If you do this, you can improve your fertility remarkably. The secret with PCOS is to figure out what the "root cause" is for *you*. Is it your insulin, your stress hormones, your thyroid, or a combination of all of them? As I mentioned in Chapter 1 (see page 23), PCOS is a syndrome, which isn't the same as a disease. A disease progresses in approximately the same way for most people, whereas a syndrome is just a group of symptoms that are given a name to help us understand the condition better. The following case study explains in more detail how this works.

CASE STUDY

Early on in my career, one of my first clients, Zoe, taught me a valuable lesson. Fresh out of functional medicine training and armed with my own success story of fixing my symptoms, I thought I'd cracked the code on PCOS. I wrote out the treatment plan that had helped me get symptom-free, I created PDFs of precisely what I did and how to implement it, and I handed them out to my patients. Any unsuccessful patient was deemed to not be following the program. Until I met Zoe.

Zoe was suffering from acne around her mouth and chin, and had been trying to conceive for two years. She had classic PCOS symptoms, so I gave her the treatment plan and organized to follow up in a month. After three months of no improvement, Zoe came to our follow-up consultation armed with spreadsheets recording everything she'd eaten, the supplements she'd taken, her workouts, sleep, and meditation sessions. She had rigorously implemented everything I had given her for three months, and yet her symptoms hadn't changed. I was stumped.

I went back to what I had learned in functional medicine training, and realized that I had been treating the symptoms (acne and infertility) without understanding the root cause. When I treated my insulin, stress hormones, and gut health (my root causes), my symptoms improved. But when Zoe did this, nothing happened.

We ordered some blood tests, and I learned a fundamental rule about PCOS that changed the course of my life and that of so many other women with PCOS: We are not the same because we have different "root causes" or systems in our body that contribute to our hormonal imbalance or PCOS symptoms.

Zoe didn't have a problem with her insulin, and so the treatment plan wasn't working. Instead, her stress hormones and thyroid weren't working correctly. I needed to treat her root cause.

The biological uniqueness of each of us is precisely the reason why a very-low-carbohydrate (ketogenic) diet that worked for a woman with PCOS who you saw on Instagram makes you feel worse when you try it. Or why the herb vitex helped another woman with PCOS get her period back, but makes your own cycles get longer, not shorter.

The type of food you eat, the exercise you do, and the supplements you take all have a specific action on your body. Similar to pharmaceutical drugs, you need to know what you're treating to pick the right medication. For example, a doctor could have two patients with the same symptoms: temperature, headache, and vomiting. But when they look at the root cause, they find that one is caused by the flu (influenza) whereas the other is from bacterial food poisoning. If they gave both patients antibiotics, the one with the food poisoning would improve because they have a bacterial infection. The flu patient has a virus, however, which won't respond to the antibiotics. In fact, the flu patient might actually get worse, as the medicine would be killing off their gut bacteria, which they need for their immune system to function correctly.

It is just the same with PCOS. For one woman, a very-low-carbohydrate diet could work wonders if she has severe insulin resistance and no issues with her adrenals. But for another, this could leave her feeling exhausted and irritable, and offer no improvement for her symptoms.

THE LEADING ROOT CAUSES OF PCOS

As I explained in Chapter 1, (see Destynne's case on page 31), figuring out what fertile ingredient(s) aren't working correctly allows you to make the right lifestyle changes to match the problem. However, we *always* need to know the root cause first, so now I'll talk about the leading ones. This isn't an exhaustive list, and by no means does it suggest that you've in any way "caused" your PCOS. I use the term "root cause" to help you understand how there are specific body systems that contribute to our hormones getting out of balance, which then results in what we know as PCOS.

The most common "root causes" I see are:

1. Insulin resistance
2. High levels of stress hormones
3. Hormonal birth control
4. Hypothyroidism

These are explored in depth below.

Insulin resistance

Insulin is a food storage hormone. When you eat, your body detects a rise in blood sugar. Your body doesn't like blood sugar to be high, as this damages cells in your brain, liver, pancreas, heart, and eyes over the long term—so it stores the sugar away in cells in your muscles and liver for later use. Insulin is the hormone that tells the cells to open up and let the glucose in. Without it, your cells would starve—which is why people with type 1 diabetes need to inject insulin to survive.

Insulin is excreted by the pancreas. It binds to a cell receptor to open the cell "door," similar to the way a key opens a door. When there is a genetic predisposition for the lock not to work, or the key has been used too much, or there is chronic low-grade inflammation, the lock starts to get a bit worn and clogged up; the key no longer fits. The body responds by producing more and more insulin until the cell door does open and the glucose can flow in. This is **insulin resistance**, and up to 80 percent of women with PCOS have insulin resistance (even those women who aren't overweight).[10]

When you have insulin resistance, it can take an hour, two hours, six hours, or even 12 hours for your insulin to get the cell door open, and in the meantime, all of your cells are exposed to the excess amount of insulin you are producing. If you have really high insulin levels all the time, this causes your body to overproduce testosterone.

In most parts of the body there are feedback loops in place—this means that if the level of something gets too high, the body shuts off its production. Unfortunately, this isn't the case with testosterone. Your body wasn't designed for the havoc that excess insulin—and other aspects of modern life—can cause, and so nothing stops the testosterone levels from getting higher and higher.

And it doesn't stop there. Hormones should be 80 percent bound up to other cells and proteins, with only 20 percent roaming free in the blood. It's the hormones that are roaming free that are generally the troublemakers: they get into hair follicles and make it fall out; get into skin glands and cause acne; or settle in hair follicles on the face and make it produce thick, dark hair where it otherwise wouldn't. Your body has a testosterone sponge, called sex-hormone-binding globulin (SHBG), that roams around and mops up excess testosterone (this is part of the 80 percent bound to cells that I mentioned earlier). Unfortunately, however, high insulin reduces the amount of SHBG and thus allows testosterone to increase in this way as well. Research has shown that those of us with PCOS have 13 percent less SHBG than other women.[11]

But it's not over yet. In what feels like a cruel turn of events, testosterone also increases insulin, making the situation worse.[12] You can think of insulin resistance as a delinquent child that has put the plug in the bath, turned on the taps of testosterone, stolen your sponges, and has then run away, calling "Catch me if you can!"

Insulin resistance can lower your chances of becoming pregnant. As I explained earlier, (see page 16), three 'fertile ingredients' are needed: a good-quality egg and sperm need to meet in the fallopian tubes, and the uterine lining needs to act as a safe nest for the fertilized egg, without collapsing. Insulin affects all three fertile ingredients because:

- Insulin resistance (and therefore high levels of insulin in your body) suppresses follicle-stimulating hormone (FSH). This means that none of your eggs develop to the right size, or they are of poor quality. Instead of continuing to try with that egg, you cut your losses and discard it (this is what forms the "cyst" on the ovary).[13]

- Luteinizing hormone (LH) acts like a switch to turn on ovulation —you can only ovulate when your LH rises and reaches a certain ratio with your FSH (2:1). But high levels of insulin increase LH too much[13] (as well as decreasing FSH), and the high ratio of LH to FSH then stops your body ovulating.[14] Around 94 percent of women with irregular cycles and PCOS have a ratio of LH to FSH that's too high.[15]

- Too much LH also reduces progesterone, which causes your uterine lining to collapse.[16] Either your egg doesn't have enough time to burrow into the lining, so you don't become pregnant, or you miscarry. Miscarriage or early pregnancy loss may be as high as 40 percent in women with PCOS compared with 10 to 15 percent in women without PCOS.[17] One study showed that 65 percent of women with high LH had a miscarriage.[18] The effect on progesterone is the likely reason why this is the case. (See also Chapter 11.)

As I described earlier in this chapter, insulin resistance in PCOS is primarily caused by our genes not interacting properly with our environment. We'll take a more in-depth look at what causes insulin resistance—and therefore what we can do about it—in Chapters 5 to 10, but here's a short insight into how it happens in PCOS.

The role of your genetics

Genetics plays a huge role in whether or not someone will develop insulin resistance. To put this into context, there are 88 known genes and genetic mutations that have already been associated with the development of type 2 diabetes, which results from insulin resistance.[19] So if you have a family member with pre-diabetes or type 2 diabetes, then you're probably genetically predisposed to develop insulin resistance. This is why your best girlfriend might live precisely the same lifestyle as you, but she doesn't develop insulin resistance and PCOS and you do. But similarly, while you don't develop breast cancer, she might because she has the BRCA1 or BRCA2 genetic mutations. This is where genetics come into play: the genes we are born with predispose us to develop certain conditions—although particular environmental factors are also needed to turn them on. We'll look at this in the next section.

The role of your environment

Studies have shown that genetic predisposition to a particular condition is only part of the story; the genes also have to be present in the right environment for us to develop symptoms.[20] We can see how this works by looking at studies of identical twins. One of these studies followed more than 4,000 genetically identical twin pairs (8,000 participants in total) with differing BMI (body mass index—a measure of body fat based on height and body weight) scores for 15 years.[21] The researchers compared the risk of heart attack, death, and type 2 diabetes between the twins in each pair. They found that even though the twins had the same genetic makeup, they weren't equally as likely to develop type 2 diabetes. The twins who did develop type 2 diabetes were more likely to do less exercise and more likely to have a higher BMI—these are the environmental components.[21]

As well as lack of exercise, other environmental factors are thought to contribute to the development of insulin resistance and type 2 diabetes. Here are just a few of them:

- What you eat—for example, a high sugar intake has been associated with increased risk for insulin resistance and type 2 diabetes.[22]
- If your mother developed gestational diabetes or if you were exposed to high levels of insulin when you were in the womb.[23]
- If your mother experienced a major stressful life event when you were in the womb.[24]
- Being overweight (although this is a murky area because we don't know what happens first—weight gain or insulin resistance).[21]

- Being older—your risk increases with age.[25]
- Poor gut health.[26]
- Lack of sleep.[27]

We go into more detail on the most critical environmental factors that you can control elsewhere in the book.

High levels of stress hormones

The second most common root cause I see is high levels of stress hormones. When you are stressed, your brain (hypothalamus and pituitary) recognizes this and stimulates your adrenal glands to produce stress hormones: adrenaline (the fight-and-flight hormone) and cortisol (produced when stress is high for a prolonged period of time, meaning days or weeks rather than minutes or hours). Another hormone, dehydroepiandrosterone sulfate (DHEA-S), is also produced by the adrenal glands. As we learned earlier, DHEA-S is a member of the androgen family, which includes testosterone. While testosterone is mostly produced in your ovaries (as well as smaller amounts in your fat tissue and liver), DHEA-S is produced mostly by your adrenal glands.

When your brain activates your adrenal glands because of stress, this causes both cortisol and DHEA-S levels to rise. DHEA-S does the same thing as testosterone: it affects the quality of your eggs; affects LH, which stops you ovulating; and it gets converted to the potent form DHT, which causes acne, hair loss, and hirsutism. Most people (and even physicians) are not aware that 50 percent of women with PCOS have excess adrenal androgens (DHEA-S).[28]

High levels of DHEA-S and cortisol affect your fertile ingredients in the following ways:

- **Egg quality**—The more DHEA-S your eggs are exposed to, the fewer good-quality eggs you'll have.[29] The number and quality of eggs you have is known as "ovarian reserve." If you don't have enough good-quality eggs (diminished ovarian reserve), your body won't be able to pick a dominant one to release into the fallopian tubes, and you won't ovulate.

- **Ovulation**—High cortisol can stop ovulation from occurring, or delay it, by inhibiting the production of LH.[30] Your body might have to try four, five, or 20 times to ovulate before it finally has enough LH to push that egg out of the sac. The result is that you might have a cycle of 40, 50, or 100 days long.

- **Progesterone**—High cortisol reduces the amount of progesterone that your body releases, meaning that the nest (your uterine lining) doesn't stay intact long enough either for implantation or to make it to the 12-week mark.[30]

What causes high stress hormones

When you hear the word "stress," you might immediately think of that feeling of being stuck in traffic when you're already running late, looming deadlines you don't have time to complete, or receiving unexpected bills when money is already tight. This is psychological stress, and it accounts for much of our high modern-day stress; however, it's only one form of stress in the body.

In the medical world, the term "stress" means anything that exceeds the adaptive capability of your body and raises your level of cortisol. This means that you could be lying on a beach in the Bahamas, sipping a piña colada, with millions in the bank, yet still have high levels of cortisol. Everyday, non-psychological stressors that raise cortisol include:

- chronic infections
- inadequate sleep
- inflammation
- autoimmune disease
- environmental toxins
- loneliness and isolation
- dieting
- too much exercise
- too much caffeine (or any, if you're sensitive to it).

If you're anything like me, you'll probably have a combination of several of these—and the more you have, the worse you'll feel. You might not feel physically stressed, but if you've got any of the underlying issues listed above, then they'll be having the same impact on your stress hormones.

It could also be that your stress response has been hardwired from when you were a child or going through puberty.[31] It is thought that if you had a stressful time during adolescence, your body may have a limited tolerance for stress. The same stress that your best friend can handle just fine raises *your* cortisol inappropriately. I see this happening in women who were élite athletes when they were going through puberty—especially in sports that emphasize low weight, like gymnastics—or if they were exposed to significant family stress, the death of a loved one, or some other trauma during or prior to puberty. Adolescent stress seems so significant that researchers have proposed that it might cause PCOS. One study reported that girls exposed to stress before or at puberty were significantly more likely to go on to develop PCOS than those who weren't.[32]

Hormonal birth control

The third root cause of PCOS is hormonal birth control (HBC). Many women develop PCOS symptoms after coming off HBC. Relatively frequently, I'll meet women who didn't have PCOS before going on HBC, but once they come off HBC to try to get pregnant they find that their cycles are now many months long, and they have acne, and they receive a diagnosis of PCOS. After making a few lifestyle tweaks, their symptoms disappear. This is referred to as "post-pill PCOS," and I learned about this phenomenon from my friend and colleague Dr. Lara Briden. If you haven't read her book *Period Repair Manual,* I recommend you grab a copy.

The reason why HBC can cause this often temporary change is likely due to the synthetic hormones present in it. HBC may increase the amount of insulin you produce by up to 20–40 percent[33]—something you probably weren't told when it was prescribed. One study looked at how HBC affects insulin and blood sugar levels in adolescents with PCOS. The study followed two groups of girls who had never been on hormonal birth control. Each group was given a different form of HBC often used to treat PCOS symptoms, such as acne and missing periods. After 12 months of being on HBC, both groups had increased insulin-resistance. A particularly alarming discovery was that after just 12 months, one group's insulin increased by 100 percent after eating—a statistically significant increase.[34] As I outlined in Chapter 2, more insulin affects all three of the fertile ingredients. Additionally, HBC may stop exercise from improving insulin sensitivity (which is the primary way that exercise helps us with PCOS).[35] This is why I'm cautious about HBC as a "treatment." While it can improve symptoms like acne and unwanted hair growth, it might be making things worse in the long run, especially for those with some insulin resistance.

Independently of the effect on insulin, HBC also causes a chronic increase in LH levels, which stops ovulation and therefore reduces your likelihood of getting pregnant.[32, 36] As you now know, if LH is too high then the ratio of LH to FSH is unbalanced and an egg won't be released.

Many of you may have been put on HBC as a teenager before your periods had a chance to become regular, or maybe they were irregular and you had some acne, and that's why you were put on it. That's okay, and it doesn't mean that you didn't have PCOS before going on HBC. HBC can mask many little issues, so you just don't know. What I'm trying to explain here is the cases, like that of Lisa (below), where everything was perfect before going on HBC and then very much not perfect after coming off it.

CASE STUDY

Lisa started taking HBC when she got married at 25; before that, she had a regular menstrual cycle. After deciding to have a family three years later, she came off HBC but her periods didn't return to their previous pattern. She went for six months without a period, and when they finally came back, they were 90 days apart. Her doctor diagnosed PCOS, and said that because she didn't need to lose weight there was nothing she could do and she would need IVF.

Lisa was living in London in the UK, and IVF wasn't funded in her area; it would cost thousands of dollars per round. To even get on the wait-list she had to try to conceive naturally for another year. Consequently, she was feeling incredibly defeated and at the mercy of the health system telling her when she and her husband could have a baby.

When Lisa contacted me, her description of her menstrual cycle immediately told me that her body was really struggling to either grow a dominant egg to size or release it, and was going through multiple attempts before it got it right. So my first testing was aimed at figuring out why. Through the testing we identified that Lisa's LH was much too high, at a 4:1 ratio with her FSH.

Once I knew what the first part of the problem was, I could look at why it was happening. Further testing showed that Lisa's insulin was slightly high. We tweaked her diet and lifestyle, and her cycle went from 90 days to 34 days in two months. She was pregnant within four months.

Lisa's case was a classic example of post-pill PCOS where just a few tweaks and a bit of time is all that's needed to help get the fertile ingredients firing again after coming off HBC.

Hypothyroidism

The final root cause of PCOS is hypothyroidism, and it is actually one of the most common "hidden" root causes. A quarter of all women with PCOS have a thyroid condition, but this mostly goes undiagnosed.[37] According to the Rotterdam criteria for diagnosis of PCOS, hypothyroidism (an underactive thyroid gland) should be ruled out before you are diagnosed with PCOS.[38] However, in my experience, this rarely happens. I regularly see women with thyroid symptoms that have gone undiagnosed for years.

Your thyroid is a gland that sits at the base of your neck and controls how quickly your body uses energy (i.e. your metabolism), makes proteins, and controls your body's sensitivity to other hormones. It does this by releasing a hormone called thyroxine (T_4). T_4 is released into your bloodstream and carried around your body to all your organs, cells, and tissue that need thyroid hormone to work correctly (which is most of them). As your body needs thyroid hormone, it will convert T_4 into the active form T_3 (triiodothyronine). **Hypothyroidism** is when you don't have enough thyroid hormone.

The three forms of hypothyroidism are:

- **Classic hypothyroidism.** If your body detects that you don't have enough thyroid hormone, it will send a message to your brain telling it to release another hormone, thyroid-stimulating hormone (TSH), to stimulate your thyroid to produce more T_4. Hypothyroidism occurs when your body can't make enough thyroid hormone to keep up with the demands of your body. If this happens, your metabolic rate will decrease. You'll likely feel cold and exhausted, and will gain weight.

- **Hashimoto's thyroiditis.** This is an autoimmune condition. Autoimmune conditions occur when your immune system becomes chronically activated, meaning activated all the time instead of just when it's needed. In the case of Hashimoto's, your body detects the thyroid gland as a foreign invader and begins producing antibodies to attack it. The thyroid gland stops functioning properly as a result.

- **Low T_3 syndrome.** This is when you have enough T_4 but it's not being converted into T_3. This can happen because you have insufficient amounts of selenium and zinc, or your body is converting T_4 to "reverse T_3" instead of T_3. Reverse T_3 (rT_3) is an inactive form of T_3. Typically, your body will convert T_4 to both T_3 and rT_3 continually, and will then quickly eliminate rT_3. But under certain conditions, more rT_3 is produced and the desirable conversion of T_4 to T_3 decreases; this can become a vicious cycle with T_4 being increasingly converted to rT_3 rather than T_3. This is common in Hashimoto's thyroiditis and other autoimmune conditions, fibromyalgia, chronic fatigue syndrome, chronic dieting, high stress, or other conditions where your body thinks you need to hold onto extra body fat and reduce your metabolism. Your lab results will show normal TSH, normal T_4, but low T_3, or even normal T_3 but high rT_3.

The effect of hypothyroidism on PCOS and fertility

Your thyroid hormone is essential for your entire health, and especially fertility. Too much or too little thyroid hormone can affect all three of your fertile ingredients. In PCOS the more common problem is hypothyroidism (too little thyroid hormone), and especially the autoimmune version, Hashimoto's thyroiditis.

1. **Hypothyroidism and Hashimoto's thyroiditis can affect the quality of your eggs.** The thyroid gland is crucial for the health of your eggs. If you don't have enough thyroid hormone, your eggs won't mature fully. Hypothyroidism also causes increased androgens, which reduce the quality of your eggs. The antibodies produced in Hashimoto's thyroiditis can also reduce egg quality.[39]

2. **You may not be able to ovulate.** The second fertile ingredient is being able to release that egg so that it can encounter sperm. If you don't have enough thyroid hormone, your hypothalamus won't be able to release LH and FSH to trigger your body to ovulate.[40]

3. **You may not be able to keep the nest in place.** When you become pregnant, your body requires a lot more nutrients and hormones, including thyroid hormone. If you already have thyroid antibodies, your body won't be able to produce the amount of thyroid hormone required, which can cause a miscarriage. This is a prevalent cause of miscarriage[41] that I discuss further in Chapter 11. Good thyroid function is also essential for your growing baby, who needs your thyroid hormone until they can take over and make their own.

CASE STUDY

Ava had struggled with her weight for all of her life, even when eating a low-calorie diet, as well as with irregular periods, hair loss, and unwanted hair growth. When she asked for more tests to find out why she wasn't losing weight, she was told that she just needed to try harder. Her doctor said, "PCOS is just an excuse for being fat."

When she was originally tested, her TSH was within the range thought to be normal at the time (although this has changed and it would now be deemed to be higher than normal), so further testing was refused. I encouraged Ava to pay for a full thyroid panel privately. Her results were pretty astonishing. Her thyroid antibodies were well above the reference ("normal") range, indicating that she was in the early stages of Hashimoto's thyroiditis.

Ava had likely been affected by hypothyroidism for her whole adult life. About 25 percent of patients with an autoimmune disease develop other autoimmune diseases, including rheumatoid arthritis, multiple sclerosis, lupus, and inflammatory bowel disease. People like Ava need to know this so that they can treat the underlying issues (imbalances in gut bacteria, food intolerances) and avoid developing these other conditions.

Ava also had insulin resistance, and when we addressed both of these conditions she saw some significant results. Over six months, Ava lost almost 60 lb (27 kg), her periods became regular for the first time in her life, her hair stopped shedding, and her facial hair growth slowed significantly.

Chapter 3
Why you shouldn't focus on weight loss

Weight gain (and inability to lose weight) is a widespread symptom of PCOS. Many of you will have been told by your doctor to lose weight to improve your fertility. However, I find that it's really unhelpful to focus on weight loss. The reason for the weight gain in PCOS is that insulin and testosterone cause a vicious cycle in the body. An increase in insulin causes the body to store fat (unused glucose in cells is converted to fat) and to overproduce testosterone. The high levels of testosterone cause further weight gain. The additional weight then makes the insulin resistance worse, and also increases testosterone as much of our testosterone is produced in fat tissue. This then causes additional weight gain . . . It is the most vicious spiral that's incredibly hard to break. This is why it's unhelpful to focus on weight loss when it comes to PCOS.

A scenario that many of you will likely have experienced is that you go to the doctor because you've been trying to conceive for many months, and nothing is happening. You're told to go away and lose some weight and keep trying. This leaves you feeling defeated, because you've been trying to lose weight for years, if not decades, with no success. You

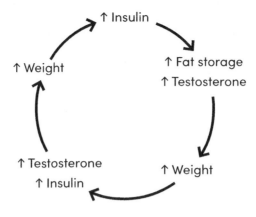

Figure 1: The insulin–testosterone–weight gain cycle

feel that not being able to conceive is your "fault" because weight, of course, is all about calories and therefore in your control.

But weight loss isn't just about the calories you eat or burn—they don't even factor into the cycle shown in Figure 1, above. While calories do play a part when it comes to reducing your waistline, they are not the *only* factor. But instead of addressing insulin and the root cause, we tend to focus just on cutting calories, which rarely works and leaves us feeling defeated. And although losing 2 to 5 percent of your bodyweight can help kick-start ovulation,[1] it isn't the calories that are stopping you from conceiving. Your hormones—insulin, thyroid, and the stress hormones—are also causing you to put on weight.

> ## Dramatic results happen when your focus shifts from calories and weight loss to the root cause and hormones.

CASE STUDY

Carmen was diagnosed with PCOS when she was 27, and was very concerned about the idea of not being able to get pregnant. Her doctor suggested that she and her partner start trying immediately and Carmen conceived quickly. However, over the years her PCOS and other symptoms (IBS [irritable bowel syndrome], anxiety/depression, and panic attacks) had worsened and her weight was also increasing. She and her partner decided to try for a second child, but after an early miscarriage, nothing was happening. Visits to the doctor yielded the same answer: "You just have to lose weight."

Carmen tried Weight Watchers and taking herbal appetite suppressants, and spent a year working one-to-one with a nutritionist focusing on a low-calorie diet. She was told to eat six small meals a day and focus on low-calorie, low-fat foods. Every two weeks she would go into the clinic to meet with her nutritionist and be weighed—but the numbers on the scales didn't shift. The nutritionist would ask Carmen what was happening, and she would produce her immaculately detailed food diary with the weights and measurements of everything that she'd eaten. Carmen was motivated to have a baby and she wasn't under-reporting, but overeating wasn't the reason why she wasn't losing weight.

Carmen felt ashamed and frustrated at her failure to lose weight and conceive. She described it as an "emotional rollercoaster." She'd feel elated when she got on the scales and she'd lost a little, and then so unhappy and frustrated when her weight went the other way. The result was that she went from restricting her food intake to saying "F**k it, it's not working anyway," and eating what she wanted before "getting back on the wagon."

Carmen also didn't shy away from natural health treatments. She received regular massages and acupuncture, and had a naturopath on her medical team for many years. She was taking a variety of herbs, and also natural progesterone. But she still felt like no one was getting to the root cause. She was still tired all the time, her depression was getting worse, she was putting on weight (despite her physically demanding job as a landscaper), and she always felt like she needed to have something sweet after every meal.

Carmen started working with me about three years after she and her partner started trying for a second baby. We quickly identified that her insulin wasn't functioning well, and her high stress was contributing to it, as was her gut health. But we put zero focus on weight loss. Although Carmen's diet was perfect for someone without insulin issues, it wasn't the right solution for her; so we overhauled that to make her more sensitive to insulin. We also focused on her sleep, and increased the vitamins, minerals, and herbs she needed to improve her insulin and stress hormones.

At the first follow-up, Carmen reported having more energy and not being tired all the time. She also felt satisfied because she wasn't starving, for the first time in years, and didn't feel like she *had* to have sugar after every meal. Her mental health was markedly better. However, her IBS was still affecting her, and she still wasn't pregnant. We did a comprehensive liver function and stool analysis to get to the root cause of that.

The results showed that Carmen had elevated beta-glucuronidase, which can reduce the body's excretion of unwanted substances, including estrogen. This meant she was reabsorbing estrogen and toxins that should have been excreted. She also had deficient levels of probiotic lactobacilli (which should make up about a third of gut bacteria). Carmen had malabsorbed meat and vegetables in her stool sample, which showed that she didn't have enough stomach acid. There was also a bacteria called *Citrobacter* present, which can lead to IBS symptoms when lactobacilli levels are low.

The beta-glucuronidase finding was especially interesting, because it showed a direct link to why Carmen probably wasn't conceiving. If she was reabsorbing estrogen, this would lead to estrogen dominance and result in low progesterone (even though she was also taking a natural progesterone supplement). I started Carmen on a plan to address this, and her body reacted super quickly to this new regimen. Within two months, Carmen was pregnant without any weight loss.

An important takeaway from Carmen's story is that we put zero focus on weight loss and headed straight to fixing the root cause. We improved her insulin and stress hormones first (the main priority), and then focused on more in-depth testing to identify any other factors that needed addressing—her liver and gut health—and it took just six months.

HOW WEIGHT LOSS REALLY WORKS

Weight loss isn't just "energy in, energy out." I see so many "experts" (read mostly male personal trainers) preaching online that a calorie deficit is the *only* thing that reduces weight, but this isn't correct. The calorie model for weight loss is incredibly outdated. It assumes that your body is like a bank account, and saving is like losing weight. If you put $2,000 into your bank account but only spend $1,500, then you've saved $500. According to this model, weight loss works this way:

- Say that your body burns 2,000 kcal in a day, and you eat only 1,500 kcal.

- Your body has to make up that 500 kcal from somewhere else, so it goes to the pantry (your fat stores) and grabs 500 calories from your fat stores to burn instead. You burn that fat, and you lose weight.

Ta-dah!

Not quite. What this model doesn't address is that the human body is not just any old bank account. It's a bank account with the most intelligent computer known to humanity working inside it. That computer is continually scanning the environment and making changes to your spending/saving without your control. The following analogy explains this in more depth.

Last week, it rained for the first time in many months. As I was leaving work, I got my mini umbrella out of my bag and pushed up the metal sliders as I burst through the door into the downpour. Instead of being protected from above by a dome of waterproof fabric, I found that the fabric was sticking to the back of my neck with a stream of water flowing delightfully down my back. I spun the umbrella around to find that half the metal prongs were broken and the umbrella had completely flopped on one side. Deeming it completely useless, I slid it straight into the nearest trash can (shuddering at the thought of the broken umbrella graveyard at the landfill). Then I sprinted across the open square, trying to keep my laptop from getting wet, and along to the outdoor store to find a new umbrella.

In there I was greeted with an array of umbrellas, from $20 replacements of what I'd had to $100 Blunt umbrellas—an incredibly designed dome umbrella with blunt edges to withstand wind and rain and with a lifetime guarantee. Given the amount I'd spent on short-lived umbrellas in the past two years alone, I decided that the Blunt was an excellent investment.

But what if I hadn't? Even though I knew that the $100 was a good investment, maybe I had a savings goal of $250/week. Say I went into the store and checked my account only to find that I had just $25.50 left to spend this week. I would have felt incredibly guilty about buying another shoddy umbrella that would break within two months, but my savings goal was my main target. So I'd buy the flimsy umbrella with $5.50 to spare, and get home still reasonably dry.

But now, what if that bank account had a computer in it that made its own decisions? It might have said, "You didn't invest that $100 on a Blunt umbrella, but I've decided this was a poor decision and overrode it. I checked the weather forecast, and it's going to rain three out of seven days next week. In fact, based on the historical rain records for your area, it will rain 57 days this winter. I also analyzed what you've spent on cheap umbrellas over the past three years, and if you had invested in a lifetime-guarantee Blunt in the first place, you would have saved $331.57. So I went ahead and purchased one for you; it'll arrive tomorrow, but given you've also spent $20 on the shoddy one, you've now only saved $155.50 this week."

How frustrating! Imagine that—a bank account that thinks it's making the best decision for you but it doesn't understand your goals. This is precisely what your body does when it comes to weight, and the way it does this is through hormones (chemical messengers). Insulin is the chief chemical messenger that is at play in PCOS.

Our body fat levels directly correlate to how long we can survive in a famine situation, so our body is inherently risk averse when it comes to

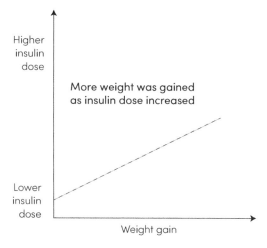

Figure 2: Weight gain with increasing insulin

shedding some of that fat. Even if you decide your goal is to lose weight, your body might override this decision if it thinks you're risking your life by doing so.

Calorie deficit (eating less than you burn) is only the first part of the weight-loss equation. But most people don't realize that there is a second part to this equation: Your body has to actually be able to open the pantry door to access that 500 kcal of stored fat to make up the deficit. What opens the pantry door is hormones, but what keeps the door closed is also hormones. Think about your pantry door at home, and imagine it's one-way: You can't put food in and take it out at the same time. This is how our hormones work.

In Chapter 2, I explained that 80 percent of women with PCOS have some insulin resistance. When we eat, instead of producing just a little bit of insulin, our body produces lots of insulin over a long period. The problem with this is that insulin is our "fat-storing" hormone, and it blocks the action of the "fat-burning" hormone. It's a one-way door: we can't be both burning and storing at the same time. The result is more insulin production and more weight gain.

How do we know this? It's pretty clear in the research. A study back in 1992 on people with type 2 diabetes who needed to inject insulin found that the more insulin they injected, the more weight they gained (see

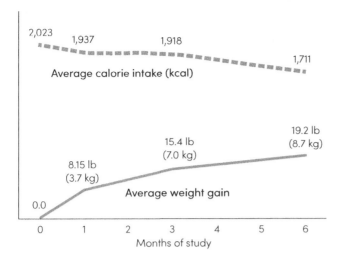

Figure 3: Calorie intake and weight gain over six months[2]

Figure 2, opposite). The same pattern was seen when blood insulin levels were graphed against weight gain—the higher the blood insulin was, the more weight was gained. The study participants gained an average of about 20 lb (9 kg), about 9 percent of their bodyweight, in six months.[2]

But the most astonishing thing was that the participants gained weight even when they reduced their calories. At the start of the study they were eating 2,000 kcal, and by the end they were eating only 1,700 kcal, as shown in Figure 3, above. Normally, to gain 20 lb or 9 kg over six months, you need to eat a lot more than usual. As you can see from Figure 3, though, this wasn't happening. It wasn't calories that were causing the weight gain—it was insulin.

While this study was on type 2 diabetes, and not all women with PCOS have type 2 diabetes, it helps us see what the body is doing when it overproduces insulin. This isn't the only study to show that higher insulin levels lead to weight gain; studies have consistently been showing this from 1990 until now.[3, 4] Conversely, lower insulin levels help with weight loss, and this is demonstrated in people with type 1 diabetes—when they inject less insulin, they lose weight. About 30 percent of women with type 1 diabetes don't inject enough insulin for this reason, even though this can be dangerous—those who restrict their insulin have a three times greater risk of death than those who don't.[5, 6]

The findings are consistent with each other. Raising insulin levels causes weight gain. Lowering insulin levels causes weight loss. In a highly enlightening study in the *American Journal of Clinical Nutrition*,[7] the researchers found that people with higher insulin levels lost less weight and gained it back most rapidly. The 50 study participants were in the obese category for bodyweight. They were put on a calorie-restricted diet of 1,200 kcal for women and 1,500 kcal for men for six weeks, followed by six weeks of weight maintenance. The results showed a vast difference in weight loss between the study participants. About one-third lost 22 lb (10 kg) over the 12 weeks, whereas another one-third only lost about 2.8 lb (1.3 kg), even though there were no differences in the participants' age, calorie intake, exercise, or any of the often-touted causes of weight gain. Those with the highest levels of insulin resistance and inflammation lost the least amount of weight during the first six weeks (only 8.8 lb/ 4 kg), and then gained almost all (5.5 lb/2.5 kg) of it back during the following six-week maintenance phase.

Studies on diet and exercise involving women both with PCOS and without PCOS showed that overweight women with PCOS made similar food choices and ate the same amount of calories (approximately 1,750 kcal/day) as lean women without PCOS.[8] There was also no significant difference in physical activity between these two groups. We can see from this that the number of calories consumed or burned goes nowhere near explaining why women with PCOS gain weight easily and have such a hard time losing it. The one thing that was different was their fasting insulin level. Women with PCOS had significantly higher fasting insulin levels than those without PCOS.[8]

These studies show that it's not overeating, or too little exercise, or lack of self-control or motivation that is causing your weight gain and inability to lose belly fat; it's insulin. And as you've learned in the previous chapters, it's also insulin that's been disrupting your three fertile ingredients and therefore your fertility.

It's not weight loss we need to focus on, it's the root cause: Your insulin levels.

This research totally reflects the experience I've had with women with PCOS. Women often tell me that they have put on something like 45 lb (20 kg) in six months without any change in their lifestyle; if anything, they were eating less and exercising more.

CASE STUDY

Tiffany joined my *PCOS Protocol* program after she'd put on 33 lb (15 kg) in the four months leading up to her wedding; she couldn't conceive because she hadn't had a period for the past two years. Like many women, Tiffany wanted to look fabulous for her wedding and started her #shreddingforthewedding campaign.

"Four months into planning the big day, my wedding dress said 'no' to me. My 33 lb (15 kg) weight gain ended with my alterations lady asking 'Did you gain weight?' as I tried to squeeze into my dream dress. I was working out twice a week and eating super-clean. My periods were starting to lessen as my stress increased like crazy. I couldn't sleep, my acne was flaring up, and I felt hopeless."

We identified that Tiffany's insulin was too high and changed her diet, exercise, supplements, and other parts of her lifestyle to make her body more sensitive to insulin and stop producing so much. The results were dramatic. In less than a month, Tiffany was ovulating (and subsequently getting her period), and over 12 weeks she lost 5 inches (13 cm) from her waist. She then went on to conceive naturally a few months later.

I see this pattern time and time again. Periods (and therefore ovulation) will be the first thing to return when you treat your root cause, and then weight loss will follow after.

OTHER REASONS NOT TO FOCUS ON WEIGHT LOSS
Disordered eating

Focusing on weight and weight loss can be incredibly damaging both psychologically and physiologically. The incidence of disordered eating and poor self-esteem are much higher in PCOS, and part of the reason for this is that we're being told it's all our "fault."

In an extensive study of 148 women with PCOS and 106 without, researchers found that women with PCOS were four times more likely to have an eating disorder, and 17.6 percent had a binge-eating disorder.[9] A focus on weight loss is at least partly to blame for why women with PCOS are more likely to have an eating disorder, and specifically a binge-eating disorder.[10]

Sometimes known as compulsive overeating, binge eating is a severe eating disorder, which is defined as recurring episodes of eating significantly more food in a short period than most people would eat under similar circumstances.[11] Binge-eating disorder feels like a loss of control when eating, and is often coupled with a compulsive (or irresistible) urge. The bingeing is often done in secret because it's accompanied by feelings of embarrassment, guilt, self-loathing, severe self-criticism, or even disgust. This can end in a vicious cycle of restricting food to compensate for the binge, which leads to more bingeing, which leads to feeling more hopeless and out of control, which leads to looking to food as a coping strategy.

CASE STUDY

Amanda, who features on my podcast in episode 4, developed binge-eating disorder after being diagnosed with PCOS and becoming really conscious of her weight and her body. In the interview, she explains how people would often comment on her weight. Or that weight would be the topic of conversation, and while this was often innocent, it had an extremely negative effect on her. She started to restrict her food intake, but would then binge uncontrollably, at least partly due to hunger and sugar cravings. The bingeing led to feelings of disgust, guilt, and self-loathing, which led to another period of restricting . . . and then, you've guessed it, bingeing again. This is a really vicious cycle.

One of the most important things that helped Amanda get through her binge-eating disorder was seeing a great counselor who specialized in disordered eating. The second was changing her diet so that she wasn't starving and craving sugar all the time. Amanda has insulin resistance, and this was making her blood sugar go up and down like a rollercoaster all day long. When her blood sugar was low, she'd suffer from intense sugar cravings and hangry attacks. She found that when she followed the diet recommendations for insulin resistance (see Chapter 7), her blood sugar stabilized, and she stopped craving sugar and being ravenously hungry.

I wrote my honors thesis on eating disorders in female athletes, so I've seen first-hand the devastating effects that disordered eating can have on women, their families, and their friends. I'm very thankful that this is finally being addressed in the international guidelines on evidence-based best practice for PCOS. These guidelines state that health professionals working with women with PCOS on lifestyle change need to consider their "weight-related stigma."[12] This is a start, although we certainly are not there yet. The guidelines go on to recommend that women with PCOS should be offered "regular monitoring for weight-related changes and excess weight."[12] *Woof.* This shows that there is still an inherent lack of understanding in our medical community about how weight gain and weight loss occur, and the damage that can be done by telling women with PCOS just to "go away and lose weight."

De-motivation

I never, ever focus on weight with the women I work with. If my clients want to lose weight, that is a totally fine goal to have. But I never ask them to weigh themselves, and in the first week of my program I ask them to unfriend their scales by throwing them away. I encourage you to do the same, for one excellent reason: We think that weighing ourselves is good motivation. If the numbers go down it will motivate us to keep going, and when they go up it will motivate us to try harder. But this isn't the way it works in real life.

Think back to a day when you stepped on the scales and that magic number had gone down. Boom—you fist-pumped, you could almost hear the trumpets sounding, and you skipped off those scales and into the day with a positive mindset and encouragement to go forth and live well like you were freakin' Mary Poppins.

But now think back to when you had been *so* "good," in calorie deficit all week, and you couldn't wait to get on those scales to receive your reward for all the hard work you'd put in. But when you stepped on, that dirty little number had gone up! What happens next? You immediately start the day feeling terrible about yourself. You try to rationalize that it was just water weight, and it couldn't be "real" because you'd been so "good." But your heart is still sinking. You step out the door and into your car, your mind still trying to work out what you'd done wrong, and you get honked by another vehicle for changing lanes in front of them.

"WTF?! I was indicating!" *Grrrr!*

You arrive at work and open up your 272 new emails, one of which is a snarky one from a client about something you'd been going above and beyond to fix for them, and which wasn't your fault in the first place. By 10 a.m. you're feeling really down. Your brain recognizes that you're feeling bad and knows that sugar will make you feel great (as it spikes serotonin, your feel-good hormone, for a few seconds). You're also short of sleep, which reduces your insulin sensitivity, so that's a double-whammy reason for your brain to want sugar.

You sit there trying to resist the sugar/refined-carb cravings, and eventually say "Well, f**k it, this diet isn't working anyway, so I might as well just eat what I want." Next minute you're off to the cafe downstairs for a sausage roll, which you wolf down before getting back to your desk. (If you're in the US, a sausage roll is a sausage wrapped in puff pastry. If you've never tried one, you're missing out!)

Your brain now goes into overdrive: "Oooooooooooh you've stuffed it up now! Oh well, you might as well ruin the rest of the day/week/month, and then you can always start again with a clean slate tomorrow—Monday, the first of the month." So next minute you're back down to the cafe for another sausage roll, two custard-filled donuts, a bag of candy AND a chocolate bar.

On Monday, you're back to getting on those scales, restricting what you eat, and inevitably repeating the same vicious cycle the next week.

How do I know this? Because I've repeated this cycle countless times during the many years that I was battling to get my PCOS under control. Those uncontrollable sugar cravings would drive me to the vending machine at 3 p.m. on the dot day after day.

This vicious cycle triggered by de-motivation means that overall we don't eat that well, and a massive factor in conceiving is having a healthy, quality egg and sperm. Bingeing and restricting cycles are inevitably going to increase the amount of insulin, testosterone, and inflammation that an egg is exposed to.

THE DANGER OF FOCUSING ON CALORIES ALONE

Focusing on low-calorie foods may make you more likely to eat insulin-stimulating foods. If your insulin isn't functioning correctly, you're more than likely to have sugar cravings that are off the charts and to feel hungry all the time—two hallmarks of high insulin. So if you focus on reducing calories while still suffering from these cravings and hunger pangs, you're going to be hunting out all the low-calorie sweet treats and foods you can find.

A quick google for low-calorie foods comes up with lists like the "22 low syn foods," which you'll be familiar with if you've ever tried the Slimming World plan. Most low-calorie diet plans or clubs have similar lists, which include foods like:

- zero percent fat Greek yogurt
- frozen mango and grapes
- fat-free cottage cheese
- high-fiber bars
- light cheese spread tubes.

While these foods might sound "healthy" and low in calories, they are hugely insulin-stimulating—even the dairy products (I'll explain more about this in Chapter 7). For women without PCOS and insulin resistance this may not matter—they might well be able to eat them and still lose weight. For you, though, it's different. When you eat these foods, your insulin will be rising and will set off the vicious cycle that I described earlier.

I find it so much more effective both physiologically and psychologically to focus on root cause rather than weight. Even if you've been told that you need to lose weight, or won't qualify for fertility treatment until you reach a certain BMI, I want you to put that out of your mind for now. Instead, just focus on identifying and treating your root cause.

Chapter 4
Conventional medical treatments

There are many amazing medical treatments to help with fertility in PCOS. I love that we can combine the best of traditional medicine and holistic/lifestyle medicine to help women conceive. However, in many cases, conventional medicine jumps straight to drugs and surgery when a holistic lifestyle treatment can often do the same job, if not better, at no risk. Because there is *always* a risk when it comes to drugs and surgery.

The 2018 international evidence-based guidelines for the assessment and management of PCOS advocate this lifestyle-first, combined approach, too.[1] These guidelines were the result of input by over 3,000 PCOS health professionals, researchers, and patients across the globe, and are designed to give best-practice, evidence-based information to health professionals working with women with PCOS. They state:

> Holistic approaches are required, and pharmacological therapy
> in PCOS needs to be considered alongside education, lifestyle,
> and other options, including cosmetic therapy and counseling.[1]

So why isn't your doctor giving you detailed information about exactly what to eat, how to chart your cycles, what vitamins and minerals you need, and whether you need to prioritize sleep over exercise for the next few months? To be honest, it's likely to be because they don't know this information because it isn't part of the conventional medical curriculum.

As I said earlier, don't dismiss the wonders of conventional medicine. We have medicines and vaccines to thank for curing epidemics such as the plague, smallpox, and influenza. Conventional medicine can save your life if you get hit by a bus or a bullet. But acute conditions such as these are not the only problems in our modern-day world. We now have epidemics of chronic, complex conditions like infertility, cancer, type 2 diabetes, and heart disease, and these can't always be cured by drugs or surgery.

However, conventional medicine is still primarily what our doctors are taught during their training and, consequently, this is what they have in their kitbag to give as treatment. They typically aren't taught about in-depth diagnostics like charting your cycle to check that your luteal phase is long enough. They aren't taught about how insulin levels can disrupt ovulation or how you can modify your diet, exercise, vitamins, and minerals to fix this. So you're unlikely to get these options from a conventionally trained doctor.

In this chapter, you'll learn about the different conventional medical treatments available and how they work, but I'm also going to inform you of the risks involved for both you and your children. In no way do I intend to scaremonger, and I definitely don't want you to feel "guilty" if you *do* need medical intervention—which many of you may. I am giving you this information merely to help you make an informed choice and to know that these are not your only options.

My motto for PCOS is lifestyle first, and then if needed, bring in conventional treatment, which includes the following.

COMMON FERTILITY MEDICATIONS
Clomifene

Clomifene (also called clomiphene or clomiphene citrate and marketed under the trade names Clomid and Serophene) is the most common fertility medication for PCOS. It works by artificially stimulating your body to ovulate. Clomifene blocks the receptors for estrogen in your brain, which makes your body think that its estrogen levels are lower than they are. This leads to an increase in the amount of FSH (the one that grows the egg to size). It's not 100 percent clear how this process works in PCOS, but it's likely that the increase in FSH improves the ratio of FSH to LH so that the LH no longer appears too high and you can now ovulate. About a week after the last dose of clomifene, ovulation will occur when a surge of LH from the pituitary gland stimulates the developing egg to mature and release.

Clomifene can be really helpful for women who aren't ovulating. Unfortunately, however, the success rate isn't particularly high in PCOS—and only 22 percent of women have a live birth after six treatment cycles.[2] This might be because one of the downsides of clomifene is that it thins your uterine lining (the nest).[3] The success rate can be increased by combining metformin (an insulin-sensitizing drug) with clomifene, or by bringing your insulin down naturally using the steps I have given in this book.[4]

Before starting clomifene, please do the following:

1. **Check whether or not you're ovulating.** Clomifene helps you to ovulate. So if you're already ovulating, taking clomifene does not increase your chances of getting pregnant.[5] It doesn't make sense to be taking a drug that affects your hormones and can thin your uterine lining, let alone outlaying for the cost of the drug, if it isn't going to help you get pregnant. Unfortunately, many women I see haven't been checked for this before being prescribed clomifene. You can easily check whether you're ovulating by following the instructions in Chapter 9 (see page 218–231).

2. **Get a basic fertility workup done for you and your partner.** While ovulation is an important part of conception, it's no more important than the quality of your partner's sperm or the ability for that sperm to reach your eggs in the fallopian tubes. As well as

a sperm analysis, get a hysterosalpingogram (HSG) to confirm that your tubes are open. There is no point pummeling your body with drugs and risking ovarian hyperstimulation if your partner's sperm isn't going to be able to do the job or get through to your egg.

The clomifene treatment process

Day 1—Your doctor or fertility specialist will tell you to contact the clinic on the first day of your period. If you aren't getting cycles, you'll likely be given medroxyprogesterone (a progesterone medication which you'll probably know as Provera) for five to 10 days at a dose of 5 mg or 10 mg daily to induce a period.

Days 2 to 3—Your doctor or fertility specialist might also perform a baseline ultrasound check to see how your eggs are growing. What they are looking for is whether your body is choosing one dominant egg to grow to maturity. This egg is usually quite easy to spot as it's much bigger than the others. If a dominant egg can't be seen, it's likely that the treatment cycle will be canceled and you will try again when your next period arrives.

Days 3 to 5—Treatment begins! If everything looks good, you'll be given clomifene to take for five days, from Day 3, 4, or 5. The standard starting dose is 25 to 50 mg.

Days 8 to 17—Clomifene gets to work! After you've finished taking the drug, its effects kick in by blocking the estrogen receptors in your brain. Your body thinks that your estrogen levels are lower than they are, and increases the amount of FSH. About a week after the last dose of clomifene, ovulation will occur when a surge of LH from your pituitary gland stimulates the developing egg inside the follicle(s) to mature and release.

Days 10 to 21—This is when treatment can really differ, depending on your specialist. Apart from telling you to have sex daily over the next week, some doctors or fertility specialists leave you to it; others monitor you with blood tests and ultrasound. The monitoring will reveal how many follicles are growing, whether the lining of your uterus is thick enough, and whether you're going to need a hormonal trigger shot (more on this below) or intrauterine insemination (see page 77). While monitoring isn't compulsory, it does have some major benefits, so if possible try to choose a fertility specialist who will do this.

It is important to check how many follicles are growing, to prevent you having twins. Clomifene can cause overstimulation, meaning that your body abnormally grows two dominant eggs rather than one. As I'll explain in the next chapter, having twins may sound great but it comes with a huge risk for you and the babies, so it really isn't desirable. I also know of a couple who got quads after clomifene treatment—just imagine! So if your doctor cancels the treatment because of multiple eggs, please listen to them and don't have sex. Or use a condom. I know it's so hard when you've been waiting for such a long time and you finally have an egg, but it's very important for your health.

The thickness of your uterine lining is also really important. Because clomifene can cause thinning of the uterine lining[6], it can make it hard for the egg to burrow in and make a safe nest for itself. Remember, the uterine lining is the cake mold, and if the mold is too thin then it's likely to split. If your uterine lining is too thin, you may be given an estrogen suppository to insert to stimulate the lining to thicken.

You may also be given a "trigger shot" of the hormone human chorionic gonadotropin (hCG). This is the hormone that's detected in pregnancy tests, and it does a similar job to LH: it signals to your body to project the egg out into the fallopian tubes to meet the sperm. This is why it's called a "trigger shot," because it triggers ovulation to occur in the next 24 to 36 hours. This is obviously super-helpful for you to time sex. The trigger shot is usually given seven to nine days after your last clomifene pill, but might be delayed if an ultrasound shows that you need more time to grow your egg to size. You'll likely be given the trigger shot to inject between 6 p.m. and 10 p.m., and be told to have sex that night (so that sperm is waiting there when the egg is released) and again in two days, if not both days. If you're using IUI (intrauterine insemination), an appointment will be scheduled for you for two days later.

Days 14 to 25—Meet the sperm! This is the time when you need to have sperm ready waiting for your egg to be released. If you're not having a trigger shot, ovulation usually occurs 5 to 10 days after taking your last clomifene pill. I recommend trying to have sex daily starting three days after your last clomifene treatment and continue until you have ovulated. This is why combining clomifene treatment with charting your cycles (see Chapter 9) is really effective. If you're charting your cycle by using your temperature, you can easily confirm when you've ovulated, even if you're not having ultrasounds.

If you're doing IUI because your partner's sperm needs a bit more assistance, you can still have sex as well—it's just bonus points. Or consider the at-home IUI that I explain in Chapter 11 (see page 265).

Days 19 to 21—This is when your doctor or fertility specialist may do a progesterone test to determine whether or not you ovulated. If you're charting your cycle by measuring your temperature (see Chapter 9) you'll already know whether you have ovulated, but if not then the progesterone test may tell you. Remember that progesterone rises after you've ovulated. In the baking analogy, it's the cake tin that keeps the batter in place so it can bake properly and not spatter all over your oven. Progesterone also makes your body temperature rise, which is why you can track your temperature to see whether you've ovulated.

Days 21 to 35—This is the big wait to see whether you're pregnant. If you're charting your cycle, you can see this from your temperature. If your temperature stays elevated for 18 days from ovulation, then this is a really good indicator that you're pregnant.

Day 35 onward—If you did successfully conceive, congratulations! Now, I'd really recommend doing another progesterone test to check that your progesterone is high enough to keep that cake mold (your uterus) in place. If you don't have enough progesterone, you are at greater risk of miscarriage. See Chapter 12 for more on this.

If you didn't conceive, I know it's a massive blow—but remember that all is not lost. You might just need a different dose. If your ovaries were overstimulated and produced two follicles, you'll likely need a lower dose. If an egg wasn't released, you'll likely try again with a similar dose or maybe have it increased. Some women need up to 150 mg of clomifene before their eggs start to grow properly.

Additionally, clomifene works more effectively if your insulin is lower—so if you've picked up this book mid-treatment and haven't yet determined your root cause, please do this first. I really encourage you to consider stopping the treatment and addressing that root cause first, especially if it's your insulin. You can always come back to clomifene treatments later, but once you've reached your maximum number of treatment cycles there is no going back. The maximum number of rounds in most countries is six, and for women over 38, it's just three. This is because too much clomifene can overstimulate your ovaries. This is a really dangerous condition that, in rare cases, can lead to death. Another reason is that if clomifene hasn't worked by round six (many fertility specialists say round three), it's very unlikely to work at all.

"Clomifene resistance" is the term used when you don't conceive within the maximum number of cycles permitted. This is generally due to your insulin or androgen levels being too high, and affects about a quarter of women with PCOS.[2] Even then, all is not lost, and it is possible to conceive naturally if you work on your root cause.

CASE STUDY

Sarah had been a competitive athlete all her life, competing in lacrosse and cross-country. However, in her later high school years she found that she was gaining weight, and her periods disappeared. Her doctor put this down to the fact that she was training heavily, and advised her to go on HBC to regulate her periods. But this never sat well with Sarah, who thought it wasn't normal for training to stop her periods when her weight was increasing.

In 2013, Sarah came off HBC, and her periods didn't return. She also had an outbreak of acne, was gaining weight, and felt constantly fatigued. She eventually visited her doctor, who diagnosed her with PCOS. "I felt incredibly lost, as they had no real treatment plan for me. The doctor just said, 'If you want to have kids, then we'll give you metformin and clomifene. But until then you just have to stay on HBC.'"

In 2015, Sarah married and she and her husband started trying for a family immediately. They tried for two years before Sarah was given clomifene. She went through six rounds of treatment without success and was told that IVF was her only option.

"I'd tried acupuncture and every herb and supplement I'd read about 'helping PCOS.' But nothing had any effect at all. I also had the glucose fasting test, but it came back within the 'normal range.'"

However, when I tested Sarah's insulin levels in 2017, it was evident these were not optimal, and she also had high levels of stress hormones. This was why she wasn't ovulating naturally and also probably why she was resistant to clomifene. I tweaked her diet slightly so that her insulin levels could come down. Instead of running 8 miles (13 km) a day, Sarah switched to weight training and lots of low-intensity walking. I also changed her supplements to help reduce her insulin levels. In addition, I had Sarah really prioritize her sleep, because as you'll learn later, sleep is crucial for your insulin sensitivity.

The results of these small changes were quite dramatic. Within one month, Sarah's cycles had returned, and within four months she was pregnant, completely naturally. But there were also other improvements for Sarah:

"I lost quite a bit of weight, my acne cleared up, my energy levels

> were so much better (I felt like Superwoman!), and I wasn't hungry all the time like I had been for my entire life!"

What happened with Sarah is what I love about treating the root cause: You see so many other changes. The big one for Sarah was her energy and hunger levels. She had no idea that her fatigue and constant hunger were symptoms of insulin resistance. This was seriously affecting her life and her ability to do her teaching job. Couple this with pregnancy fatigue and then newborn fatigue, and it's a recipe for one burnt-out momma.

When you treat the root cause, you see resolution in so many symptoms that you may not have even known were related.

Side-effects of clomifene

Some of these can be a bit nasty, sorry! Because clomifene blocks your estrogen receptors, it tricks your body into making more estrogen. So you're going to get all the symptoms of high estrogen. Think of it as your mom going through menopause meets your worst teen angst PMS ever: incredible moodiness, hot flashes (flushes), bloating, vaginal dryness, weight gain, and sore boobs.

Metformin

Metformin (trade name Glucophage, among others) is the next most commonly used medication for PCOS and fertility. It's not a fertility drug, but it does address the root cause—insulin levels—to help your body ovulate naturally. Metformin is an insulin-sensitizing drug, causing the body to produce less insulin. The research supporting this effect is really positive, and metformin has been shown to reduce HbA1c, a marker of insulin resistance, by 1.5 percentage points.[3] As you know from Chapter 2 (see page 39), a lower insulin level helps all your fertile ingredients.

I've seen a couple of women who have addressed their insulin with my five-step plan and also taken metformin and conceived. But when it comes to the research supporting metformin as a fertility drug, it isn't particularly strong. Metformin is generally used in combination with clomifene to stimulate ovulation. In one large study,[2] 626 women with PCOS who were struggling to conceive took metformin alone, or clomifene alone, or a combination of the two. Only 7 percent of the women in the metformin group had a live birth, compared with 22 percent in the clomifene-only group and 26 percent in the combined clomifene and metformin group.[2]

However, if you are already ovulating and therefore don't need clomifene, metformin may really help to reduce your risk of miscarriage. But this isn't the only way to reduce your risk—see Chapter 12.

If you are taking metformin, you'll also need to ensure that you're taking vitamin B_{12} or B complex, as metformin leaches vitamin B_{12} from your body[7] (more about this in Chapter 5). And while it's great that metformin addresses the root cause (insulin), it isn't without its risks. The way metformin increases insulin sensitivity is by damaging the mitochondria—the little "motors" inside the body's cells that produce energy. Similar to the way the motor in a car takes fuel and oxygen and makes energy to propel the car forward, the mitochondria take glucose from food, and together with oxygen convert it into ATP—energy you can use. Metformin makes the mitochondria inefficient so they can't produce as much energy.[8] Instead, the cells use glucose to make lactate, a process that provides the body with much less energy. This is likely to be why many people report feeling really tired when they take metformin. Another downside is that metformin can cross your placenta into the baby, which means if your mitochondria can be damaged, so can your baby's.[9] I explain more about the potential risks of this in Chapter 5.

Letrozole

Letrozole (trade name Femara) is a less-well-known fertility drug, but the evidence is showing that it may be much better than clomifene for stimulating ovulation. The 2018 international evidence-based PCOS guidelines recommend that letrozole be the first choice of fertility treatment over and above clomifene.[1]

Letrozole wasn't designed as a fertility drug; it was developed to treat postmenopausal breast cancer, but it was found to trigger ovulation if used in the same way as clomifene. Both drugs block estrogen and trick the body into producing more, so that you ovulate. But instead of blocking the estrogen receptor as clomifene does, letrozole inhibits the enzyme (aromatase) that converts testosterone into estrogen.

Letrozole is more effective than clomifene, especially in PCOS. An analysis of randomized controlled trials, which together involved over 2,000 women with PCOS, concluded that taking letrozole resulted in significantly more women ovulating compared with taking clomifene.[10] However, like clomifene, if you're already ovulating then letrozole probably won't increase your chances of getting pregnant.

If you're working with a fertility specialist who wants to put you on clomifene, query this and point them to the 2018 PCOS guidelines, which state that letrozole is the better option;[1] I've included a link to these in the Resources section at the end of this book.

The treatment process for letrozole is very similar to the steps outlined above for clomifene. The side effects of letrozole aren't much better than those of clomifene, unfortunately; dizziness and fatigue are two of the most commonly reported.

Gonadotropins

Gonadotropins are synthetic forms of LH and FSH (the hormones that grow your eggs and then release the dominant one), and are injected into you to stimulate your body to ovulate. Because gonadotropins are hormones, they are stronger drugs than letrozole and clomifene, and so are used as a "second-line" treatment—i.e. when letrozole and clomifene haven't worked for you (and your doctor or fertility specialist has checked out all the most common reasons why those drugs might not have worked, like blocked fallopian tubes).[1] Where gonadotropins could be the most helpful is where you have a high LH level that just won't come down.

The injections start on Day 3 or 4 of your cycle, to grow your egg, and last up until Days 12 to 14 of your cycle. During the course of injections you should be monitored via ultrasound to check that your eggs are growing to size and that there is only one dominant follicle. Once your fertility doctor can see a large egg, you may receive a trigger shot of hCG as with clomifene (see page 69).

Gonadotropins are sometimes used in combination with IUI (see below), or with natural timed sex.

Progestin

If you haven't had a period, or haven't had one in many months, you may be given a progestin (a synthetic form of progesterone) to help stimulate your menstrual cycle. The most common brand used is Provera. The idea is that after you have bled, you'll ovulate in the next cycle and can conceive, or you can have an ovulation-inducer like clomifene or letrozole.

However, a study published in 2012 showed that this didn't actually work in practice. When researchers compared women with PCOS who either received or did not receive progestin, they found that women who received a dose of progestin followed by ovulation induction ovulated in 30 percent of cases.[11] But only 7 percent of these women conceived. The women who didn't receive progestin ovulated 27 percent of the time, but nearly 28 percent of these women were able to get pregnant.[11]

Immune-modulating medications

In Chapter 11, I explain that another really common reason why you may not be getting pregnant is that your immune system isn't making your uterus particularly habitable for an egg to implant in. This is especially the case if you have endometriosis or an autoimmune condition like Hashimoto's thyroiditis as well as PCOS. It is important to check out all the factors in Chapter 11 to find out what else could be affecting your fertility.

While the practice is still not particularly common, some doctors are now prescribing medications that help calm the immune system to improve egg quality and make the uterus a better place to call home. These medications include low-dose lymphocyte (white blood cell) immunotherapy, which has been shown to help some women who have had recurrent miscarriages.[12] Naltrexone is another drug that can help reduce autoimmune markers when used in low doses.[12] It is a relatively "new" drug to be trialed on women with PCOS, but an early trial showed that it significantly improved ovulation rates in women with PCOS who were resistant to clomifene.[13] Low-dose aspirin has also been successfully used to help women with high inflammation to conceive.[14] Please don't try this at home, though—if it's used in the wrong context and the dosage isn't correct, it can increase the risk of bleeding.

Hormonal contraception

This is the most common medication given to women with PCOS to "regulate" periods. I won't talk about it here; if you're trying to conceive, then you're probably not going to be on HBC. However, if you are reading this in preparation for conception, then check out the detailed information in Chapter 13.

ASSISTED REPRODUCTIVE TREATMENTS

If medications aren't successful, you'll likely be referred for assisted reproductive treatments, of which there are many.

Intrauterine insemination (IUI)

This is one of the "lower-tech" treatments. In very basic terms, instead of letting the sperm find their own way up to your cervix and into your uterus after sex, a fertility specialist will take your partner's sperm and manually insert it into your uterus, bypassing the cervix. Charming no, but sometimes very necessary; and IUI is much cheaper and gentler than IVF (in-vitro fertilization).

It's not actually quite as simple as I've described. First, your partner's sperm will be sifted to remove any dead semen, white blood cells, and seminal fluid. This is an important first step because the seminal fluid contains prostaglandins, which your cervix would normally filter out.

Prostaglandins can cause cramping in the uterus.

Before trying IUI, it's critical to know your "root cause." If you're not ovulating, then IUI alone isn't going to help you as it doesn't stimulate ovulation. If you are ovulating (either naturally or with the assistance of clomifene or letrozole) but your partner's sperm isn't optimal, then IUI is likely to be very helpful.

The other situation where IUI can be helpful is if you don't have a lot of cervical fluid, which may be more common in PCOS.[15] Cervical fluid is discussed in Chapter 9. Your cervical fluid helps get sperm up through your cervix and into the uterus. If you don't have much cervical fluid, the sperm won't make it into your fallopian tubes before they die, so are very unlikely to make it to date night with your egg.[16]

The good news is that some data from fertility centers show that IUI can increase pregnancy rates in PCOS from 20 percent without IUI to 25 percent with IUI.[17]

In-vitro fertilization (IVF)

In IVF, eggs are extracted from your ovary (or donor eggs are used) and then fertilized with sperm from your partner (or a donor). After the eggs have matured for a few days, one or more embryos are inserted into your uterus. Understandably, IVF is the most invasive fertility treatment, but is an incredible treatment for those who need it.

The first stage of IVF is to stimulate your body to make eggs that can then be retrieved. This is generally done by giving you injections of gonadotropins (see page 75). A hollow needle is then inserted through your cervix to suck out the eggs (don't worry—you'll be given some drugs for the pain!). The more eggs they can collect, the more likely it is that you'll get some embryos (eggs fertilized by sperm).

Your partner then provides some sperm, which is mixed together with your eggs in a Petri dish and left to allow the sperm to fertilize your eggs. If your eggs and sperm do get together, you'll get some embryos after about three to five days. But if your doctor is concerned that the sperm won't be able to fertilize the eggs, the sperm might be injected directly into the eggs.

Once you've got some embryos, a small tube is inserted into you so that the embryos can hydro-slide down into your uterus. If all goes well, the embryos will implant in your uterine lining about six to 10 days later.

The success rates of IVF for women with PCOS are very similar to those for women without PCOS.[18] If you have PCOS and no other immune issues (like endometriosis), then you'll likely find that IVF isn't necessary. It's called a second-line treatment and is only used if ovulation stimulation doesn't work.

SURGERY

There are a couple of surgical treatments that are offered to women with PCOS to help improve their chances of conceiving.

Laparoscopic ovarian surgery

Laparoscopic ovarian surgery, also known as ovarian drilling (OD), can trigger ovulation in women with PCOS, often with great success. A surgeon uses a laser to puncture each ovary three to eight times, and in 74 percent of cases the women will ovulate naturally in the following three to six months, with up to 50 percent then successfully conceiving.[19, 20] It is not known exactly how OD works (it could be due to increased ovarian blood flow), but the drilling improves the hormonal profile, which then improves your fertile ingredients. The procedure is a bit invasive, so is generally only used if letrozole or clomifene doesn't work.

The consensus given in the 2018 international PCOS guidelines is that "Laparoscopic ovarian surgery could be a second-line therapy for women with PCOS, who are clomiphene citrate resistant, with anovulatory infertility and no other infertility factors."[1]

Bariatric surgery

While not specifically a fertility surgery, bariatric surgery (gastric bypass, gastric sleeve, etc.) is sometimes offered to women with PCOS who haven't been able to lose weight through diet and exercise to qualify for IVF. This surgery is incredibly successful for some women, with the weight loss helping to improve their insulin. However, the surgery needs to be combined with lifestyle changes (see Chapters 6 to 10) to keep insulin levels down over the long term. I have seen many cases of women being able to become pregnant after bariatric surgery, but equally many who haven't because one or more of their fertile ingredients are still not right. There are also no long-term studies of the effect of the surgery on you or your baby. My concern would be around getting enough calories, vitamins, and minerals after surgery and during pregnancy due to the much reduced amount you are able to eat.

In terms of its use for fertility, the consensus from the 2018 international PCOS guidelines is: "Bariatric surgery should be considered an experimental therapy in women with PCOS, to have a healthy baby, with risk to benefit ratios currently too uncertain about advocating this as fertility therapy."[1]

Chapter 5
The downside of the current medical approach

To help you make an informed choice, this chapter outlines some of the risks involved with the current medical approach to PCOS and fertility. As I said in the previous chapter, I love that we can combine the best of conventional medicine and holistic/lifestyle medicine to help you conceive. However, in almost all cases I see, that conventional medicine jumps straight to drugs and surgery when holistic lifestyle treatment may actually have done the same job, if not better, at no risk. The oath of all medical practitioners is to "Do no harm," and the evidence shows that medications sometimes cause harm, so why would we not want to avoid this and make you and your child healthier at the same time? It seems totally obvious to me.

LACK OF FOCUS ON THE ROOT CAUSE

One of the biggest problems arising from the way that PCOS and fertility are treated at the moment is that the root cause isn't investigated, which can put the health of both you and your child at risk. The medical goal is just to get you pregnant, and this may not always consider whether you or the baby will be healthy in the process.

Although the treatment pathway differs slightly between countries if you have PCOS and are struggling to conceive, your doctor is typically your first stop to ask for help. They'll first look at your weight, and if your BMI is over 30 you'll be told to go away and lose weight before they can do anything further. In my experience, there isn't much guidance given on how to achieve this except to eat less (but everything in moderation—no fads of course), and exercise more. You'll also likely be given a prescription for metformin (an insulin-sensitizing medication, see page 73). If your BMI is below 30, you may also be given the drugs clomifene (see page 66) or letrozole (see page 74) to help to get your body to ovulate.

At no point in the typical pathway does anyone sit down and thoroughly analyze your situation to understand your root cause and educate you on how to fix it. This isn't a criticism of your doctor—they are generally doing the best job they can. The real problem is that:

- They don't have training in root cause analysis; and
- They don't have the time to do this thoroughly (15–20 minutes per appointment compared with the hour or so I spend looking over a client's lab results and intake paperwork before I even meet them).

For example, if you're a fertility patient, whether or not you have PCOS, it's highly unlikely that anyone will sit you down and check that you're actually timing sex correctly. Conception can only occur on about six days out of your cycle. This might be mind-blowing news for any of you who have been led to believe that you can get pregnant on any day of your cycle and have been taking hormonal contraceptives to protect yourself from that. In fact, you can only conceive when you are in your fertile window—the time leading up to ovulation. (I explain this in detail in Chapter 9.)

You may believe that ovulation happens on a certain day in your cycle; for example, you might have been told that you ovulate on Day 14. But in fact, even with a 28-day cycle only 10 percent of women ovulate on Day 14.[1] The day that you ovulate can dramatically change from month to month, even if the length of your cycle is always the same.

CASE STUDY

Karen, a general-practice doctor (MD) from the UK, and her partner had been trying to conceive naturally for years and had used IUI to conceive their first child. She was interested in my *Eggducated* program, in which I teach women how to identify the signs and symptoms of when they are fertile (the days before ovulation), so that they can time sex accordingly.

Karen had always believed that she ovulated on Day 14 (14 days from the start of her period). After going through the program, she found that she actually ovulated on more like Day 17, and so was completely mistiming sex.

Just two months after starting the program, she conceived successfully. Given that Karen is a medical doctor, she likely had more training than most of us in reproduction—and even she didn't have the right information. How likely is it that your doctor will be able to give you the correct information or pick up any problems there might be?

Karen's story illustrates what we see in the research. Dr. Kerry Hampton, who was my fertility lecturer, carried out some incredibly interesting research in Australia. She surveyed 262 couples who were attending assisted reproduction clinics and had been trying to conceive for at least a year. Although 83 percent of these couples had read information about ovulation and how to time sex correctly, and 62 percent had tried to follow the guidelines they had read, only 13 percent could accurately identify when they were fertile.[2] These findings were repeated in a New Zealand study involving over 1,000 women,[3] and in a study in India, where the researchers found that 85 percent of women didn't know their fertile/ovulation period—they thought they were fertile the entire cycle.[4] Missing the fertile window is only one example of a root-cause diagnosis;

testing for insulin resistance, hypothyroidism, and autoimmune antibodies is also very rarely done.

Reset your expectations

This is where I need your help. I know that when you decide you want to try for a baby, a switch flicks and you want it to happen now. Especially if you are in your thirties and are worried about that ticking biological clock. By the way, there is no judgment here. We can't control when we meet a partner we want to reproduce with, and I completely support women prioritizing their careers. I'm never going to say (or think) that you've been "delaying" having a child.

What I am very aware of is that when you decide you want that child, it can become an all-consuming desire. You don't want to have to wait six months or a year for it to happen. But here's where I need you to ask yourself this:

- Is my goal just getting pregnant?

OR

- Is my goal having a healthy pregnancy without developing gestational diabetes, and a baby that's going to carry to term and also be given the best possible chance to become a healthy adult?

I think you will be answering yes to the second question.

So, I want you to reset your expectations—to accept that this might be a six- or 12-month process. To not automatically jump or push your doctor for the fast or easy option, but instead take your and your child's health into consideration. While not all of it is in your control, and I absolutely don't want you to feel guilty if you use medical help, I do want you to be informed so that you know you have the best chance of a healthy pregnancy (and a healthy baby).

> Reset your mindset on your goal—not just getting pregnant, but also long-term health for you and your child.

RISKS OF NOT TREATING THE ROOT CAUSE FIRST

As I've been using insulin as an example throughout this book so far (and given that 80 percent of all women with PCOS have some insulin resistance), I'll now give you an example of how untreated insulin resistance increases your risk of complications.

Insulin resistance means that you're going to have more insulin in your body. Elevated insulin affects all three of your fertile ingredients, which is likely the reason why you aren't conceiving. If the elevated insulin isn't addressed, and instead you're given a medication like clomifene, then you're still going to have high insulin and also high testosterone levels because the insulin is driving that up.

What's the big deal? Your health and that of your child. That's a big deal.

How your health is affected

If you have high insulin during pregnancy, you have a 24 percent increased risk of pre-eclampsia[5] (high blood pressure and protein in your urine, which can be life-threatening to you and the baby), and a 40 to 46 percent risk of gestational diabetes[6] (more about this in Chapter 12). You're also going to be at greater risk of miscarriage because progesterone is crucial for keeping your uterine lining intact, and if you have high insulin you will have lower progesterone.

If you're then using clomifene, studies have shown that you have an increased risk of miscarriage, both after six weeks and before six weeks.[7] Your ovaries are also more likely to be hyper-stimulated by clomifene and release more than one egg, which can result in up to a 9 percent increased risk of having twins[8] (see page 91 for why this isn't a desirable outcome.) And finally, you're more likely to be resistant to clomifene if you have high insulin levels.[9]

How your baby's health is affected

Research shows that babies exposed to high levels of insulin in the uterus are also more likely to develop a metabolic syndrome (obesity and insulin resistance)[10]. They may also be at greater risk of developing autism.

High levels of testosterone (among other hormones like cortisol) have been associated with autism in both male and female children, and we know that many PCOS root causes increase testosterone levels.[11] It's thought that exposure to high levels of androgens in the uterus changes the way the brain develops, which produces a brain that's very similar to the brain of an autistic person.[12]

When researchers looked at exposure to high androgens in the uterus, they found that women with PCOS had a 35 percent higher chance of having a first-born child with autism, and this was after taking into account other factors that could potentially cause this, like diabetes, complications in childbirth, and the mother's psychiatric state.[12] This isn't the first study of this kind, either. Swedish researchers in 2016 found that maternal PCOS increased the chances of having a child with autism by 59 percent.[13] Be aware that this is just a correlational study—the researchers looked historically at the correlation between PCOS and having a child with autism. The results don't prove that high androgens cause autism; the cause might be something that the researchers didn't think to account for. To categorically prove that high androgens cause autism, we would need a study that involved a group of women who were all exactly the same, then increase testosterone levels in half of the group and see how many of their children had autism. As you can imagine, there are some pretty major ethical issues associated with this, so it is unlikely to happen.

In addition, even if there is indeed a link between androgen levels and autism, keep in mind that the risk is still minor. The risk of having an autistic child is quite low, only 1 to 2 percent in women who don't have PCOS. Even though the risk increases by 35 percent in women with PCOS, that's still only a 1.35 to 2.7 percent chance.[13] Very importantly, there is a lot that you can do to reduce your androgen levels—by changing the way you eat, sleep, move, and live—and this could possibly reduce any potential risks. The major thing to focus on is that if you prioritize addressing the root cause, you'll be improving both your health and the health of your baby.

RISKS ASSOCIATED WITH FERTILITY TREATMENTS

In the previous chapter, we looked at some of the risks involved with not treating the root cause underlying why you're currently not getting pregnant. Now, let's look at some of the risks of the various fertility treatments.

Potential risks of metformin

When I was diagnosed with PCOS, the first thing I asked my doctor was what I could take to "fix" it. She gently explained that there was no pill or surgery to cure it, but there was a drug that could help. Metformin would help with insulin resistance and weight loss, and, better yet, it was a "safe" drug with no major side-effects. Sign me up! I thought that metformin was the wonder drug. I had a quick look online to see what its side-effects were, and read diarrhea, loose stools, fatigue, and muscle soreness, but no long-term effects. I thought, "Small price to pay for finally being able to lose some weight!" And when I lost about 11 lb (5 kg), more than I had ever been able to lose previously, I was ecstatic.

However, it turns out that there are some much more serious side-effects of metformin that aren't so widely publicized.

Mitochondrial damage

As I explained earlier (see page 73), metformin makes your body more sensitive to insulin. As this means treating the root cause (the insulin), it's definitely one of the better treatments, but its damage to the mitochondria is where the issues lie. There have been very few studies on the safety of metformin in pregnancy, which is quite disconcerting given that we've known for some time that it does cross the placental barrier and, therefore, can affect the baby.[14] The results of a study published in 2018 are most alarming. In this study, a randomized controlled trial (RCT), which is the gold standard in scientific research, 182 women with PCOS from Norway were given either 2,000 mg of metformin or a placebo, and were then followed for many years to track the outcomes for their children.[15] The researchers took measurements at birth, 18 months, two years, and four years of age. They expected that the babies that were exposed to metformin would have better insulin levels and body weight at four years old, but found the opposite—the babies exposed to metformin in the uterus had a higher BMI and were almost twice as likely to be overweight or obese by the time they were four years old (32 percent of the study group), compared with their peers who weren't exposed (18 percent). The researchers had taken account of factors such as the mothers' insulin and weight levels. The weight itself is not the issue, but it is a sign that metabolism and insulin function have been damaged.

This isn't the only study to report these findings. A 2020 review of all the research in this area found that metformin was associated with an increased bodyweight and metabolic derangements in babies exposed to metformin in the uterus.[16]

Vitamin B_{12} deficiency

Metformin also leaches vitamin B_{12} and folate—the naturally occurring form of folic acid—from your body;[17] it has been reported that an average of 6 percent to 30 percent of patients could be deficient in vitamin B_{12} due to metformin use.[18, 19] If you're trying to conceive, I bet you've had it drilled into you how important folic acid is and why it's included in the prenatal vitamins you are advised to take (there is more on this in Chapter 7). Folate and vitamin B_{12} both help to form the neural tube around your baby's spine; deficiency results in an increased risk of neural tube defects in unborn children.[20] One study found that mothers with a vitamin B_{12} deficiency were two to three times more likely to have a baby with neural tube defects than mothers with no deficiency.[20] With new research showing that pregnant women actually need triple the current recommended dietary allowance (RDA) of vitamin B_{12},[21] it's going to be very hard to achieve that if your body is losing most of what you're taking in.

Given this information, you might expect that vitamin B_{12} levels would be checked in all women who have been prescribed metformin. However, in my experience this rarely happens. I recently conducted an online survey of women with PCOS, and found that almost 75 percent of the women who had been prescribed metformin had neither had their B_{12} levels checked or been advised that they might need to take a B_{12} supplement. Although this is not journal-level research, it certainly reflects what I'm seeing with my patient base.

If you are taking metformin, please get your vitamin B_{12} levels checked, and follow the guidelines for optimal B_{12} intake in Chapter 10.

Effect on gut bacteria

Gut bacteria are essential for good immune function and proper weight regulation. Read any forum on metformin and you'll find plenty of stories from women who are having to base their everyday lives around the nearest toilet just in case they have an "incident." However, there is much more going on than just loose stools, because metformin seriously affects the microbiome (community of bacteria) living in the intestine.

An incredible 100 trillion bacteria live inside our intestines, and studies have shown that our gut is responsible for 70 percent of our immune system's functioning.[22] We also know that these bacteria directly control the calories that we extract from food and, therefore, aid weight regulation. It's no wonder, then, that if these bacteria are disrupted, weight loss gets even harder.

Effect on resistance exercise

Resistance exercise can be really beneficial for women with PCOS because it makes us more sensitive to insulin, thereby lowering the insulin in our bloodstream.[23] Metformin stops this from happening. In one recent study, 53 people who did not have type 2 diabetes were split into two groups, with one group taking metformin (1000 mg twice daily) and the other group taking a placebo. Both groups did an exercise program for 12 weeks, involving three bouts a week of 45 minutes on a treadmill, elliptical or bike at 85 percent of their maximum heart rate.[24] The researchers found that metformin diminished improvements in not only muscle mass but also cardiorespiratory fitness and insulin sensitivity—the one thing that metformin is supposed to help with! This is not the only study to have results such as these. Another 2019 study found that people taking metformin had significantly less growth in muscle mass compared with people doing the same exercise but not taking metformin.[25] Additionally, earlier studies have found that metformin can lower the exercise-induced improvements in cardiovascular fitness and insulin sensitivity.[26, 27]

Lack of long-term studies

Lastly, there have been no long-term studies on the health of women who have been on metformin for, say, 10, 20, 30-plus years. We just don't know what's going to happen to your body if your mitochondria are compromised for that long. This is why I'm cautious about using metformin as a long-term option—especially as there is another alternative that has been shown in studies to be as effective, if not more effective. This is changing what you eat, how you exercise, and taking some supplements.[28, 29] In some cases it might be absolutely necessary for you to take metformin, but I always recommend trying the least risky option first.

Potential risks of clomifene

We covered some of the risks involved in taking clomifene, an ovulation-inducer, in the previous chapter. However, the story is more complex when you dig a little deeper.

Risk of uterine cancer

A survey of over 15,000 women found that those who were treated with clomifene had an overall higher incidence of cancer.[30] This was especially the case for uterine cancer, but the research also reveals higher risks for breast cancer and non-Hodgkin lymphoma. Note that this wasn't a randomized controlled trial, so it is not possible to say that clomifene was definitely the cause, but it is likely enough that it needs to be investigated further.

Risk of ovarian hyperstimulation

Ovarian hyperstimulation syndrome (OHSS) is more common in PCOS with all fertility treatments, including clomifene (especially in combination with gonadotropins) and IVF.[31] In OHSS, the blood vessels in your ovaries react abnormally to hCG and begin to leak fluid. This fluid swells the ovaries and sometimes leaks into your abdomen, which can be lethal. In PCOS the prevalence is about 5 to 16 percent.[31] The risk can be managed in fertility treatments by starting with a more conservative dose.

Risk of multiple births

It is well known that a common result of fertility treatments such as ovulation induction (i.e. clomifene) or IVF is an increased risk of multiple births.[32] For every 20 pregnancies conceived via clomifene, one will result in twins.[33]

This might seem like a wonderful outcome—two (or more) for the price of one? Fabulous. However, apart from the practical aspects of getting through those first few daunting years with not one but two (or three, or even five) screaming babies, the risks to you and your children are pretty daunting. Pre-eclampsia (high blood pressure and protein in the urine), gestational diabetes, preterm birth, and small fetal growth are all well-known risks.[34]

Risks for your baby's health

In a study of over 30,000 children, researchers found that children conceived after ovulation induction (i.e. clomifene) had poorer health and were more frequently hospitalized and for longer periods than those conceived without treatment.[35] They also had more long-term illnesses, were more likely to be on long-term medication, and more likely to be hospitalized later in life.

Risks of IVF

If clomifene and metformin treatments aren't successful, IVF is generally the next step (as in Sarah's case, see page 71). Again, in most cases that I've seen, root-cause investigation isn't completed at any of these steps.

As mentioned above, it's well known that a common result of IVF is an increased risk of multiple births. Although some countries have reduced the risk of multiple births by requiring single-embryo transfer, multiple transfers are still common in many parts of the world, including the US, the UK and Europe. The Centers for Disease Control and Prevention (CDC) in the US showed that approximately 46 percent of IVF pregnancies were twin (or higher-multiple) births,[36] and in the UK and Europe it was nearly 20 percent.[37]

An extensive analysis of the studies done on babies born after fertility treatment found that they were more likely to be born preterm, be low weight at birth, have a higher rate of abnormalities, and be more likely to be stillborn.[38] Concern has also been raised about the long-term health of children born through IVF. Otherwise healthy children conceived by IVF may have higher blood pressure, adiposity (overweight or obesity), glucose levels,[39] and more generalized vascular dysfunction than children conceived naturally.

It's also important to understand that fertility treatment is big business and is expected to hit a market size of US$36 billion by 2026.[40] Fertility clinics and their staff have endless skills in reproductive techniques and medications to help you conceive, and for this we are so grateful. Their metric of success is getting you pregnant, but as I've outlined to you already, I think we need to move away from just achieving a pregnancy and instead focus on making sure that you stay pregnant, and have a healthy pregnancy and a baby that grows into a healthy adult.

I'm also concerned how unregulated the fertility world is. Neither the American Society for Reproductive Medicine nor the European Society of Human Reproduction and Embryology has guidelines on the use of IVF.[40] This means it's unlikely that someone is going to go through your medical history and say "No, you don't need IVF, you just need a few more months of timing sex correctly and working on making your body more sensitive to insulin. Here you go, here's the exact plan of how you do that, and a fertility educator to teach you how to identify when you're fertile." This was shown to be the case in the study I refer to on page 211; 56 percent of those women waiting for fertility treatment didn't need it, they just needed help to time sex when they were actually fertile.

WHEN FERTILITY ASSISTANCE IS FANTASTIC

As I've said many times, I am not anti-medications or anti-fertility treatment. However, it's important to know that these drugs and treatments don't come without some risks to you and your child. Also, your health is going to be vastly improved by treating your root cause first—then, if you still need fertility assistance, that's exactly the right time to use it.

CASE STUDY

In 2017 I met Cassie. In our first consultation, she told me that she'd been overweight since she was a young teenager and had never had regular periods. At boarding school she'd been put on a special low-fat diet of steamed fish and vegetables, which obviously wasn't appealing for a teen. Cassie was diagnosed with PCOS as an older teenager and told to lose weight if she wanted her symptoms to improve.

Every trip to the doctor was torture, as almost all of her condition was attributed to her weight. Fast-forward to university and post-university, and Cassie's weight continued to climb, despite trying every diet under the sun.

After getting married, Cassie and her husband decided to try for a baby, but as no periods were in sight this was somewhat difficult. After a year of trying, they were referred to a reproductive endocrinologist who told Cassie that she wasn't eligible for any treatment until she lost a significant amount of weight, and set her up with an appointment for bariatric surgery.

She tried Slimming World and was filling up on "zero-point" diet sodas, grapes and pre-cut pineapple, and fat-free yogurt. Her intentions were good, but even though she was in calorie deficit these foods spiked her insulin dramatically, and it was rising higher and higher. Cassie's weight loss was minimal, and her periods didn't return.

After seeing her blood test results I knew that Cassie's insulin wasn't optimal, and it was preventing her ovulating and was causing her body to store rather than burn fat. I tweaked her diet, exercise regimen, supplements, and other lifestyle factors to make her more sensitive to insulin. We didn't focus at all on calories, or ever even mention weight; we just worked to improve her insulin.

Cassie's body responded by losing a staggering 57 lb (26 kg) in less than six months, and she got her periods back after only three months. The reason why Cassie hadn't been successful before was that she had never been told that the root cause of her weight gain was insulin, and that making her body more sensitive to it was the key to losing weight. Instead, like so many others—including me—she'd been told that weight loss was a simple equation of eating less than you burn (calories in, calories out).

Her energy levels and moods were also so much better, and she was a self-confessed "nicer person to be around." Her periods became regular for the first time in her life . . . but month after month went by with no baby. We investigated endometriosis, Hashimoto's thyroiditis, and many other reasons. Cassie went back to her fertility specialist, who was astonished at the staggering amount of weight she'd lost and confirmed that she was now eligible for fertility treatment. After a few rounds of treatment, Cassie conceived her adorable baby girl.

FIVE-STEP PLAN FOR A HEALTHY PREGNANCY, CHILD, AND YOU

Chapter 6
Step 1—Identify the root cause(s)

Now that you know why it's so important to treat the root cause, your first step in improving your fertility is to understand yours. As we discussed in Chapter 1, PCOS is a syndrome, which means it's different in all of us, due to a combination of our genes not playing nicely with our environment.

The key is to find out which systems and hormones aren't functioning properly (the root cause) so that you can improve them. Even though all of us with PCOS have the same condition, the systems in our bodies that aren't working properly can be vastly different. This is why there isn't one "PCOS diet" or supplement. It's the same reason why there isn't one fuel for all cars—it depends on whether your motor is gas, diesel, or electric. If there was one easy solution for everyone, you wouldn't be reading this book as you'd already have the answers.

Think about your PCOS symptoms as being like the layers of an onion with loads of eye-watering layers. There's the flaky outside skin, then the fleshy layers underneath.

Think about your symptoms, for example not getting pregnant, as the outside layer: the dry, flaky one. We don't know what's causing those symptoms, so we peel back that layer to expose what's underneath: the first fleshy layer. What we find here is that some or all of your fertile

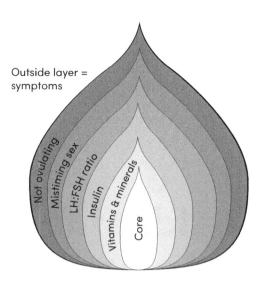

Figure 4: Peeling the layers to get to the root cause

ingredients aren't working properly; for example, you're ovulating late so you're mistiming sex or your nest (uterine lining) isn't staying intact for long enough.

But again, we don't really know *why* you're not ovulating, so we peel off another layer. We do some testing and find that your ratio of LH to FSH isn't right, so the egg is being released late, and when it finally does get released, the second half of the cycle is too short and the egg doesn't get a chance to burrow into the lining to become a viable pregnancy. We also find that your testosterone is too high, which is affecting the quality of the egg.

But we still don't know *why*, so we peel back another layer to find which systems in your body aren't working properly. For example, your body might be overproducing insulin, and this is causing your LH to be a greater than the ideal 2:1 ratio.

We ask *why* again, and peel back another layer of the onion to get to the core. What is it about your environment that's disrupting your systems (in this case, your high insulin)? What are you eating? Do you have enough essential vitamins and minerals? Are you sleeping enough? And can we optimize your exercise?

This is what I mean about getting to the root cause or the "core."

Even though each case of PCOS is unique, there are a handful of really common "root causes:"

- insulin issues
- hormonal birth control (HBC)
- adrenal issues
- inflammation and thyroid.

I'll also investigate your partner's sperm, because although it has nothing to do with your PCOS, it has 50 percent to do with whether you conceive or not, so it's definitely part of your fertility "root cause." When you have PCOS, so much of the emphasis is put on *you*, but it could be that your partner's sperm is suboptimal and is also part of the problem.

There usually isn't just one "root cause." Our body systems work in synergy, so it makes sense that if one system is disrupted, then others will be too. For example, it's very likely that if your adrenal glands (which produce your stress hormones) are overworked, then your insulin also won't be optimal. Stress hormones cause your body to dump glucose into the blood, and over time this can result in problems with your insulin.

CHECK YOUR INSULIN

Insulin is the first thing that I check because up to 80 percent of women with PCOS (including lean PCOS) have some insulin resistance.[1] When researchers used the most sensitive tests for insulin resistance, they found that insulin resistance was present in 75 percent of lean PCOS cases and 95 percent of overweight PCOS cases.[2]

You may not know that your insulin isn't working properly because it's unlikely that correct tests will have been done. Or maybe you've been prescribed the insulin-sensitizing drug metformin, but don't know why. Due to the high prevalence of insulin resistance in PCOS, many doctors will just assume that you have insulin resistance without further testing, and will prescribe metformin (especially if you're struggling with weight gain). But as we explored in Chapter 4, if you knew you could achieve the same outcome just by changing the way you ate and moved, you'd probably do that instead and avoid any side-effects or risks.

Anna, who we've already met, got married in 2015 and came off HBC to try to conceive. However, her periods didn't return for six months, and when they did, they were up to 90 days apart. She also had acne around her chin and jaw, which she hadn't experienced since being a teenager (before HBC), and had slowly gained about 20 lb (9 kg) over the past three years, mostly around her stomach. After a year of trying, Anna went back to her doctor, who diagnosed her with PCOS and prescribed metformin.

Three months later, Anna conceived. She was ecstatic. Like me, she thought that metformin was a wonder drug. Her pregnancy went well, and she had a beautiful daughter. But Anna struggled enormously with crippling fatigue when her daughter was born. She couldn't shift any baby weight because the fatigue was so bad she couldn't exercise.

By the time her daughter was nine months old, Anna's periods hadn't returned, the acne was still there, and her fatigue was still severe. She was dreading returning to work, so she decided to sign up for my *PCOS Protocol* program. She soon learned that her insulin wasn't functioning properly, and changed her diet, supplements, and exercise accordingly. Within just eight weeks, the fatigue had resolved, and her clothes were feeling much looser around her waist. Her periods had also resumed again.

Anna was horrified that she hadn't been told what the actual problem was. She'd googled metformin and knew that it was often used to help conception in women with PCOS, and also that it was a diabetic drug. She hadn't been diagnosed with diabetes or pre-diabetes, so she'd just assumed that she'd been given it for fertility, and had no idea about the way it helped. She felt so let down; if she'd just known, she could have easily changed her lifestyle. Not only could she then have conceived naturally, but she might have had a much easier postnatal phase and reduced her risk of developing type 2 diabetes later in life.

Most women with PCOS have insulin resistance, but it's missed because the right tests aren't being performed.

Common tests for insulin resistance

The common tests for insulin resistance are HbA1c and fasting blood glucose, but these tests are not sensitive enough to pick up the early stages of insulin resistance. If you remember the insulin analogy from Chapter 2 (see page 38), you'll remember that it's like a key that fits into a receptor (the lock). Insulin should be able to open the lock within a few minutes, but if you have insulin resistance, it might take it 30 minutes, an hour, two hours, four hours, six hours, or 12 hours to open the door.

Tests like fasting blood glucose and HbA1c may pick up on when insulin is taking, say, 12 hours to get the lock open; but not 30 minutes, an hour, or even two hours. A study in 2014 found that HbA1c will not identify even 45 percent of people with full-blown type 2 diabetes.[3] Similarly, fasting blood glucose is not sufficiently sensitive to pick up pre-diabetes, partly because the current "normal" upper limit of 100 mg/dL (5.55 mmol/L) is much too high. In another study, researchers found that many of those with fasting blood glucose levels between 91 and 99 mg/dL went on to develop type 2 diabetes.[4]

Even the oral glucose challenge, where you have to drink a horrible sugary drink (if you know, you know!) and have your glucose measured in the three hours afterward, won't pick up early changes in insulin because they measure your glucose, not your insulin. One study showed that the oral glucose challenge test did not identify up to 50 percent of people with diabetes.[5]

The consequence of these insufficiently sensitive testing methods is that one-third of people with pre-diabetes or diabetes go undiagnosed.[6]

The best test for insulin resistance

The most sensitive test for insulin resistance is called the "insulin challenge" or "insulin assay."[6] This is similar to the oral glucose challenge, but measures your insulin instead. The insulin assay has been shown to pick up on 75 percent more cases of diabetes or pre-diabetes than the oral glucose challenge.[5]

The 2018 PCOS international evidence-based guidelines state that all women with PCOS planning to get pregnant should be offered an oral glucose challenge.[7] As I've said above, this can miss up to 50 percent of people with diabetes, so ask if your insulin can be measured at the same time. If this isn't possible, at least an oral glucose challenge is better than an HbA1c.

> For those of you who are lean and have been told by your doctor that your insulin levels are okay, please don't think that this doesn't apply to you. In my view, "lean PCOS" is a pretty useless term—all it tells you is that you have PCOS and don't have weight gain as a symptom. Up to 75 percent of women with lean PCOS also have insulin that isn't functioning properly.
>
> Additionally, up to 50 percent of women with lean PCOS may have reactive hypoglycemia.[8] Reactive hypoglycemia is a drop in blood sugar about 1.5 to 5 hours after eating. This drop can result in symptoms such as fatigue, dizziness, lightheadedness, and increased hunger. You might recognise this feeling as being 'hangry.' Your doctor likely won't know this, and may dismiss any issues of insulin if you're lean, or only measure HbA1c or fasting blood glucose.

Unfortunately, there is still a huge amount of stigma when it comes to weight and insulin resistance/diabetes. It's still thought that being overweight *causes* insulin resistance. This isn't the case at all, and leaves so many "lean PCOSers" not getting the treatment they need.

In Chapter 3, I explained why weight loss in PCOS was rarely about calories, and more likely due to high levels of insulin. But weight gain is only one symptom of insulin resistance, and not having it doesn't mean that your insulin is working optimally. It's like a heart attack and nausea. Nausea can be a sign of a heart attack, but not all people who are having a heart attack have nausea. Just because they don't have nausea, it doesn't mean that they're not having a heart attack.

Remember, Lisa, who I introduced to you in Chapter 2 (see page 45)? She'd come off HBC a year earlier and hadn't got her period for six months. When they did return, her periods were over 90 days apart. She'd been to visit her doctor, who'd diagnosed her with PCOS and said that because she didn't need to lose weight, there was nothing that she could do and she would need IVF. But, in fact, her insulin wasn't functioning properly.

In the following chapters, I'll explain how you, like Lisa, can "tweak" your diet, find the right exercise for you, and change your supplements along with some super practical, easy-to-follow guidelines to get back to a picture of health and able to conceive naturally. But for now, what I need you to understand is that fixing the root causes is the big domino, and if you nail this, all your symptoms will fall down like little dominos.

And if you ask for the insulin assay test and your doctor doesn't know what you're talking about, know that this is not unusual—and keep asking. Most doctors won't know what you're talking about when you ask if you can have an "insulin assay." It's not a common test, even though the research has shown it to be much more sensitive than other tests. The reason that the insulin assay is not commonly used is probably due to cost: it currently costs about five times as much as an HbA1c.

Danah, a doctor, who I introduced you to in the book's introduction (see page 14), is a great example of this. She continued to follow her gut instinct that things didn't feel fine to find her root cause. This is why you need to have both your doctor and a specialist in PCOS and lifestyle changes on your health team.

As the insulin assay isn't a commonly available test, I've created a simple test plus workshop to help you understand more about these root causes. This is what we do at the start of the *PCOS Protocol* program, and you can access it on my website under "Root Cause Identifier & Workshop." Here I can help you order your own tests in many countries, including the UK, US, and Australia.

But it's not all about lab tests—your symptoms also tell us a lot, too. How you sleep, your hunger levels, your sugar cravings, and many more simple symptoms can tell us so much about your insulin, your stress hormones, inflammation, or thyroid issues that might be contributing to your PCOS. One of these symptoms alone isn't very meaningful, but when grouped together they tell us so much.

HAVE YOU RECENTLY COME OFF HBC?

Many women develop PCOS symptoms after coming off HBC. In my practice I often see clients who have had completely regular periods and no other signs or symptoms before going on HBC. However, after coming off it, their periods don't return for six months, and when they do, they're 90 days or more apart. The reason for this is twofold:

1. HBC disrupts the communication between your brain and your ovaries, which stops ovulation (this is how it prevents you from getting pregnant). For many women, this communication (and periods and ovulation) resumes after they stop taking HBC, but for some it doesn't, and they get diagnosed with PCOS. The problem lies with the two hormones, luteinizing hormone (LH) and follicle-stimulating hormone (FSH), or, more accurately what the ratio of these two is. A ratio of LH and FSH of about 1:1 is what kicks off ovulation. If the ratio of LH to FSH becomes greater than 2:1, ovulation may not occur.

2. HBC may make you less sensitive to insulin. Studies have shown that HBC can reduce your insulin sensitivity.[9, 10]

If you remember from Chapter 2, when we did some testing on Lisa we found that her LH and FSH ratio was greater than 3:1, and when we looked at why this was, we found that her insulin wasn't functioning properly (see page 46). When we tweaked her diet and supplements, her periods returned to a 30-day pattern within two months, and within four months she was pregnant.

HBC relieves symptoms but doesn't treat the root cause

The effect of HBC isn't just isolated to those who had no issues previously; it also exacerbates any previous symptoms. Many of us were put on HBC at an early age because our periods were irregular and/or we were struggling with acne. The way HBC improves acne is by increasing the amount of sex-hormone-binding globulin (SHBG). SHBG is like a sponge for testosterone. So instead of turning the tap off to stop the basin from overflowing, you're just throwing more sponges in there to mop up the water. Not only is this inefficient, but when we take HBC away, there is also going to be a massive spike in androgens (the testosterone family). We know that high androgens can increase insulin resistance,[11] so when you come off HBC your insulin sensitivity may have decreased, and then you're hurled a bunch of testosterone to make it even worse.

Due to this increased insulin resistance, it's no wonder that women develop PCOS symptoms after coming off HBC, or their symptoms get much worse for about six months. If you've just come off HBC and have been diagnosed with PCOS, it's most likely that insulin has some role here, so follow the recommendations for insulin root cause in this book.

COULD IT BE YOUR ADRENALS?

After insulin, the next thing to check is your adrenal glands, which produce your stress hormones. Don't think "That can't be me, I'm not stressed" or "I'm no more stressed than any of my friends, and they're all pregnant." That's not how your stress hormones work in PCOS.

Dehydroepiandrosterone sulfate (DHEA-S) is a member of the androgen family, related to testosterone. While testosterone is mostly produced in your ovaries (as well as in smaller amounts in your fat tissue and liver), DHEA-S is produced in your adrenal glands. Your adrenals are the little pyramid-shaped glands that sit on the top of your kidneys and are responsible for producing your stress hormones—adrenaline and cortisol, but also DHEA-S, the androgen one. Most people (and even doctors) are unaware that 50 percent of women with PCOS have excess adrenal androgens (DHEA-S). Take note, especially if you're lean! If you're lean, you're much more likely to have high DHEA-S.[12]

DHEA-S does the same thing as testosterone. It affects the quality of your eggs; it drives up LH, which stops you ovulating; and it's converted to the potent DHT (dihydrotestosterone), which causes acne, hair loss, and hirsutism.[13]

What causes higher levels of adrenal androgens

Our brain detects when we are under stress, and it releases something called adrenocorticotropic hormone (ACTH). ACTH travels through our blood to the adrenal gland and tells it to produce more DHEA-S. Like testosterone, DHEA-S is really good in small amounts—it gives us sex drive, and improves mood and feelings of wellbeing. The problem comes when we produce too much.

Women without PCOS might produce, say, two units of DHEA-S in response to the ACTH, but in PCOS our response is super-exaggerated.[14] We're more likely to produce, say, 10 units. So the kind of stress that wouldn't have much effect on other women has a massive effect on your symptoms. You could say that your body's reaction to stress is over the top.

How stress can affect fertility

High amounts of DHEA-S affect our fertile ingredients in two ways:

1. If exposed to too much DHEA-S, our eggs don't develop properly.
2. It increases LH, causing the ratio of LH to FSH to get out of balance.

Aside from the effect that DHEA-S has on your fertility, stress can seriously disrupt your menstrual cycle, even if you don't have PCOS.

If you've ever tracked your periods (I cover this in Chapter 9), assuming that you've had a regular cycle at some point in your life, you might have noticed that your period was often late after you'd had a significantly stressful month. Maybe the loss of a loved one, or exams, or a boss beyond unreasonable. Whatever it was, if you've had a late period, stress was likely the culprit.

This "stress effect" has been proven by researchers. In a study of 166 female college students, stress was found to significantly increase the likelihood of having a cycle of 43 days or more.[15] Women who were more stressed (e.g. had started a new job, or got married) or who simply had a lot going on (family, work, and social commitments) were up to twice as likely to have long cycles compared with women who reported minimal stress during their cycles.

Covid-19 has provided a really interesting example of how stress can disrupt our cycles. There were reports of irregular cycles from women in my *PCOS Protocol* program, and I'd also noticed that my own ovulation was delayed by about 10 days. I was intrigued by this, as I didn't really think I was stressed. My job had stayed the same; my team and I had just moved our laptops from our office to home, and if anything I had more time to go for walks and relax than I ever had before as there was literally nothing else to do.

So I conducted a very unscientific poll on social media. Of the thousand woman who responded, 70 percent said that their cycle had been disrupted (either shorter or longer) during the first two months of Covid-19. Even women who were on HBC reported irregular bleeding. While this isn't a scientific study, it does highlight how in tune we are to our environment. Our brains are experts at scanning our environment and picking up when things don't look right. So while you might think that you are stressed, or "busy," but this is "just your normal," your brain might not agree with you there.

While this can be super-frustrating when you're trying to conceive, it's actually a survival mechanism. As Lisa Hendrickson-Jack says in her book *The Fifth Vital Sign*, "It's helpful to consider that your ovaries are incredibly intelligent and will protect you from the added stress of a potential pregnancy during an already stressful time."[16]

CASE STUDY

Heidi was in her late twenties when she suddenly developed crippling anxiety for no reason. She also started getting acne for the first time, and her periods became painful and irregular. She went to a dermatologist for the acne, who put her on HBC. This helped for a while, but then Heidi's symptoms started to slowly creep back and get worse.

She came off HBC in 2016 in the hope of getting pregnant, but instead she couldn't get out of bed for six months because of intense exhaustion and brain fog. She also didn't get her period for this entire time, and her acne was so bad that she didn't feel comfortable leaving the house.

Heidi was finally diagnosed with PCOS and was put on a cocktail of medications to regulate her cycles—which left her feeling really sick. Her endocrinologist was perplexed when she didn't conceive and concluded that there "was something wrong with her head." She was (naturally) shocked at that answer and asked about lifestyle changes, which the endocrinologist quickly dismissed.

Heidi didn't have any issues with her insulin, but instead she had high stress hormones and inflammation. Within a month of eating fewer inflammatory foods (see Chapter 7, page 168), and reducing her stress levels (see Chapter 8, page 186), Heidi's periods had returned and were regular for the first time in her life. Within 12 weeks, her exhaustion and brain fog also disappeared, as did her acne. Most importantly for Heidi, she felt that she was now out of "victim mode" as she realized that there were changes she could make to improve her symptoms.

Tests for stress hormones

You may have had your blood cortisol measured and everything looks fine, even though you have all the symptoms of high stress hormones. This is most likely because blood cortisol isn't a very accurate measurement of the levels of cortisol in your body. It is better to test for saliva and urinary cortisol and cortisone levels, which are much more accurate, especially for more mild changes.

For the women I see, I test for these straight after waking and then about five further times during the day to reveal their daily pattern of cortisol, and also how their body is breaking down cortisol. It also shows me their levels of DHEA-S (the adrenal "testosterone") and how their body is metabolizing that too. This gives me so much more insight than just a one-off blood DHEA-S test.

> It is possible to have both high insulin and high DHEA-S. In my "Root Cause Identifier & Workshop," we identify whether your symptoms are indicating that stress and insulin are affecting you. Stress can exacerbate insulin resistance and also drive up DHEA-S.

How stress can affect your insulin and blood sugar

One of the main roles of your stress hormones is to get you out of danger *fast*. But they can't do that on their own. To run fast, jump, fight, or flee, you're going to need some energy to make your muscles work, and this energy comes in the form of glucose. As your cortisol rises, your body also releases glucose into your bloodstream (which is why it is called a glucocorticoid).

This is all very well if your body does need to run, jump, fight, or flee. But most of our stress comes not from these physical threats, but from physiological threats like too much coffee, tight deadlines, or traffic. Your body doesn't need to use the glucose that's been released into your blood, and so it has to be taken up again by your cells. If you have some insulin resistance, then your insulin can't get the glucose back into the cells quickly, which causes more insulin to be released. When this is repeated day after day, it can exacerbate insulin resistance.

I experienced this firsthand: my combination of the high-stress lifestyle of overtraining, undereating, and lots of gels and sports drinks was the perfect storm for high insulin and high DHEA-S. It was important for me to focus not just on my diet to improve my insulin, but also on my stress levels. The diet side was easy for me, the stress a whole lot harder. The most significant source of stress for me by far was over-exercising. Not only was my training and competing part of my identity, it was also a way I thought I could stop my weight from completely spiraling out of control. It took me many years to finally agree to back off training entirely for a few months; but when I did, this is when I saw my ovulation return to normal again.

Dimity had always had painful periods and acne, and had been on HBC from the age of 15 years to control it. Before that, she had been on isotretinoin (an anti-acne medication) for three separate rounds (with minimal improvement). In her late twenties, Dimity was finally diagnosed with endometriosis and then PCOS due to her irregular periods, acne, weight gain, cystic ovaries, and elevated testosterone. She'd also always had a larger build than many of her friends:

"In my teens it was somewhat manageable, but even as a teenager I was aware of it and attempted to do things (e.g. Weight Watchers, not eating, excessive exercise). After I left university in 2004, my weight skyrocketed, but it wasn't until 2011 that I got serious about losing weight. I joined a gym, went five days per week, and had one or two personal training sessions a week. I also followed the gym eating plan (very low calories), and I did lose about 33 lb (15 kg). In 2013 I got engaged; I kept up the gym and eating plan, but I didn't really lose anything more, and I was super-frustrated. I was working my butt off, sometimes going to two classes per day or doing cardio/weights along with PT sessions. During 2015 and 2016, my eating got lax; I was stressed (both work and life) and I put on weight, but never went back to my previous higher weight."

When I first saw Dimity in 2018, she was trying to conceive but wasn't getting anywhere with her doctor, who told her to lose weight.

"When I asked questions about how I could address the root cause of my PCOS, I got nothing. I got told to lose weight and there was no answer other than finding what eating works for you (with no further guidance), exercise more, or eat low-GI, skip breakfast, try high-protein or high-fat, a low-calorie meal delivery service or diet shakes [all of which she'd already done]. I asked for additional help, for referrals to specialists (especially dieticians), but just got told that PCOS was not a specialty area."

Understandably, Dimity was feeling very despondent. One of the most important things we did was to identify that her insulin wasn't working properly, and this was part of her PCOS root cause. It was causing her to gain weight and make it very hard to lose, and it was affecting her energy and her fertility. The second part of the solution for her was recognizing that it wasn't just her diet that was contributing to her high insulin, but also her stress hormones.

Dimity is a super-busy psychologist, flying all over Australia, but even though she was talking every day to others about what stress does to the body, she had no idea just how much it was affecting her PCOS symptoms. This became clear to Dimity when we started using a glucometer to test her blood glucose after eating. A self-confessed data nerd, Dimity was fascinated by not only what she ate but also how stress affected her blood glucose. She conducted a mini-trial on herself one week, where she ate the same thing every day and measured her blood glucose. She found that on days when she was stressed, her blood glucose skyrocketed; but on the days when she wasn't, her blood glucose stayed well within the normal ranges.

This was the first time she could really see the damage stress was doing to her physical health, not just her mental health. It gave her the motivation she needed to really take her stress management seriously. It also all started to make sense to her. Dimity remembered a time a few years back when her stress levels had increased dramatically due to work, life, and the ill-health of a loved one, and her weight ballooned way beyond what would be considered "normal" for virtually no change in diet.

We changed Dimity's diet to help her insulin, and focused on stress management and getting her to prioritize sleep. Within just a couple of months, she'd noticed significant improvements in her energy and sleep, and she was pregnant.

See the Resources section for the link on my website for Dimity's podcast.

CHECK YOUR THYROID HORMONES—EVERYONE!

As I explained in Chapter 2 (see page 46), hypothyroidism is a condition where thyroid hormone is low, and it is extremely common in PCOS. Up to a quarter of women with PCOS have a thyroid condition, and it can seriously affect your ability to get pregnant.[17]

When you get diagnosed with PCOS, your doctors should have ruled out hypothyroidism—but this rarely happens. As well as increasing your androgen levels, hypothyroidism can also affect fertility on its own. Studies have shown that low thyroid hormone, even if it's within the medical reference ("normal") range, can stop you from conceiving.[18] Additionally, just having thyroid antibodies present, without having actual hypothyroidism, has been associated with infertility and reduced response to fertility treatment.[19]

As I said earlier, it's really important to make sure that your thyroid is functioning properly before you get pregnant—not just to assist conception but also for the health of your baby. During pregnancy your requirements for thyroid hormone skyrocket,[20] as your baby also needs thyroid hormones. Not having enough thyroid hormone may lead to miscarriage or neurodevelopmental delays for your baby.[21] A fetus isn't able to produce any of its own thyroid hormones before 12 to 14 weeks of gestation, so it needs to get all its thyroid hormone from you.[22]

Hypothyroidism plus other root causes

Hypothyroidism often goes hand in hand with insulin resistance, and also chronic stress. Hypothyroidism can aggravate insulin resistance—so you really want to get this sorted or you'll struggle to reverse your insulin resistance.[23]

Studies have shown that just a small increase in thyroid-stimulating hormone (TSH) levels, even within the reference range, still increases the amount of insulin we produce, and may be associated with insulin resistance and metabolic syndrome.[24] They've also shown that treating hypothyroidism helps improve insulin resistance.[25] If you do have insulin resistance, your thyroid could be stopping you from improving your insulin sensitivity, so make sure you get it checked out.

Symptoms of hypothyroidism

Many of the symptoms of an underactive thyroid gland are very similar to PCOS symptoms, which is why hypothyroidism so often goes undiagnosed. For example, you gain weight because your thyroid controls how fast or slow your metabolism is. If you have an underactive thyroid, then your metabolism will be slower, causing weight gain even on a low-calorie diet. Other symptoms shared by PCOS and hypothyroidism include:

- hair loss
- slow metabolism
- low mood and depression
- fatigue and muscle weakness
- high cholesterol
- low temperature when charting your cycles (see Chapter 9, page 218).

Diagnosing hypothyroidism

If you have got some of the symptoms listed above, then either do my "Root Cause Identifier & Workshop" or get down to your doctor and get tested. Hypothyroidism is diagnosed via a blood test. Unfortunately, the test for TSH, most commonly used to look for hypothyroidism, is not very accurate. TSH is produced in your brain and tells the thyroid to produce thyroid hormone. If too little thyroid hormone is produced, then your body will increase TSH to try to produce more of it. It would, therefore, be expected that TSH levels are a good indicator of whether or not the thyroid is functioning well. However, it's not quite this simple in practice.

TSH does not detect autoimmune conditions. You can have a completely "normal" TSH and have sky-high thyroid antibodies, which is very common in autoimmune Hashimoto's thyroiditis. (Ava from Chapter 2, see page 48, is a great example of this.) As I mentioned earlier, pregnancy requires more thyroid hormone than normal, so many women with already high antibodies develop hypothyroidism during pregnancy.

This is why it's important to test at least for TSH and thyroid antibodies, if not a full thyroid panel.

It is also really hard to know what the "normal" level of TSH is. The current "normal" range is between 0.5 and 5.5 mU/L in most countries. However, how "normal" is actually determined is questionable. A group of people, who may or may not have a thyroid condition, is selected at random. Their thyroid hormone levels are measured and then graphed, giving a bell curve. The range of values that 95 percent of the group fall within is then called the normal range. I don't know about you, but I'd just call this "common"—not normal or, in other words, optimal.

When the National Academy of Clinical Biochemistry (NACB) measured thyroid hormone levels in a group of people with normal thyroid function and graphed the results, they found that the 95 percent range was *much* smaller—between 0.4 and 2.5 mU/L.[26] Interestingly, this is the level that's been shown to help in improving conception rates and reducing miscarriage rates.[27]

Important tests for thyroid function

The following are all the tests your doctor or fertility specialist would need to conduct to conclude that your thyroid was not negatively affecting your fertility. Note that the laboratory ranges can vary by region and laboratory from the ones given below; check your results against the reference range given by the laboratory.

Thyroid-stimulating hormone levels

When thyroid hormone in the bloodstream is low, the body detects this and signals the pituitary gland to increase its output of TSH—thyroid-stimulating hormone. The increased levels of TSH stimulate the thyroid gland to release more thyroid hormone. If the levels of thyroid hormone are high enough, TSH is not released.

There are two reference ("normal") ranges for TSH to know about:

- Laboratory reference range: 0.45 to 4.5 mU/L
- Functional reference range: 0.4 to 2.5 mU/L[24, 25]

The laboratory reference range is much too high, especially for pregnancy. A review of the research in 2015 showed that even when patients weren't technically hypothyroid but did have higher TSH levels, giving them thyroid hormone to help them reduce their TSH to below 2.5 mU/L significantly increased the conception rate.[27]

If your levels are above 2.5 mU/L and you also have high levels of thyroid antibodies, talk to your doctor or fertility specialist about how this could be affecting your fertility and whether a trial of thyroid hormone replacement is possible. This is, of course, in addition to the lifestyle treatments described in this book. If your doctor or fertility specialist is unwilling to look at the research I've talked about above, seeing someone with more functional medicine or integrative medicine training might be a better option.

Treatment for thyroid conditions can involve thyroid hormones, nutritional supplements, amino acids, and herbal medicines—depending on which type of thyroid condition is present. Naturopathic treatment for thyroid is often integrated with conventional thyroid medications when needed, to optimize response and improve fertility.

Thyroid peroxidase antibodies

Thyroid peroxidase (TPO) is an enzyme that helps convert the thyroid hormone T_4 to T_3, and TPO antibodies inhibit this enzyme. If TPO antibodies are present in your body, you will be less able to convert T_4 into T_3. If this is the case, you'll likely experience many of the symptoms of low thyroid hormone, as well as potentially having reduced fertility.

The laboratory reference range differs by country, and there is no functional reference range, so compare your levels with the normal range given on your test results.

Antithyroglobulin antibodies

Thyroglobulin is a protein made in the thyroid gland which is essential for producing thyroid hormones. Antithyroglobulin antibodies (TGAbs) act against this thyroglobulin protein. As the protein is inside the thyroid gland, an antibody attack can destroy the thyroid gland.

The laboratory reference range differs by country, and there is no functional reference range, so compare your levels with the normal range on your test results.

> Elevated TPO antibodies and/or TGAbs indicate that you have the autoimmune condition Hashimoto's thyroiditis. As you'll learn in Chapter 12, autoimmunity and antibodies can cause fertility issues by making your uterus uninhabitable.

Free T_4

Thyroxine or T_4 is the thyroid hormone produced by your thyroid gland, and this test establishes the amount of it that's floating free in your blood, and not bound to carrier proteins. It makes up 80 percent of the thyroid hormone in your body, but is inactive in the T_4 form. Its major function is to be converted into the active form, T_3. The thyroid hormone replacement drug levothyroxine is in T_4 form.

Reference ranges for free T_4 are:

- Laboratory reference range (can vary by region): 0.82 to 1.77 ng/dL (10 to 12 pmol/L)
- Functional reference range: 1–1.5 ng/dL (8.5 to 15.2 pmol/L).

Free T_3

Triiodothyronine T_3 is formed when an enzyme in the body converts T_4 into T_3, which is the active form of thyroid hormone. The level of T_3 is one of the most important ways to judge thyroid function. Often you can have adequate T_4 levels but your body isn't able to convert it into T_3 (often due to TPO antibodies attacking the enzyme that does this). T_3 accounts for 20 percent of the thyroid hormone in the body, and this test measures the amount circulating free in the blood, not bound to carrier proteins.

Reference ranges for free T_3 are:

- Laboratory reference range: 2.0 to 4.4 pg/mL (3.53 to 6.45 pmol/L)
- Functional reference range: 2.5 to 4.0 pg/mL (4.61 to 5.38 pmol/L).

Reverse T$_3$

When your body detects that your T$_3$ levels are sufficiently high, it converts excess T$_4$ into a compound called reverse T$_3$ (rT$_3$) to protect you from the effects of too much thyroid hormone. But sometimes the body gets the wrong message and converts too much T$_4$ into rT$_3$, resulting in low T$_3$ levels. This is why rT$_3$ should be included in your thyroid panel, although in some countries (like New Zealand) you can't get a test for rT$_3$.

Reference ranges for rT$_3$ are:

- Laboratory reference range: 9.2 to 24.1 ng/dL

- Functional reference range: Same as laboratory range.

If you're in the US, UK, or Australia, I can help you order your own tests through my "Root Cause Workshop" if your doctor won't do a full panel. A printable PDF giving all these ranges is included in my *PCOS Protocol* program.

GET A SEMEN ANALYSIS

The second part of Step 1 is for your partner—get a semen analysis done to ensure that all is well there. An extensive review of the research on fertility found that 40 to 50 percent of all infertility is due to male factor infertility.[28] This makes sense: it takes two to toe-wrestle. However, this step is often missed out, especially when you have a condition like PCOS that is known to affect fertility. All the focus is on you. But even if your fertile ingredients aren't quite there yet, this doesn't mean that your partner's automatically are. There is no point in spending the next six months improving your diet and lifestyle to get ovulating again, while he's kicking back and eating junk food, only to find that his sperm needs some work and he could have focused on this at the same time as you.

We know that sperm quantity and quality are in decline generally. One study in 2017 reported that sperm counts in the Western world have reduced by almost 40 percent in the past 40 years,[29] so it is likely that your partner's sperm isn't optimal.

Improving sperm quality can be done months, if not years, before you start trying for a baby.

> ## Just like your cycles reflect your general health, the same goes for your partner and his "boys."

The great news is that he can change the reel and improve his sperm quantity and quality. The earlier you do this, the better: just like with our eggs, the quality of sperm doesn't get better with age. The more time you have to fix any issues before age hits, the better. Plus, fertility is one of the best motivators around for getting off the couch and onto the treadmill while you watch *Game of Thrones*.

Optimal qualities for sperm

Sperm is classified by:

- **Concentration**—How many sperm are there per milliliter?
- **Motility**—Can they swim, or are they flailing around like a three-year-old with a mask and snorkel?
- **Morphology**—What percentage of sperm are "normal," and what percentage are misshapen (have two heads, two tails, a tail like a tree stump, a Connie Conehead, etc.)?

Naturally, what we want is lots of sperm per milliliter, that are good swimmers and have normal-looking bods. They don't have to be so perfect that they could appear on the cover of *Sports Illustrated*; they just need to be normal-enough-looking to do the job.

The World Health Organization (WHO) states that male factor infertility is occurring when:

- concentration is below 15 million sperm per milliliter
- motility is below 40 percent, and
- morphology is 4 percent or below.[30]

A morphology of 4 percent means that 4 percent of the sperm are normal-looking. The other 96 percent are abnormal. Talk about setting the bar just off the ground! A successful pregnancy requires sperm of normal motility and morphology in sufficient numbers, so if you only have 40 percent of the sperm in every ejaculate having sufficient motility and 4 percent normal bodies, it leaves a very few optimal ones to work with.

What we really want to know is whether your partner's sperm levels are optimal, not whether he's able to just about sidle under that WHO limbo stick. A study published in the *New England Journal of Medicine* (a highly regarded, aka very "medical" journal) reported that optimal sperm parameters are:

- a minimum of 48 million sperm per milliliter
- greater than 63 percent normal motility, and
- greater than 12 percent morphology.[31]

If you don't want to do the math, that's about triple the WHO levels.

Just like the thyroid and insulin levels we discussed previously, we want the sperm to be *optimal*, not just "common." When you have had the semen analysis done, don't accept just being told that the levels are "normal" or "okay." Ask for the actual results and compare them against the optimal levels above.

How to improve sperm quality

Pass this book over to your partner to read now; I want to talk to him directly. (No one likes being told what to do by their partner, whether it's picking your hair out of the shower drain or cutting down on those beers to help your sperm.)

Firstly, if your sperm levels are suboptimal, don't feel bad. I know that this can come as a blow, but it can be improved and it certainly doesn't mean that you won't be able to father a child. Just like your partner and her cycles, you can improve your sperm quality with a few tweaks to how you're currently living.

Secondly, regardless of the result of your semen analysis, you want to adopt as many of these habits for healthy sperm as possible. It's not just about having enough sperm to "do the job." It's about making the healthiest baby possible. Your baby's DNA is made up of half the chromosomes from your sperm and half from your partner's egg. We know that the messages coming from our DNA can be altered by environmental factors (this is called "epigenetics"). So, the healthier your sperm and her egg, the healthier your baby will be.

Many factors affect sperm production, just like many factors affect your partner's egg production. We're not as clear about how to detect the "root cause" of suboptimal sperm as we are with PCOS, so you might need to adopt a few techniques to cover your bases. Below I'll outline all the research I've been able to find on what affects sperm quality. Don't try to adopt all these at once, as you'll likely not achieve any of them. Instead, I'll cover them in order of what I think are the most important, then you can pick a maximum of three per month to focus on.

Quit smoking

I know this can be a tough habit to kick, but it is *really* important for the quality of your sperm. When researchers looked at the quality of sperm in over 1,700 smokers and non-smokers, they found that the concentration and motility of sperm in smokers were reduced by about 17 percent when compared with the sperm of non-smokers.[32] Vaping isn't any better, unfortunately. Although the research on vaping is limited to animal studies, researchers have found that just low-dose nicotine, the amount you would get from using nicotine patches, was enough to reduce all markers of sperm quality.[33] You get a lot more nicotine in a puff from a vaping device than you do from a nicotine patch.

Quit recreational drugs

Don't buy into the "grass is greener" hype. When it comes to your sperm, research has shown that men who smoke marijuana more than once a week have 29 percent lower sperm concentration than those who don't.[34] And the effects are worse if you also use other recreational drugs. A combination of smoking marijuana more than once a week, combined with other recreational drugs, reduced sperm concentration by 52 percent.[35] While this was a correlational study only, the findings have been supported by other studies.[35]

We don't exactly know how marijuana affects semen quality and hormone levels, but we do know that the active component of cannabis, THC, binds to human cannabinoid receptors, which have been found not only in the brain but also in testes and sperm cells.

Cool testes = happy testes

The process of sperm production is dependent on temperature. Your testes need to be a few degrees cooler than your core body temperature, which is why they hang outside of your body.[36] Spending time in hot baths or hot tubs, or even taking long, hot showers, can all increase the temperature of your testes. As can sitting down for long periods, and wearing tight briefs.

Here are a few simple lifestyle swaps that can really improve your sperm quality:

- If you sit a lot at work, take regular walks around the office, and stand up at your desk. If your work won't get you a standing desk, get your own tabletop desk converter (you can now buy quite cheap cardboard converters online in many countries), or (worst case) a couple of strong cardboard boxes on top of your desk will do the trick.
- If you drive for a living, take regular breaks and wear loose clothing.
- Wear loose boxers instead of tight briefs.

Tone down the alcohol or take a break from it

Alcohol affects sperm just like it affects your partner's eggs, and this effect isn't just limited to heavy drinkers. In a study involving Danish men, just 5 units of alcohol (that's 60 g or 2.12 oz, equivalent to 2.5 pints of normal-strength beer or 4.2 standard drinks) per week has been found to reduce sperm quality, and this was even more pronounced in those drinking 25 units or more a week.[37] The more you drink, the worse it gets: men who drank more than 40 units a week decreased their sperm quality by 33 percent compared with the light drinkers.[37]

Eat real food

Diet is an important part of improving sperm quality. Although there isn't much research into this, the few studies that do examine the role of diet and food intake on sperm quality conclude that diet plays a key role.[38]

I could go into a lot of detail about what to eat for optimal sperm production, but that's really outside the scope of this book. The easiest and most basic advice is the following:

- Aim for at least 80 percent, ideally 90 percent, of your diet to come from unpackaged, unmanufactured food.

- Focus on getting 2 cups of vegetables at every meal (even breakfast). A quarter of your plate should be carbohydrates like legumes, potatoes, sweet potatoes, or rice, and a quarter should be protein like eggs, fish, poultry, and red meat.

- Eat organic fruit and vegetables. If you can't afford this or they aren't available, focus on the Environmental Working Group's "Dirty Dozen,"[39] the fruit and vegetables with the highest pesticide levels. For the rest, wash them thoroughly with a mixture of four parts water to one part vinegar. Pesticides aren't water-soluble (otherwise they'd just wash off in the rain), so you need the vinegar to help remove them.

Other easy (and important) changes

The following are all simple lifestyle changes that could make a real difference to the quality of your sperm:

- Walk more, lift heavy things, and move fast occasionally—but don't overtrain. Exercising is great, but when it gets to the level of two hours a day, five days a week, it's been shown to reduce your sperm quality.[40] If you are a competitive athlete, this might be a hard change to make. I understand—I too had to get my head around the fact that my level of training was contributing to my PCOS symptoms. Just remember that this doesn't mean you'll never be able to train or compete again, but if fertility is your goal and your sperm is suboptimal, then you may need to back off for a few months.

- Keep tech on the desk, not on the downtown lads—don't put your laptop on your lap. This is counterintuitive given the name, but your laptop should always be on your desk. Similarly, your cellphone should never be in your pants pockets. Having said that, I do live in the real world: I know there will be times when this is unfeasible. But aim for 90 percent of the time out of your pockets. When driving, at work, or walking, take your phone out of your pocket and keep it in the console, on your desk, in your man bag, or even just in your hand.

- Swap out your toxic products for non-toxic options. Most plastics, pesticides, and other toxins are harmful to us because they mimic estrogen. As a man, you're probably well aware that having extra estrogen (the "female" hormone) isn't a great thing for your boobs or your sperm. Our hormones work by acting like a key that fits into a lock. Estrogen mimickers copy the shape of the estrogen 'key' and fit into the estrogen receptor lock, making our body think we have more estrogen in our body. This isn't healthy for your partner either, so follow these simple guidelines:

  - Swap your plastic bottles and food storage for glass, ceramic, or metal.

  - Never heat food in plastic—always transfer it to ceramic or glass.

  - Don't handle till receipts: most of them have a ton of BPA in them.

  - Get rid of any fragrances in your personal care/home/office/car. I'm especially talking about aftershave/cologne, perfumed deodorants, those "air fresheners" you plug into your car air-con vents or hang around the rearview mirror, fragranced diffusers, air fresheners, and soaps. All fragrances are estrogen mimickers. You can swap these for essential oils instead if you want a fragrance.

Prenatal nutrients for your sperm

Just like your partner needs to ensure that she has optimal nutrient levels to assist conception and also support a pregnancy, you also need optimal nutrient levels for your sperm. These are important for anyone trying to conceive, but especially important if your semen analysis results were suboptimal. While I strongly encourage you to get all of these vitamins and minerals from your food, you may also need to be prescribed some supplements if your levels of certain nutrients are a bit low and they can't easily be obtained from food.

When it comes to sperm health, antioxidants seem to be especially important. These are molecules that help counteract oxidative stress in your body. Oxidative stress occurs when you have more free-radicals than your body's natural antioxidant defenses can cope with.[41] This oxidative stress can lead to oxidative damage in sperm. It is caused by poor nutrition, stress, over-exercising, environmental toxins, smoking, alcohol, and drugs—pretty much everything I listed above.[42]

Below I'll outline some of the key research-backed nutrients for improving sperm quality.

Selenium and vitamin E

Selenium is an essential mineral, meaning that it must be obtained in our diet as we cannot make it. It is also a powerful antioxidant, and combined with vitamin E has been shown to improve sperm quality. One study involving 690 infertile men gave one group of them vitamin E and selenium supplements for three to four months. The results showed a 56 percent improvement in either sperm motility, sperm morphology, or both, and 10.8 percent reduction in spontaneous pregnancies compared with the group that didn't receive the supplements.[43]

> **Best food sources of selenium:** Brazil nuts, fish and seafood, legumes
>
> **Best food sources of vitamin E:** Seeds, nuts, leafy greens

Folate and zinc

Folate is a B vitamin (B_9) that is essential for the development of your sperm. You might have heard of folic acid, which is the synthetic form of folate that is used in dietary supplements and fortified foods and drinks, but 30 percent of people have a gene mutation that means they can't use folic acid (see also Chapter 10). This affects fertility for both men and women. Zinc is the second most abundant metal in the body after iron, and is another powerful antioxidant.

One study of 103 men with sperm concentrations of less than 20 million sperm/milliliter found that just supplementing their diet with a combination of zinc and folate increased their sperm count (those with normal morphology) by 74 percent.[44]

Best food sources of folate: Liver, legumes, leafy greens, avocados

Best food sources of zinc: Meat and shellfish, and smaller amounts in lentils and legumes

Coenzyme Q_{10}

Coenzyme Q_{10} (CoQ_{10}) is an enzyme that has a critical role in energy production. If you've ever gone down the Google rabbit warren and found yourself watching videos of sperm swimming frantically up a vagina, you'll know that they look like a mob of ravenous snakes chasing a baby iguana across a desert. As it turns out, the whipping action they make with their tails requires a lot of energy, so if they don't have enough CoQ_{10} they'll be a bit sluggish. As CoQ_{10} is also a powerful antioxidant, if you're using it all to mop up after oxidative stress, you aren't going to have enough to help your buddies swim fast.

In a large study, nearly 300 infertile men (with sperm parameters below the WHO guidelines, and with fertile partners) were given CoQ_{10} supplements for 12 months.[45] The researchers reported that by the end of the 12 months, they had seen more than a 100 percent increase in sperm density and motility, and more than a 70 percent increase in sperm with normal-looking bodies (morphology). This means that 48 percent of the men who had previously been "infertile" according to the WHO guidelines now had "normal" sperm parameters.[45]

Best food sources of coenzyme Q_{10}: None, it's an enzyme your body makes, so you might need a supplement

N-acetylcysteine

N-acetylcysteine (NAC) is a precursor to the amino acid cysteine, which is needed to produce the "mother of all antioxidants:" glutathione. You might have heard that vitamin C is a good antioxidant, but glutathione does much more than vitamin C does. One study investigated supplementing NAC along with selenium (see above), for 26 weeks.[46] The researchers found that this combination significantly improved all semen parameters.

> **Food sources of NAC:** NAC is found in proteins such as meat, fish, and poultry, with smaller amounts in dairy products, legumes, nuts, and seeds

Vitamins A and D

Deficiencies in both vitamin D and vitamin A have been associated with poor sperm quality. We make vitamin D when the sunlight hits our skin, and vitamin D deficiency is super-common if you live far from the equator, have darker skin, or have chronic inflammation. With inflammation, the receptors in your skin don't work properly which means you can still be vitamin D deficient despite living near the equator and being out in the sun all day.[47] If you carry more bodyweight, your vitamin D will also be less available for your body to use.[48] Men have vitamin D receptors in their testes and reproductive tract, which shows how important it is for sperm production. Men with vitamin D deficiency have been found to have poorer sperm quality.[49] Vitamin A is also essential for sperm production, and deficiency has been associated with reduced sperm production and infertility.[50]

Both vitamin D and vitamin A are stored in our fat. This means that if we have too much we don't just pass the extra out in our urine; high doses can lead to the buildup of toxic levels. Vitamin A can potentially be toxic (it may lead to osteoporosis) if you don't have enough vitamin D.[51, 52] For this reason, I'd recommend that you get your vitamin D levels tested before supplementing with vitamin A, and supplement with a cod liver oil that contains both vitamin A and vitamin D, instead of a vitamin A pill.

You won't be able to get too much vitamin D from sunshine or fatty fish, but you can from high-dose supplements.[53] However, if your vitamin D levels are low, you may want to look at supplementing until the levels have risen. The optimal level of vitamin D (measured as the metabolite, 25-hydroxyvitamin D or 25(OH)D) is very different from the laboratory reference range, which indicates a clinical deficiency.

> **Optimal vitamin D (25-hydroxyvitamin D):** 35–60 ng/mL (or 87–150 nmol/L)
>
> **Sources of vitamin D:** Sunshine, fatty fish, vitamin D fortified foods, cod liver oil
>
> **Sources of vitamin A:** Liver and organ meats, cod liver oil, eggs, yellow and orange vegetables, cod liver oil

How long will it take to see results?

Sperm production takes about 75 days, so the health of your sperm is a reflection of what you were doing 10 weeks ago.[54] However, it's more than likely that you'll need to keep up these changes for six months or more if your sperm are suboptimal. If you look at many of the studies on supplements and sperm that I've talked about above, you'll see that the studies are typically done for 6 to 12 months. This is why I recommend picking three goals for the first month, and then building on the good habits you'll get into.

Chapter 7
Step 2—Address your diet

Now that you've identified your "root cause(s)" in Step 1, you can be more targeted about which lifestyle factors you need to focus on. If you don't want to wait for your doctor to order tests, or you're struggling to get what you need, then join my "Root Cause Identifier & Workshop" or do the full *PCOS Protocol* program.

Diet is an important lifestyle factor. Nutrition can have an enormous effect on your fertility, so I'm breaking this step into two parts:

1. What to include in your diet to improve your health, the quality of your eggs and your fertility—regardless of the root cause.

2. Special dietary considerations to address each of the "root causes" that could be affecting your fertility.

WHAT TO INCLUDE IN YOUR DIET

Here, I will go through the top three guidelines I give to everyone with PCOS and trying to conceive, regardless of their root cause.

Aim for 10 servings of vegetables a day

Vegetables are powerhouse foods. I don't believe in "superfoods," but if I did, then vegetables would be it. They are packed with fiber, vitamins, and minerals, which are all great for improving your insulin, reducing inflammation, and enhancing egg quality. Fiber not only helps you feel fuller for longer, but it's also what you need to help feed your gut bacteria—the most undervalued and under-recognized organisms in the twenty-first century. We've only recently started to see studies that link dysregulated gut flora with obesity, diabetes, autism, and depression, in addition to autoimmune diseases like type 1 diabetes and Hashimoto's thyroiditis. Only now are gut flora getting the attention they deserve. So much so, that many experts believe the study of gut bacteria in the twenty-first century will be on a par with the study of antibiotics in the twentieth century.

The current guidelines in most countries are "five-plus a day" of both fruit and vegetables. However, this is much too low for optimum health. Also, I don't include fruit, because if you have insulin resistance some fruit can be quite insulin-spiking; I'll talk more about that in the special guidelines for those of you with insulin resistance.

The reason I give such a big target—10 servings of vegetables a day— is to give you something to aim for along with a feeling of abundance. Many of the other guidelines are about reducing certain foods, which can leave you feeling like "poor me, I can't have this or that." If, instead, you put your focus onto how you can fit all those vegetables into your day, it can completely change your mindset. Up to 80 percent of women with PCOS (including me) have unwanted weight gain as a side-effect. Most women I've worked with (like me) have had a long history of dieting, often with patterns of extreme restricting and constant hunger and then the inevitable binging. The power of a change in mindset away from restriction and into abundance cannot be underestimated.

CASE STUDY

Destynne, who you have already met, joined my *PCOS Protocol* program in 2019 and has a very similar story to mine. At high school, she was a pole-vaulter and was always very aware that she was much bigger than the other girls on the team. Just like distance runners, pole-vaulters are famous for their slim figures, crop-tops, and briefs, so when you don't quite fit that mold, you become hyper-aware of it. For Destynne, this started a long history of dieting and restricting calories and various foods, and subsequently feeling like a failure when it wouldn't work, or she'd inevitably succumb to her food and sugar cravings.

In her podcast, she talks about the experience of doing the "beach body" diet and her coach telling her that she needed to quit sugar for a week to give her body a "cleanse." But every time she tried to just cut sugar cold-turkey, she'd get massive sugar cravings and end up having sugary BBQ sauce on her food, chocolate, or even fruit, which she felt was a failing. She then tried different supplements, going plant-based for a year, and finally doing triathlons. Seeing all the female triathletes with their slim bodies had her thinking: "This must be it; I just haven't been training hard enough or long enough. If I do triathlon, I'll look like these women."

Just like everything else she'd tried, it didn't work. And none of these things helped with her other symptoms: irregular periods and unwanted hair growth. While weight had been an ongoing issue for Destynne, she didn't realize that it was due to PCOS until she went through fertility challenges. She and her partner tried for three years to conceive, with no success from the fertility drug clomifene.

"One of the most important things I realized in the *PCOS Protocol* was it wasn't my 'fault' or 'lack of self-control.'" Her insulin wasn't functioning optimally, and this was why she was angry all the time, was constantly craving sugar, finding it so much harder to lose weight than other women. But the most important thing was realizing that she didn't have to restrict her food intake anymore. She didn't have to always be starving and craving sugar. Just changing her breakfast took her off the blood sugar rollercoaster. "Realizing that I didn't have to restrict anymore, and not focus on what I couldn't have but instead focus on getting as many vegetables in there as possible, was huge for me."

Destynne's body responded very quickly. After only a month, her cycles returned and she started ovulating again; by the following month, she was pregnant with her son completely naturally, after three years of trying.

While Destynne lost weight, she also realized this wasn't important to her anymore. What was far more important was seeing how good she could feel. Realizing that she didn't have to collapse in a heap of brain fog after 1 p.m., unable to be productive. Realizing that she could be free from hunger and sugar and generally just thinking about what you aren't going to eat, and the massive amount of space that takes up in your brain. And realizing that feeling grumpy and moody wasn't just "her," but a sign of her insulin not functioning optimally. All of these things far outweighed the importance of weight.

See the Resources section for the link on my website to Destynne's podcast.

How increasing vegetable intake can improve your fertility

Vegetables are great for helping to improve our micronutrient intake and are full of fiber, which is crucial for our gut health and also helps to blunt our insulin response.

It increases nutrients and antioxidants

Vegetables are full of antioxidants, which are great for fertility. In studies on IVF retrieval, researchers have found that the level of antioxidants in the fluid around the eggs influences the quality of those eggs, and, therefore, how many eggs can be retrieved.[1] They concluded that a focus on increasing antioxidants three months before egg retrieval could increase the number of good-quality eggs retrieved.[1]

It improves your insulin

Vegetables are high in fiber, which can help improve insulin issues. A high intake of fiber has been shown to significantly reduce insulin and testosterone in women with PCOS, and also to improve menstrual cycle length (from over 50 days to a normal cycle length of 30 days) within 3 months.[2] This is likely to be partly due to the "filling" aspect of fiber, which means that you eat less, and partly because it stops your insulin rising so high. However, it has been reported that fewer than 10 percent of Americans (and I would predict those living in most other Western countries) get their daily recommended uptake of fiber.[3]

Research shows that a higher intake of vegetables is associated with a lower risk of type 2 diabetes,[4] and given that insulin resistance can lead to type 2 diabetes, this is super-important! Even at just three servings a day, it is estimated that you have a 16 percent reduced risk of heart disease, an 18 percent reduced risk of stroke, a 13 percent reduced risk of cardiovascular disease, a 4 percent reduced risk of cancer, and a 15 percent reduction in the risk of premature death.[5] This same study, involving a systematic review of the current research, has shown that if you increase your veg intake to seven to eight servings a day, the risks are reduced even more: You have a 30 percent reduced risk of cardiovascular disease, a 28 percent reduction in stroke and cardiovascular disease risk, a 12 percent reduced risk of all cancers, and a 25 percent reduced risk of all causes of mortality.[5] And the common factor in all of these conditions is insulin resistance.

Let's think about that for a minute . . . If you just get seven to eight servings of veg a day, you reduce your risk of dying by a quarter! (And in many cases, the numbers are even better for 10 servings.)

It improves gut health

The natural plant fiber in vegetables will also improve your gut bacteria. We have 100 trillion microorganisms in our bodies, i.e. about 10 times more bacteria than we have cells. Something that large cannot be ignored, and for a good reason. Bacteria aren't all bad—the problems lie in having too much of the wrong type of bacteria, or not enough good bacteria. The **microbiome** is the name given to the bacteria, yeast, fungi, and protozoa that live throughout your body, in your gut, nose, throat, mouth, skin, and urogenital tract.

A healthy microbiome is one that has loads of different species, and lots of each one!

Think of your gut as being like a vegetable garden. What constitutes a healthy garden? An abundance of varieties of vegetables (e.g. tomatoes, cucumbers, herbs, zucchini/courgettes, broccoli, cauliflower, cabbage, etc.), and lots of them. Whereas if your garden only had, say, one species, like parsley, it wouldn't be very useful. There is only so much you can do with parsley.

Similarly, you're not going to be able to make a salad for the tribe with one tomato and one spinach leaf. And even worse is when your garden gets overgrown with weeds (bad gut bacteria). To increase the variety and quantity of veg in your garden, you need to feed and water it. The same goes for your gut.

Your gut bacteria live in your large intestine (bowel). Your large intestine comes after your small intestine, which is where you absorb most of the nourishment from your food. If you only eat food that you can absorb, then your gut bacteria will starve. It's like the big brother who eats all the food, leaving nothing for the little brother. So we need to eat food that resists digestion in the small intestine—and that's fiber!

Studies of women with PCOS have shown that we have fewer good bacteria and more bad bacteria than normal.[6] Poor gut bacteria cause inflammation and insulin resistance,[7] and we already know that both these factors contribute to or exacerbate PCOS.[8] So, help your gut bacteria by eating more vegetables for fiber.

Note that one of the most common treatments for PCOS, hormonal birth control (aka the oral contraceptive pill), could be making gut bacteria worse. One study found that women taking HBC were more likely to have *Candida* (yeast) overgrowth and periodontal disease than those not taking it.[8]

What a serving is

A serving of vegetables is 2¾ oz (80 g), which is approximately half a cup of cooked denser cruciferous vegetables or one cup of raw leafy greens.

While 10 servings might seem excessive, don't think that you're a failure if you don't reach this quota. Of course the aim is to increase how much veg you eat, but the hidden tactic is to get you thinking about all the food you *can* have instead of what you can't. If I'd started this chapter off with a big list of everything that wasn't so great for insulin, by the end of it you'd be feeling deprived. Focusing on what you *can* have also has the effect of "crowding out" all the other food that isn't so great for your insulin—if you focus on trying to get those servings of vegetables in, there's actually very little room left on your plate for bread and pasta (both of which spike your insulin). While eating 10 servings a day can be a stretch, it is possible; and like the age-old quote, if you aim for the stars, you'll land on the moon. If you aim for 10 servings, you'll likely get seven or eight—which is a whole lot better than the average in the US, which is only 1.7 servings of vegetables a day.[9]

The best vegetables to eat

You want mostly non-starchy vegetables. Starch is the major source of carbohydrate in veg. The common rule of thumb is that vegetables that grow above the ground are non-starchy (have less carbohydrate), and those that grow below the ground are starchy (have more carbohydrate). There are a few exceptions to this rule. For example, onions and radishes grow below the ground but are non-starchy. Pumpkin grows above the ground but is considered starchy.

The list of non-starchy vegetables opposite isn't exhaustive—I've barely even touched on many of the Asian greens available, and there may be many other veges in your part of the world that you won't find on this list. But just google those, and you'll find out whether they're considered starchy or non-starchy.

GET MORE OF THE OTHER STUFF YOUR BODY NEEDS TO MAKE QUALITY EGGS

After increasing vegetables, my second piece of 'general' nutrition advice is to get more vitamins, minerals, amino acids, fats, and cholesterol. Your eggs and hormones need all of these to work properly. Almost every

Common non-starchy vegetables

alfalfa sprouts

amaranth or Chinese spinach

artichoke

artichoke hearts

arugula (rocket)

asparagus

baby corn

bamboo shoots

bean sprouts

beans (green, wax, Italian)

beets

broccoli

cabbage (green, bok choy, Chinese)

capsicum (bell peppers)

cauliflower

celery

chayote (choko)

chicory

Chinese spinach

cucumber

eggplant (aubergine)

fennel

garlic

greens (beet or collard greens, dandelion, kale, mustard, turnip)

herbs (basil, cilantro/coriander, parsley, rosemary, thyme, etc.)

jicama

kohlrabi

leeks

lettuce (endive, escarole, romaine, or iceberg)

mushrooms

morning glory (water spinach)

okra

onions (green, red, and white)

palm hearts

pea pods (snow peas)

peppers (capsicum) (green, red, yellow, orange, jalapeño)

purslane

radishes

rapini (broccoli rabe)

rhubarb

rutabaga (swede)

salad greens (arugula, chicory, endive, escarole, lettuce, radicchio, romaine, spinach, watercress)

sprouts

squash (summer, zucchini)

sugar snap peas

Swiss chard (silverbeet)

tomato

turnips

water chestnuts

watercress

yard-long beans

zucchini (courgette)

process in your body needs vitamins and minerals to act as co-factors during a reaction, including making your eggs. Most vitamins and minerals are called "essential" because they can't be made by your body—you *have* to get them from your food. This means eating a wide variety of foods, including foods from animal sources.

While you can get many of the vitamins and minerals your body needs to work properly from vegetables, you can't get *all* the nutrients you need from plants. Some we can only get from animal sources (e.g. vitamin B_{12}), and others (e.g. iron) are absorbed much more easily from animal sources. Unfortunately, supplements are not as good as real food. As we'll explore later, nutrients like vitamins and minerals are much better absorbed when they come in food form. Lily Nichols says in her book *Real Food for Pregnancy* that "Nutrients work synergistically. Nature is not stupid. And a supplement is rarely superior to what is available in real whole food." [10]

Getting all the nutrients you need is especially important for fertility and pregnancy. Remember, the goal isn't just to get pregnant—it is also to have a healthy pregnancy and a baby that grows into a healthy adult. Once you get pregnant, your requirements for many nutrients triples to grow the organs, tissue, and bone to form your baby. If you don't have enough nutrients, your health or that of the baby may be compromised. For example, recent research shows that you need to triple the recommended dietary allowance (RDA) of vitamin B_{12} to have optimal levels during pregnancy. [11]

This is part of the reason why I tell women "If you've gone vegan for your health (and fertility), this probably isn't the best choice." Let me make things clear: If you are vegan, I respect your choice. But if you come to me for advice on what's optimal for you, I'm going to tell you straight up that I don't think a vegan diet is optimal for *most* women with PCOS. There are two reasons for this:

1. If you have insulin resistance, your body will likely not be able to tolerate as many carbohydrates, or types of carbohydrates (as I'll explain in the section on insulin later in the chapter). We cannot

change the physiology of how food is made up—plant foods contain mostly carbohydrates, and animal foods contain mostly protein. If you remove all animal foods from your diet, you have to get your protein from plant sources, and that typically comes with more fats and carbohydrates. Most people with insulin issues can tolerate some whole grains, legumes, lots of vegetables, and nuts and seeds. But they likely won't be able to eat a lot of refined carbohydrates without their blood sugar and insulin spiking. This might make your diet very restrictive. My goal is to give you the widest variety of foods that you can eat to make it more sustainable, and this is why veganism concerns me.

2. Many of the nutrients that you need for your hormones to function properly, your eggs to develop optimally, and then grow human tissue (i.e. a baby) come only from animal sources or are better absorbed from animal sources. You can only get vitamin B_{12} and pre-formed vitamin A from animal sources. You may have heard that you can convert beta-carotene from yellow and orange vegetables into vitamin A, but that's not true for all of us. Many women, myself included, have a genetic defect which means that we have up to a 70 percent reduced ability to convert beta-carotene into vitamin A.[12]

Additionally, minerals like iron are much better absorbed from animal sources. About 30 percent of heme iron from animal sources is absorbed by the body compared with just 10 percent from plant-based non-heme iron.[13] (And I'll discuss in Chapter 10 why you'll need even more iron when you do get pregnant.) Just like vitamin A, there are many women with a genetic variation that reduces their ability to absorb iron by up to 50 percent,[14] and they need much more than the recommended intake to get optimal blood iron levels. So anyone telling you that you can get all your nutrient needs from plants alone isn't really telling you the whole truth—you may not have the genetics to allow this to happen.

I know that this may come as a blow for many of you, and your immediate reaction will be one of defense. All I ask is that you hear me out and keep an open mind. You're an adult, and you can do whatever you want. But presumably you're reading this book for fertility guidance and support, so that's what I'm here to give you. I don't mean that you have to start eating meat, and it doesn't mean that you can't eat *mostly* plants. What I ask is this: What would it take for you to add some free-range eggs to your diet? This might just be what you need to get the nutrients you need and have a diet that is sustainable for you.

CASE STUDY

Francesca joined my *PCOS Protocol* program after being diagnosed with PCOS after she came off the contraceptive pill at 30. The diagnosis meant it all started to make sense for her as to why she had struggled to maintain a super-lean physique as a dancer and performer, even when training four to five hours a day and eating only an apple, while her colleagues seemed to have no problems even when eating takeout every day. Francesca's LH levels were sky-high, and consequently her cycles were really long. She also had terrible sugar cravings and mood swings, to the point where neither her partner nor her golden retriever dog wanted to be around her.

In the first week of the protocol, Francesca found that her insulin was a little high, and this was likely causing her LH to be high. So the diet changes we implemented were focused on bringing down her insulin. Francesca was leading a vegan lifestyle, but, although we gave her lots of vegan food options, ultimately she found it too restrictive to both improve her insulin and be completely vegan. So, she incorporated some free-range eggs and then fish into her diet.

As those of you who are vegan will know, the decision not to be vegan is not a simple one. Francesca was eating this way for health, sustainability, and animal rights reasons. This was part of who she was, and changing her diet was almost like asking her to change her identity. But she knew what her ultimate goal was:

"I had to make a really important decision and swallow my guilt a little bit. But I knew what my goal was, my goal and my dream at that point was 'I want to be able to fall pregnant.' I did my research, I went to farms, I got the best eggs I could find, I went and tried to buy really quality bits of fish and read where they were caught, and didn't get any farmed fish." One of the most helpful things was recognizing that this change didn't have to be forever. "I just had to say to myself 'Right, when you have a baby or you fall pregnant or you've given birth, you can go back to the way you were eating before. If it really means a lot to you, you can start to go back to being a wholefood plant-based vegan, but at least you have a healthy baby. This doesn't have to be forever . . .' and I just had to swallow it and that was it."

One of the hardest things for Francesca was what other people would think. "I was feeling morally guilty and worried with my vegan friends—what would they think of me if I ordered an omelet?" But what she found was that her friends totally respected her choice: "When I spoke about the reason WHY I'm doing it— they'd all seen how distraught I was when I found out I had PCOS— not a single person questioned me, not even my friends who were vegan."

And these changes really worked for Francesca. After just one month of the *PCOS Protocol* changes and improving her insulin, her cycles dropped to just 30 days, then 29 days, then 28 days, and then the next cycle she got pregnant. While I'm not saying that all vegans need to eat animal protein to get pregnant, Francesca found that being insulin-resistant and being vegan wasn't a sustainable combination for her.

Remember that you don't need to justify any of your dietary choices. As Francesca says: "You're never going to please everyone—you just have to do what's right for you. You don't have to justify it to anyone."

REDUCE ALCOHOL

My third piece of general nutrition advice is to significantly reduce or eliminate alcohol. You may think the same way as Alexa, who said: "I don't see why I should give up alcohol. I'm not getting pregnant, and if I do get pregnant, I'll likely be pregnant and breastfeeding for the next three years, so I want to make the most of now."

I had to laugh. On one level, I couldn't argue with her rationale. Why would anyone give up alcohol when there's nine to 20 months of pregnancy and breastfeeding sobriety ahead? And that's not counting the months it takes to actually get pregnant.

But while alcohol might give you a great time, it's likely not so great for your fertility. The evidence is far from clear-cut, but there is enough to suggest that if you have trouble conceiving, then try cutting out alcohol. Not just you, but the father too (see Chapter 6, page 121). Early research (in the 1970s) showed that a night out can cause an acute increase in estrogen in women, so it makes sense that alcohol could affect our fertility.[15] Similarly, alcohol has been shown to produce fewer cells in male ejaculate,[16] problems with sperm motility, and increased numbers of abnormal sperm when consuming as little as three standard drinks (about 5 units of alcohol) a day for a man weighing 175 lb (80 kg).[16, 17]

An interesting study done with couples going through IVF looked at the amount and timing of alcohol consumption and the effect on live birth rates. The researchers found that women who drank just under one standard drink per day (0.6 fl oz alcohol) in the month before IVF had a 13 percent reduction in the number of eggs retrieved.[18] They also had an almost three times higher risk of not getting pregnant and were twice as likely to miscarry. For men, this amount of alcohol per day increased the risk of not achieving pregnancy by 2.28 times in the month before IVF, and 8.32 times in the week before IVF.[18] Most shockingly, couples where the men drank during the week before sperm collection were 38 times as likely to have a miscarriage as couples where the man did not drink at this time.[18]

While this study focused on couples going through IVF (a very controlled environment and therefore easy to study), the same likely applies to natural conception. If you know you are coming into your fertile window (see Chapter 9), then this is an especially important time for both of you to abstain from drinking. This also extends to cigarettes and recreational drugs, even cannabis. In Chapter 6 (see page 120), I explained that cannabis, cigarettes, and recreational drugs all have a massive effect on sperm health, and that includes to your egg health, too.

ADDITIONAL GUIDELINES TO TREAT YOUR ROOT CAUSE

In this part of the chapter, you'll find targeted nutritional guidelines to help you treat and heal the root cause of your PCOS.

EXTRA GUIDELINES FOR SUB-OPTIMAL INSULIN

If your insulin isn't working properly, nutrition is going to be crucial to bringing down your insulin and allowing you to ovulate again. The aim is to eat foods that don't cause your body to release too much insulin, to avoid your insulin spiking and/or staying too high for too long.

What do I mean by insulin spiking? Look at the dashed line in Figure 5 below, which shows what your insulin *should* do if everything is normal. When you're fasting (not eating) your insulin should be less than 30 microunits/ml, i.e. it should be within the gray area in the graph. It should then rise quickly after you've eaten, within half to one hour, and then come back down to your pre-eating level within about three hours.[19]

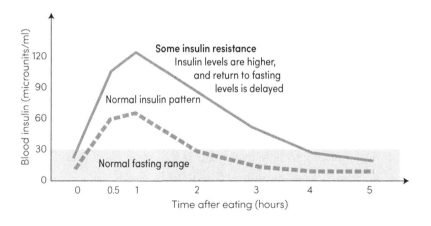

Figure 5: Normal insulin pattern and insulin resistance

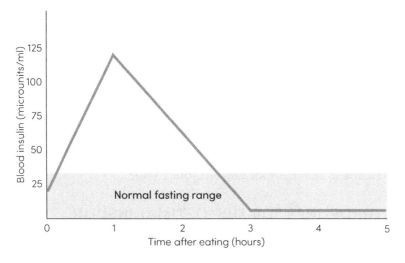

Figure 6: Reactive hypoglycemia

However, if your body has become a bit resistant to insulin, it will oversecrete insulin when you eat. The solid line in Figure 6 shows what happens in this case. As you can see, you would be secreting far more insulin (twice the amount at its highest peak), and it then takes four to five hours to return to baseline instead of three hours. With this pattern of insulin secretion, you would likely have "normal" HbA1c and fasting blood glucose levels, but you can see that the insulin isn't behaving normally.

Alternately, insulin goes high and then comes down too low. This is called reactive hypoglycemia and results in what you likely know as a hangry attack. When your insulin has gone too low, you'll feel ravenous within a couple of hours of eating; you'll feel shaky, jittery, and, well, hangry. Up to 50 percent of women, especially those with lean PCOS, have reactive hypoglycemia.[20]

When your body is a bit resistant to insulin (as it is for 80 percent of us with PCOS), this can cause insulin to rise too high or stay too high for too long. One way to help avoid this is by eating food that doesn't stimulate insulin release as much. To do this, follow the steps I've outlined below.

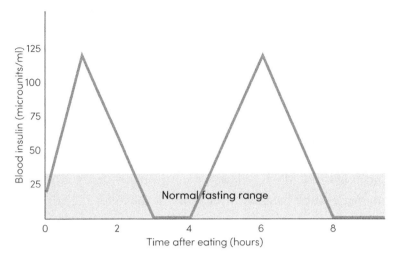

Figure 7: Insulin and blood sugar rollercoaster

Change your breakfast

I really hate clichés, but breakfast really is the most important meal of the day if you have insulin resistance! What you eat for breakfast sets up your blood sugar for the rest of the day. If you start the day with an insulin-spiking meal, your blood sugar is going to be on a rollercoaster for the rest of the day. This is what leads to those intense sugar cravings and the feeling that you have to eat every two hours or you'll have a hangry attack. This rollercoaster is what's shown in Figure 7.

A typical breakfast of cereal (especially one that uses refined grains and is sweetened) and low-fat dairy products is very insulin-stimulating.[21] When we eat these foods, our insulin will rise quite high, it will eventually be able to get the lock open, and all the glucose will flood in to the cells. The result for many of you will be that your blood sugar will drop significantly, and about two hours after breakfast you'll be ravenous again. Not the hunger that comes on gradually and you think you could eat sometime soon. No, it will be the kind of hunger that if you don't get something to eat in the next 30 minutes, you're going to be a hangry, shaky, jittery mess. So, you'll have a snack mid-morning, and your blood sugar will increase; then you'll have lunch—but by 3 p.m. that blood sugar will be going down again and the sugar cravings will hit you like a brick wall. You won't be able to think about anything other than the vending machine, the store, or that baking chocolate hidden in the back of your pantry. It's very likely that more sugar cravings will hit you after dinner, and you'll find it hard to think of anything except what sweet thing you're going to have. This is a blood-sugar rollercoaster, and it's an awful ride to be on.

The best way to deal with this is not to get on the ride to start with. Instead, have a less insulin-stimulating breakfast. Through working with many women with PCOS as well as experimenting with my own body, I've found that eating a breakfast which follows the following principles has remarkable results:

- High in protein
- Low in carbohydrates, i.e. no grains, legumes, starchy vegetables, or fruit (except berries).

You can add some fat in there, too. I have no specific recommendations around fat, but find that some women do better with more and others with less.

At the end of this chapter I've given you a few recipes for breakfast that follow these guidelines; these are things like smoothies, and protein

Source	Quantity	Protein amount
Protein powder	1 scoop	10–30 g (depends on the brand)
Chia seeds	1 oz/30 g	4.7 g
Pumpkin seeds	1 oz/30 g	8.5 g
Tuna	4 oz/100 g (raw)	30 g
Salmon	4 oz/100 g (raw)	30 g
Smoked salmon	4 oz/100 g	23 g
Mackerel	4 oz/100 g (raw)	25 g
Ground beef (90% meat, 10% fat)	4 oz/100 g (raw)	25 g
Chicken breast	4 oz/100 g (raw)	20 g
Lean lamb	4 oz/100 g (raw)	25 g

Figure 8: Protein content of different foods

pancakes and waffles, as well as egg recipes. So I'm sure you'll find something you like.

Firstly, you need to find a protein source that you want to use to get a significant amount of protein. As you can see from the table opposite, most protein comes from animal sources. If you're vegetarian or vegan, I'd recommend using a protein powder for now. In my *PCOS Protocol* program I go into more detail about breakfast and specific recommendations for vegetarians and vegans, but there wasn't room in this book.

If you're used to a cereal-and-milk type of breakfast, it will be easiest for you to start with smoothies. But then I'd encourage you to try to introduce a couple of savory breakfasts. This will help move your palate to a more savory one and reduce your sugar cravings.

> I'm not advocating for a high-protein diet all round. Protein does still stimulate insulin—about half as much as carbohydrate does—and it's important to take this into consideration when we're trying to keep insulin low.[22] As you'll see below when I go on to talk about lunch and dinner, I recommend a larger amount of protein for breakfast and a smaller amount at lunch and dinner.

The reason why having a high-protein breakfast is such a successful strategy is partly to do with how it reduces your insulin, hunger, and cravings for sugar, and partly with how a bigger breakfast helps your hormones and fertility. Researchers have found that a big breakfast increases fertility in women with PCOS.[23] They followed 60 women aged 25 to 39 over 12 weeks. All of the women were allowed to consume 1,800 kcal a day, but half of them ate their biggest meal at breakfast time while the other half ate their biggest meal at dinner time. The results were as follows:

- The women who ate their biggest meal at breakfast time decreased their insulin levels by 53 percent compared with the dinner-time group, whose insulin levels remained virtually unchanged.

- The women who ate their biggest meal at breakfast time also reduced their testosterone levels by nearly 50 percent compared with the start of the study; the testosterone levels of the dinner group didn't change.

- The most crucial change was in ovulation rates. By month three of the study, almost 50 percent of the women eating their largest meal at breakfast time *ovulated* compared with only about 20 percent of women in the dinner-time group.

The reason why changing just the timing of when you eat can have such a big impact on hormones and ovulation is because your hormones, including luteinizing hormone (which triggers ovulation under normal conditions), follow a circadian rhythm (like our sleep and wake cycle does).[24] This rhythm has been disrupted in many women with PCOS,[25,26] but eating a larger breakfast can "reset" the rhythm.[24,27]

The time of day you eat also significantly contributes to how much insulin you secrete. Your body secretes more insulin and stores more fat after meals eaten later in the day compared with meals eaten earlier in the day.[28,29] Given that we know that high levels of insulin stimulate your body to produce more testosterone, which disrupts ovulation, lowering insulin can help improve testosterone levels and therefore ovulation.[30]

Another reason why I've found this strategy to be so effective is because what you eat, especially for breakfast, makes all the difference to how hungry you are the rest of the day. Higher levels of protein consumed at breakfast (compared with lunch or dinner) makes you feel fuller and satisfied, not just in the morning but also throughout the day.[31] It does this by reducing the amount of ghrelin, the "hunger hormone" that your body releases.[32,33] If you're like me and are hungry by 10 a.m. after having breakfast, this is absolutely life-changing. I can't tell you how liberating it is not to have to be constantly thinking about food all the time.

A note about skipping breakfast

Intermittent fasting (eating all your meals within a window of less than eight hours) has become extremely popular in the past few years, particularly skipping breakfast and eating two more-substantial meals. Intermittent fasting has been widely reported to help improve insulin sensitivity. However, I'm not a massive fan of those with PCOS skipping breakfast, for two reasons.

Firstly, as we've learned from a study I described on page 145,[24] in PCOS a good breakfast is really important for bringing down insulin and testosterone and improving ovulation. This is important not only for fertility but also for your long-term health. Secondly, I've seen how intermittent fasting can trigger restricting/bingeing cycles, which makes me wary of it given the high prevalence of disordered eating in PCOS. Some studies have found that up to 23 percent of women with PCOS suffer from disordered eating.[34]

Along with having your big breakfast, what I do encourage for improving insulin is having a 12-hour gap between dinner and breakfast the following morning, and eating less often throughout the day.

Eat less insulin-stimulating food for the rest of the day

You may have heard of the glycemic index (GI), which measures how fast your blood glucose spikes after eating. If it's a high-GI food, it spikes high and fast; if it's a low-GI food, it releases sugar into the blood more slowly. However, we want to look at what happens to *insulin*, given that this is the problem when it comes to our hormones and fertility.

The **insulin index** is actually much more accurate when it comes to the foods that stimulate insulin the least. It measures how much insulin your body releases in response to a normal serving of a food (this is called the insulin demand of that food). The pioneering researchers in this field are the same ones who developed the glycemic index, so they know their way around the body's metabolism. Unfortunately, it's a costly thing to research, so even though this concept has been around since the first study was published in the *American Journal of Clinical Nutrition* in 1997, since then only 135 foods have been tested.[22, 35] However, enough research has been done to tell us what some of the more insulin-stimulating foods are.

Some of these might be surprising. For example, a small, reduced-fat blueberry muffin spikes your insulin over three times more than a medium-sized potato, while a low-fat fruit yogurt is more insulin-stimulating than white bread.[36] It turns out that different carbohydrates stimulate insulin differently, and protein also stimulates your body to release insulin as well.[22] In fact, fat is the only nutrient that doesn't trigger an insulin response. Non-starchy vegetables also don't cause much of an insulin rise. This does not mean that carbs and protein are bad—it's more about being careful about the amount and types you eat so that your insulin doesn't spike too high. The research has shown that using insulin demand information has helped people with diabetes manage their condition much better.[22]

So, my second recommendation is to aim to make lunches and dinners that contain low-insulin-spiking foods. I've found that the best way for most people to do this is make up their lunches and dinners in the following way:

- Start by choosing a combination of LOTS of non-starchy vegetables.
- Then pick ONE protein source. This could be beef, fish, chicken, prawns (shrimp), or vegetarian options like lentils and beans, tofu, tempeh, etc. Aim for a palm-sized amount if it's a thick cut (like a beef or tofu steak), or a hand-sized amount if it's a thin cut of, say, fish.
- Then pick ONE carbohydrate source. Aim for whole-grain sources like whole barley (this works well in soups), quinoa, buckwheat, or wild and black rice, instead of refined versions like flours. Whole grains like barley don't stimulate insulin much, while refined barley flour bread does. Beans and legumes are carbohydrate sources that are low-insulin-stimulating, as are starchy vegetables like sweet potato, parsnip, and pumpkin.
- Lastly, pick ONE fat source. Fat can be great for preventing an insulin spike. I like to choose those that are full of omega-3 fats, like topping a salad with flaxseeds, walnuts, or other nuts and seeds. Or having a side of guacamole, or finishing dinner with a chia seed dessert. I'm also a big fan of making quick dressings to add lots of flavor to my meals.

In my *PCOS Protocol* program we spend an entire week talking about lunch and dinner. There is a lot of detail to go into in terms of refining your carbohydrate intake for *your* body, so if you want more help, come join us there.

Choosing foods this way doesn't mean you have to have meat and three vegetables. It could be:

- Vegetable and bean stew
- Vegetable and lamb korma curry with rice
- Chicken fajita burrito bowls with homemade refried beans
- Bun-less burgers with lettuce in place of the buns, extra salad, and some sweet potato wedges
- Cajun chicken salad, then an apple with nut butter for dessert.

The options are pretty endless!

This is where the "pretty-good plate" comes in. I used to call it the perfect plate, but I now avoid perfection when it comes to eating and lifestyle. Perfection is both unnecessary and unobtainable, and the opposite of perfect is imperfect, so you're setting yourself up for failure. If you feel like you've "failed," you're not likely to want to continue. Instead, think about having a "pretty good" plate. It doesn't have to be a perfect ½ cup of quinoa—you can just eyeball it and know whether it's about right.

Note that unless you have type 2 diabetes, going totally carbohydrate-free isn't necessarily better for insulin resistance. Most women with PCOS fare better with some carbohydrate—you just need to choose the kinds that are less insulin-stimulating.

CASE STUDY

Before joining my *PCOS Protocol* program, Amber had tried so many different ways of eating, including a very, very low carbohydrate (ketogenic) diet. Lots of women on her social media accounts seemed to be doing that, so she really hoped it would be her answer to her continual weight gain, missing periods, and unwanted hair growth. Amber had always struggled to keep her weight down, and it seemed to balloon after coming off HBC.

As an accountant, Amber was super-analytical about recording everything she ate and her total carbohydrates. But at the end of two months on the ketogenic diet, she'd lost only an ounce (25 g) of weight and felt constantly exhausted and unwell.

Amber's tests showed that her insulin and stress hormones weren't working properly, but her insulin resistance wasn't wildly out of control. So I got her to start eating some more carbohydrates, one from the carbohydrate column at each of lunch and dinner. She was extremely reluctant to do this as she thought it would make her gain more weight, but the opposite actually happened. After six months, Amber was eating more carbs than she had for years (low-insulin-stimulating carbs, of course), and was down about 20 lb (9 kg)—the most she'd ever been able to lose. She also had far more energy, wasn't exhausted all the time, and her hair growth had started to slow, too.

Reduce sugar

Sugar is not only a carbohydrate, but also the most potent insulin-stimulating carbohydrate there is. By far the most insulin-stimulating food that has had its insulin demand measured is jellybeans.[37] So when it comes to eating less-insulin-stimulating foods, it is vital to cut out sugar.

Sugars (refined and unrefined, and all varieties) contain small carbohydrate molecules, meaning that they can cross from your stomach to your bloodstream very quickly and make your blood sugar rise rapidly. Your brain detects this steep rise in blood sugar and signals your pancreas to release more insulin. So to keep your insulin down, you'll want to significantly reduce your sugar intake. You might be balking at the prospect of having to reduce sugar in your diet (especially if you are getting intense sugar cravings), but if you follow the steps above—especially changing your breakfast—you'll soon find that those sugar cravings lessen significantly, and when you aren't craving sugar then it's much easier to reduce it.

Sugar-containing foods to avoid

As well as actual sugar, both refined and unrefined, these are the typical sources of sugar you might think of:

- sweetened beverages and sodas (soft drinks)
- cookies, cakes, and baking
- ice cream, candy, chocolate, etc.

However, some apparently "healthy" foods also contain sugars that spike insulin:

- Fruit juice—yes, even if you juice it yourself. When you juice fruit, you remove all the fiber from it (fiber helps reduce insulin) and you also consume much more than you would if you were eating the whole fruit. One cup of orange juice uses about 3–4 medium-sized oranges. Most people wouldn't sit down and eat eight oranges, but it's very easy to drink two glasses of orange juice.
- "Healthy" treats that are sweetened with dried fruit, maple syrup, agave nectar, brown rice syrup, etc.

So-called "healthy" sugars are just as insulin-spiking as "standard" sugar. They include (but are not limited to):

- coconut sugar
- dates and other dried fruit
- honey
- molasses
- raw sugar (it's still sugar!)
- treacle.

Opt for natural sweetener alternatives

Cutting out sugar doesn't mean that you can't have sweet treats; it just means choosing a good sugar alternative. I recommend a natural sweetener such as stevia or monkfruit extract as a sweetener for things like your protein powder. These are both derived from plants, as opposed to being manufactured chemicals, and therefore are likely a better alternative. They are a lot sweeter than the same quantity of sugar, and so you need a lot less to get the same sweetness. For baking cookies and brownies, I recommend sugar alcohols in granular form; these have similar properties to sugar and will work better in baking. Two of my favorites are erythritol and allulose. They are often sold combined with stevia or monkfruit to increase the sweetness, but if you buy plain allulose it's about the same sweetness as table sugar. If you have a dog, please avoid xylitol as it's extremely toxic to dogs.

I also recommend trying to move away from sweet food altogether. Your palate can be trained, and if it's used to getting sweet foods every day it will still want sweet foods every day—I've seen this happen in so many cases. If instead you follow all the recommendations I've given you, you're more likely to find it easier to rid yourself of those pesky sugar cravings.

You can train your palate to be more savory quite quickly, just by eating fewer sweet foods for a few weeks. The less sugar you eat, the less likely you are to want sugar. This is why I recommend that you try to introduce some savory breakfasts into your diet. The more often you start the day with a savory meal, the easier it is to stay away from sugar during the day.

Treats

Treats are more than welcome—but they should be just that, a once in a while type of thing. The exception to this would be some very dark chocolate, i.e. 90 percent cocoa mass. This is actually very low in sugar, and a square or two of this a day is perfectly fine. I've provided a few recipes later on in the book for you to use as treats. These have a lot less sugar than conventional treats or desserts, so are easier on your insulin.

Artificial sweeteners

I'm wary of artificial sweeteners. These are chemical compounds that make food taste sweet but without the associated calories. Some of the most commonly used ones are:

- acesulfame potassium—Sunnett, SweetOne
- aspartame—NutraSweet, Equal
- neotame
- saccharin—Sweet'N Low, Sweet Twin, Sugar Twin
- sucralose—Splenda.

While the research is not yet definitive, there is increasing evidence that artificial sweeteners may not be great for us and our gut bacteria. There is a lot of emphasis on artificial sweeteners being "safe" for human consumption. While I agree that a can of diet cola isn't going to kill you tomorrow, I am very interested in whether a can a day of diet cola or the sucralose in your protein powder is going to support your long-term health or possibly hinder it.

In 2014, researchers explored why, after almost half a decade since artificial sweeteners entered our food supply, rates of type 2 diabetes and obesity had gone up. The researchers took a group of rats and added artificial sweeteners (saccharin, sucralose, or aspartame) to their drinking water, and compared them with three other groups of rats that had sucrose (table sugar), glucose, or nothing added to their water. After 11 weeks of exposure, the rats that were fed artificial sweetener had developed significant insulin resistance compared with not just the rats that had had plain water, but *also* those that had been fed the glucose or sucrose![38] Interestingly, when the researchers looked at underlying reasons for their results, they found that the rats fed artificial sweetener had developed significantly different gut bacteria.[38] As I mentioned in the section on vegetables earlier in the chapter, gut bacteria are hugely important when it comes to all aspects of our health, including insulin sensitivity.

In 2018, another experiment on artificial sweeteners involved feeding normal sugar to one group of rats and acesulfame potassium to another group.[39] The results showed that the blood vessels of both groups of rats were impaired (this contributes to the development of diabetes and obesity), but via different mechanisms. The artificial sweetener changed how a rat's body processed the fat to get energy, and the sweetener also built up over time with higher amounts leading to considerable damage.[39]

Although we can't translate what we learn from rat studies to humans directly, these findings still give a lot of insight into how artificial sweeteners could be affecting our bodies. This is why I'm much more interested in helping you avoid sugar cravings altogether than having you "fill up" on diet cola all day.

CASE STUDY

Kellie-Anne had struggled to keep her weight down and her sugar cravings in check ever since she hit puberty.

"I've always been the type of person who gains weight even looking at a cookie, never mind finding it very difficult to just have one or two."

This was exacerbated when she came off HBC after getting married, to try to conceive. She gained about 30 lb (14 kg) in just a few months, even though her diet hadn't changed and she was working out with a personal trainer. The gaps between her periods were also anywhere between 28 and 90 days, and she wasn't having any luck getting pregnant.

After doing a lot of research, she suspected PCOS and went to her doctor, asking for some testing to be done. Her testosterone was found to be in the "normal" range, and therefore the diagnosis wasn't clear-cut. However, she did have non-alcoholic fatty liver (a marker of insulin resistance), and was told that she was pre-diabetic. This should have been a clear sign to Kellie-Anne's doctor that PCOS was likely the culprit, but instead she had to pay for a private ultrasound to confirm the diagnosis.

After Kellie-Anne joined us in the *PCOS Protocol* program, one of the first changes was that she stopped craving sugar. "It's literally like magic when you eat the right food during the day to stabilize your blood sugar, you just don't crave the sugar and don't have to keep trying to resist it."

She dropped 20 lb (9 kg) in 12 weeks and lost 5¼ inches (13.5 cm) off her waist. Her blood sugar levels normalized, her skin got clearer, her unwanted hair started to fall out, and, in her words: "I no longer bloat up like a beach ball." Her periods also regulated, and she was able to conceive naturally a year later.

See the Resources section for the link on my website to Kellie-Anne's podcast.

Eat less low-fat dairy

One of the significant findings relating to the insulin index was seeing how much dairy (especially low-fat dairy) spikes insulin. Low-fat dairy is low on the GI list, so foods like skim milk and low-fat yogurt have been encouraged for those with type 2 diabetes. Diabetes UK recommends switching to skim milk and having 3½ oz (100 g) of zero-fat Greek yogurt for a great snack.[37] But when we look at the insulin index, we see that low-fat yogurt is more insulin-stimulating than white bread.[22]

Why? Well, cow's milk is designed to grow a baby calf into a half-ton beast. The average cow is at least five times the size of the average human, and so its milk contains the growth hormones and protein it needs to do this. Subsequently, cow's milk contains a lot of IGF-1 (insulin-like growth factor) and branched-chain amino acids (BCAAs)—both of which are highly insulin-stimulating. This may be why, for decades, natural health doctors have seen a correlation between dairy and acne. Researchers have now found "stronger evidence" for a relationship between skim milk and acne.[40] The BCAAs and IGF-1 stimulate your insulin, which produces more testosterone, which subsequently tells your skin glands to overproduce oil, resulting in acne.

If you fancy some cheese on a Friday night for your after-work snack, opt for the harder cheeses as these contain fewer BCAAs and are less insulin-stimulating. If you're struggling with acne as well as infertility, however, you might choose to quit dairy altogether for the meantime.

THE PHYSIOLOGICAL AND PSYCHOLOGICAL COMPONENTS

An important part of changing your diet isn't about the food itself, but more about your relationship with food. Having now worked with thousands of women with PCOS, I can emphatically say that we cannot talk about changing the way we eat without addressing our relationship with food and our previous history of dieting and lifestyle change. I've found that women who have some insulin resistance along with unwanted weight gain generally have a history of dieting and some ingrained beliefs about food and habit changes. For a successful life change, you need to leave that sort of thing behind.

Arguably the most important part of what we do in the *PCOS Protocol* is investigating how to approach a lifestyle change. If you've ever "dieted" before, you will likely believe that when it comes to eating and lifestyle change, it's an all-or-nothing approach—you're either dieting strictly, or all bets are off and you're eating everything and anything you want. This is a bizarre phenomenon—nowhere else in our lives do we have this attitude. When we're learning a new sport or activity, we don't expect to be perfect from the first day. We expect there to be a learning phase, and we'll likely take a few steps forward and then maybe a couple back. But overall, if we keep trying, then we'll get better over time. Similarly, when we start a new job we expect there will be a learning curve. Imagine going to work on your first day, and throwing in the towel and going back to your old job because you didn't know absolutely everything on the first day. This would be a ridiculous way to behave, so why do we do this when it comes to eating?

At least part of the reason is because we perceive that eating is entirely within our control. So, if we eat something that isn't within our plan or "diet," then that's due to lack of self-control—our fault—and we've failed. This couldn't be further from the truth. There are so many reasons why what we are driven to eat is not within our control. The blood-sugar rollercoaster is a great example of this. It's a purely physiological reaction. A dip in blood sugar sends a signal to your brain that you need to raise blood sugar. Your body responds by sending you significant hunger signals. If you don't respond immediately by eating something, it sends inappropriately large hunger signals—"GET YOUR HANDS ON ANYTHING THAT RESEMBLES FOOD NOW!" Your body recognizes that the quickest way to raise blood sugar is to eat sugar, so it also sends signals to your brain that you need sugar. This is why you have those mid-afternoon sugar cravings. It's not due to a lack of self-control.

Scientists have found that lack of sleep has a similar effect. In one study, 23 healthy young adults were deprived of sleep for a night and then had their brains scanned. They were then allowed to sleep well for a night and their brains were scanned. When the participants were sleep-deprived, their brain activity was reduced in the area that governs the ability to make complex decisions (the frontal lobe), but was increased in the area that governs rewards. The result was that the participants favored unhealthy snacks and junk food more when they were sleep-deprived than when they were not sleep-deprived.[41] This shows that when we're sleep-deprived, our brain seeks out food that is rewarding or pleasurable, and we're going to have much less capacity for making better food choices.

Then we have the psychological component of eating. We are typically brought up in cultures that use food to celebrate, and often to commiserate. Birthdays, weddings, religious and cultural festivals, graduations, and other milestones are all marked with food. Many of us were also brought up being given sweet foods as treats or bribes for being "good." I'm sure you were told one or more of the following: "If you eat your vegetables, you'll get to have dessert." "If you're good and put your head under at swimming lessons, we'll stop on the way home and get a treat." "Wow, you got 100 percent on your spelling test! Well done, we'll go out to the cafe and celebrate." "Oh, you're upset because your injection hurt . . . There's a good girl, here's a lollipop to make it better."

This is not your parents' fault. They were merely trying to reward and reinforce good behavior, and food is an easy reward. However, this does tend to instill in you a belief that food is the answer to everything. So it's completely natural that when you're feeling upset because perhaps your boss or a client yelled at you, your brain is going to want to make you feel better, and it does this by sending you a signal to go and get something "rewarding" to eat.

Food choices are *not* entirely governed by self-control. The food choices we make are both physiological (e.g. lack of sleep, low blood sugar) and psychological (sadness, embarrassment, anger, happiness). We need to retrain our brain that food is not the fix-all for all our emotional needs, and this retraining process can take some time. There will be many times when you revert back to the old behavior, and that's okay.

I've found that the following three things are key to improving our relationship with food.

Get it out of your head that you're on a "wagon"

> **Wagon.** *Noun. A vehicle with four wheels, usually pulled by horses or oxen, used for transporting heavy goods, especially in the past.* (Definition from *Cambridge Advanced Learner's Dictionary*)

When in the past 30 or 40 years have you ever been on a horse-drawn wagon? NEVER is my guess, so why do you think you're on one now? I totally understand why—this is precisely what I thought I was on, and every minor "slip" would lead to a total and utter catastrophic "fall" from the wagon. This "all-or-nothing" mindset was incredibly damaging to my physical and mental health. The self-berating that would accompany one of these falls would be so vicious that my self-esteem would take a hammering. Here are a few key tips to help with this:

- Don't make any food a "forbidden fruit." Unless you have an allergy or intolerance to a food, or it's contributing to inflammation or autoimmunity, have it every so often, say once a month. Have a dessert once every two weeks, and damn well enjoy it! Build it into your date nights with your significant other or friends; savor it, enjoy it, and feel zero percent guilt, because you don't need to.

- If you eat something that you don't think was the best choice, take a moment to reflect on *why* you did that. Was it because you were tired, upset, or emotional, or were you actually hungry and there was nothing else around? What could you do next time to make a better choice? If you're tired and emotional, can you take a short walk and calm down, can you call someone or go talk to a colleague, can you go get a cup of tea? If it's because there's nothing else around, could you put something in your bag to have on hand in similar situations?

- Focus on the *next* meal. If you feel like you've slipped up, don't beat yourself up; just jot down an objective view of what happened. Then write down what great choice you can make for your next meal.

- Make one small change a week or every two weeks; this is what we do on the *PCOS Protocol*. If you make one small change at a time and keep building on these, you're less likely to feel like it's all or nothing.

Learn what it feels like to be hungry and to be satisfied

You might be thinking, "You've told us about breakfast, lunch, and dinner, but what about snacks?" The first question I'd ask you is, do you need one? Many women with PCOS who have struggled with weight have been told to eat "six small meals to boost your metabolism." As you've now learned, however, weight and your other PCOS symptoms, including fertility, are more likely driven by your insulin. To make your body more sensitive to insulin, it's actually better to eat less frequently, i.e. three meals a day. A study on people with type 2 diabetes showed that insulin sensitivity and weight loss were significantly better when the participants ate two meals a day (breakfast and lunch) compared with the standard advice of "six small meals." [42] I'm not saying only eat two meals, and I don't want you to be inflexible and think that you can only eat three times a day—instead, listen to your body and relearn what actual hunger signals feel like.

One of the great exercises we did at university was to relearn what it was actually like to feel hunger, and also to feel "satisfied" but not overstuffed. After going from living at home where my mum dished up dinner and controlled my portions, to living on campus at halls of residence (which essentially provided an everyday buffet), I'd forgotten what it was like to feel satisfied. This was exacerbated by my blood sugar crashes (hangry attacks). I was terrified of being hungry, as I knew that if I didn't eat something soon I'd be a shaky mess within an hour. So I got very good at never letting myself get hungry. As I started to get my blood sugar in balance, though, I needed to relearn what hunger and satiety felt like. Many of the women I've worked with have needed to do this, too.

It's an easy skill to relearn, and using the guides in the following chart can help you do this. We cover this in detail in my *PCOS Protocol* program.

10	Extremely stuffed, nauseous
9	Stuffed, very uncomfortable
8	Overfull, somewhat uncomfortable
7	Full but not uncomfortable
6	Satisfied, but could eat a little more
5	Starting to feel hungry
4	Hungry, stomach growling
3	Uncomfortably hungry, distracted, irritable
2	Very hungry, low energy, weak and dizzy
1	Starving, no energy, very weak

Figure 9: Hunger and satiety scale

When to eat

It is best to eat when you reach 3 or 4 in the table above. Try not to let yourself get to a 1 or 2—if you get too hungry, you are more likely to reach for a sugary quick-fix than to choose a better alternative. The one exception I'd make is breakfast. You might not feel particularly hungry for breakfast when you wake up, especially if you hadn't been eating breakfast normally. I would ask that you ignore this and still eat your breakfast, including a good amount of protein, within an hour of waking.

When to stop eating

It is best to stop eating when you reach a 6. It takes 20 minutes for your body to register that you're full, so if you stop eating at 6, you'll often find that you're full soon after. When I started doing this, I was worried that I'd be hungry later, so I'd eat until I was at 6 and put the rest in the fridge. I'd then go for a walk or do something to keep busy for 30 minutes. And 99 percent of the time, I wasn't hungry enough afterward to eat the rest of the meal. It's good to use this as a "security blanket" initially; after a while, you'll get better at knowing how much you need to serve yourself. If you're eating out, use the same technique. Finish at a 6 and ask for a takeout container immediately. Then you'll know that if you're still hungry you can eat some more later.

If you find that you're getting hungry and needing to snack between meals, add a bit more fat to your breakfast and lunch—maybe half an avocado, a quarter cup of nuts and seeds, or two tablespoons of mayonnaise made from olive oil, or nut butter. This further blunts the insulin response, which keeps you feeling fuller for longer.

Get joy from things other than food

When I was going through the process of changing my diet a few years ago, I realized that food was bringing a lot of joy into an otherwise crappy day. I was working for a software company in a job that, in hindsight, just wasn't right for me. Couple this with an abysmal boss who was more concerned about her hair than she was about her team, and the result was many, many unhappy days. Getting home and sinking my teeth into a few of my "healthy" bliss balls (full of sugar in the form of dried fruit!) was the perfect antidote to a terrible day. So it was hard to learn that far from this being a healthy choice, it wasn't great for my insulin. I realized that my brain was crying out for a feel-good boost, and I needed to find other ways I could get this that didn't involve sugar.

I sat down and made a list of all the things I did purely for pleasure— things that didn't involve food or drink. And the list consisted of zero items. Nothing. Nada. Zip. That was when I realized how many things I used to love doing, like team sports, doing craft projects, or reading fiction, I'd let slide. I now exercised for weight maintenance. It wasn't that I didn't enjoy it most of the time, but it wasn't purely for pleasure. I was reading for self-improvement, to get myself out of this body that was rebelling against everything I tried to do, and out of the job I hated. I would never get home and take a relaxing bath, or go to a jewelry-making course, or learn a new activity just for fun. Everything was so serious.

So I made a concerted effort to change. I made a list of everything that I used to love, that brought me joy, or things that I thought would. I got back into sewing and started some projects. I started reading (fiction) again every night, and actively sought out unputdownable books. I organized walks (not runs) with friends after work, just for fun; I learned to kitesurf, mountain bike, and ski, and organized weekends away with friends based around these activities. With all this, combined with stabilizing my blood sugar and all the other dietary changes I was making, I didn't need sugar so much, and I was a whole lot happier.

So I'd like you to do the following exercise. Over the next few weeks, note down in a journal the times when you're eating when you're not hungry, or eating something you know isn't the best choice for your insulin. Then ask why—what was it? Boredom, loneliness, nothing else to eat, sadness? After a while you'll start to notice a pattern. If it's boredom, find a ceramics or photography class and ask friends if they want to join you; or start a social sports team or plan some cool hike you want to do, and use these activities as motivation to get training with some friends. Finding things that make you happy is only going to become more important as you go through your fertility journey. In preparation for writing this book, I spoke to lots of women who'd been trying to conceive for a long time. They told me that having hobbies and activities that injected fun into their lives with people they loved was crucial. Having something to focus on other than just fertility was incredibly important.

> I know that all these steps might seem like a lot to consider, but when you get into it it's actually quite easy. On page 185 there is an example of what a day could look like for someone with suboptimal insulin, combining all the guidelines around breakfast and increasing vegetables and a wide variety of foods for different nutrients. I have so many stories about women who were able to conceive naturally after they addressed their insulin. The case study below is another one!

Sara, who is on episode 9 of my podcast (see the Resources section), was on HBC from a young age. She came off it after getting married, and for 12 months she and her partner tried without success to conceive. Sara thought it was probably time to visit her doctor, who prescribed a round of clomifene. This was unsuccessful, so she and her partner were referred to a fertility clinic, which immediately ran a whole bunch of tests to look for genetic markers of infertility.

During this process, Sara and her partner felt like everyone was jumping in headfirst, without taking a step back to check some of the basics—for example, were they even timing sex correctly? As Sara said, all they had was "third-grade knowledge" of how to get pregnant. Luckily they sought a second opinion, and their new doctor diagnosed Sara as having lean PCOS. Although her only plan for how Sara could conceive was still just IUI and IVF, her approach was slightly more holistic. Concerned about Sara's emotional and physical wellbeing, the doctor recommended that she see an acupuncturist for relaxation. Sara said, "This recommendation changed my whole path," as it opened her up to the functional medicine world of treating the root cause.

As Sara was lean, no one had suggested before that she might have PCOS. Given that one of the common symptoms of PCOS is weight gain, Sara's friends and husband had a hard time believing the diagnosis. Sara dived into reading everything she could about PCOS, and a couple of months later joined my *PCOS Protocol* program. Through this, Sara found out that her insulin wasn't working optimally, which was a big surprise to her.

Sara was already living a really healthy lifestyle. She didn't eat a lot of sugar or manufactured food, and she was working out regularly. But through the *PCOS Protocol* she now learned that if your blood sugar isn't working optimally, even "healthy" food can spike your blood sugar.

On the podcast, Sara tells the story of when she was traveling one day and didn't have a lot of healthy food to choose from, so she grabbed a watermelon and an apple for lunch and then tested her blood glucose every hour afterward. She was shocked at what she found. Her blood glucose, which should have returned to the fasting level well within three hours, was still elevated four hours later. "It totally shifted my mindset about what is healthy for me."

Sara implemented the recommendations—not just about food, but also around sleep, exercising enough (but not too much), reducing caffeine, meditating, and also charting her cycles. After only 16 weeks, she conceived naturally.

GUIDELINES FOR ADRENAL-ONLY ROOT CAUSE

If you're one of the 20 percent of women with PCOS who do not have any insulin resistance, but instead purely adrenal PCOS, then you have very different guidelines to follow. You still need to follow the general guidelines of increasing your consumption of vegetables and nutrients, and reducing alcohol intake to improve egg quality. Your eggs start developing three to six months before you ovulate, and during this development time you want to make sure you have lots of nutrients and antioxidants to help improve egg quality.[43] But there are also some extra guidelines.

Don't cut carbs

So much of what you read online about PCOS and diet revolves around carbohydrates, and for a good reason—up to 80 percent of women with PCOS have some insulin resistance. But if you are one of the 20 percent who don't, then a low-carbohydrate diet won't benefit you, and it could potentially be a risk — especially a ketogenic diet (which has become incredibly popular among those with PCOS).

Reducing carbohydrates may help some women with insulin resistance get their period back. However, it can have the opposite effect for those with adrenal-based PCOS. Researchers found that women actually need carbohydrates to ovulate[44] and get periods. Consuming too few carbohydrates disrupts LH, which is the hormone that releases the egg (ovulation; see Chapter 1, page 28). If you have adrenal PCOS, at least 30 percent of your calories should be coming from carbohydrates. To measure this easily, download an app like Cronometer or FatSecret and record all your food for three days. The app will show you a breakdown of how many calories you're consuming (helpful for the next recommendation) and how many of them are carbohydrates.

Check: Are you eating enough?

As well as sufficient carbohydrates, sufficient body fat and calories are incredibly important when it comes to ovulation and signaling to your brain that it's okay to bring a baby into the world. If your brain detects that you are not eating enough, or that you don't have enough body fat to support a pregnancy, it won't allow you to ovulate. This is an incredibly important survival mechanism. Why would we want to bring a child into a world where there isn't enough food to keep both you and it alive?

In the LH study I mentioned above,[44] a group of women with regular periods were randomly assigned to one of three groups. Group one reduced their available energy by 10 percent, group two by 20 percent, and group three by 30 percent. Group three's energy intake was around 1,300 to 1,400 kcal a day. The results showed that group three's LH was significantly disrupted (therefore affecting the second fertile ingredient). It didn't pulse like it should to trigger ovulation. The women in this group got irregular periods and/or their luteal phase (the third fertile ingredient) was too short. They didn't lose much weight, but their energy availability reduced. This shows that disruptions to your fertility are less about your bodyweight and more about how much you're eating. I routinely see women eating around 1,300 to 1,400 kcal a day, not because they intend to or want to lose weight, but because they just don't realize they are not eating enough and think that they are eating healthily.

Katie was naturally very lean. She had been married for a couple of years and they were starting to think about having a baby, but her periods were nowhere to be seen and hadn't ever been regular. After I did some investigation, I found that Katie didn't have any insulin resistance, her stress hormones were high, and I suspected that she wasn't eating enough.

She was doing a spin class in the morning, not for weight loss but to keep fit and help with mental clarity during the day, as she was a lawyer. She was having a protein smoothie and a banana for breakfast as she ran out of the gym to work in the morning (200 kcal), a chicken salad for lunch (300 kcal), an apple in the afternoon, and then grilled salmon, vegetables, and sweet potato for dinner, with a couple of squares of dark chocolate for dessert. The total for this is unlikely to even get to 1,300 kcal—which isn't enough for a non-active woman, let alone someone doing an hour of high-intensity spin class plus walking on average 10,000 steps a day. But Katie just didn't realize that she was eating so little. She'd always had a similar diet, and didn't feel as if she was restricting food. But while she didn't feel as if she was starving herself, that's the way her body was interpreting it, and consequently she had never really had a regular period. Katie started tracking her food intake, and sure enough it was about 1,300 kcal a day. I asked her to increase this by 100 kcal per day each week until she hit at least 2,300 kcal. She was very hesitant, because she didn't want to put on weight, and also because she really didn't feel like she could eat any more food.

I explained that we needed to make her body feel 'safe' in order for her to ovulate. This meant indicating to her body via increased calories that there was no famine and things were A-okay on the food front. And in some cases, that this might mean that a bit of weight may need to be gained. We know from studies on athletes in low-bodyweight sports that a reduction in bodyweight can be a major trigger for the body to stop ovulating.

I started increasing the amount of fat in Katie's diet, as that gives the most amount of calories for the smallest amount of food. She added a couple of tablespoons of almond butter to her morning smoothie and made it using some canned coconut milk. Next, she added some dressing to her salad, then ate some coconut yogurt with her apple in the afternoon, and, lastly, had some more dressing on her dinner. Sure enough, within two months of increasing her food intake, Katie's periods returned and she started ovulating again.

If you aren't getting a period, or your luteal phase is short, then download one of the apps I mentioned earlier (Cronometer or FatSecret) and check how much you are eating. Active women who aren't trying to lose weight and are trying to conceive need about 2,100 kcal a day. By active, I mean walking 8,000 to 10,000 steps a day. If you're not doing this, then start! You need activity just as much as food, and we'll talk about this later.

I often see women who haven't got their periods back after doing a physical (aesthetic) competition like a bikini competition, or high-intensity exercises like cross-fit or ultra-endurance events. With many of these sports come extreme leanness, and extreme leanness and optimal fertility don't play nicely together. Many of these women lose their period and then get diagnosed with PCOS, although in many cases it's actually hypothalamic amenorrhea (HA)—which I talk about in detail in Chapter 11. Regardless of the diagnosis, if you've lost your period after losing a lot of weight, you will probably need to eat a lot more than you think to get it back. How much you need depends on whether you're still training. If you're no longer training, then it's likely to be 2,500 kcal (or maybe more) per day. If you're still training and competing, then it's your total daily expenditure plus another 500 kcal.

The best way to eat more is to gradually increase your intake by 100 kcal a day each week to give your body a chance to recognize and adjust to the larger amount of food. Yes, some women may put on a little bit of weight and/or body fat (although some don't), but your body needs to know that it's not in a famine situation and has enough body fat stores to support a growing fetus. You need to signal to your body that it's safe, by increasing your calories. Getting pregnant while maintaining your current leanness may not be possible if you're not ovulating. If you're really struggling with the idea of gaining some body fat, then I strongly encourage you to seek help from a counselor who specializes in eating, body image, and disordered eating.

GUIDELINES FOR INFLAMMATION/THYROID ROOT CAUSE

I often see women with high levels of insulin and/or adrenal hormones who also have hypothyroidism and/or another inflammatory condition like endometriosis. If this is you, please follow the guidelines for insulin as well as the guidelines below for inflammation/thyroid. If you just have hypothyroidism and/or another inflammatory condition, then follow the guidelines below only.

Reduce inflammatory foods
Gluten

If you have the autoimmune version of hypothyroidism, Hashimoto's thyroiditis, it's especially important to remove gluten from your diet for a while. People with one autoimmune condition are more likely to have multiple autoimmune conditions.[45] If you have Hashimoto's thyroiditis, I'd recommend that you get tested for celiac disease (another autoimmune condition) because these often go hand in hand.[46]

If you don't have celiac disease, you can still benefit from going gluten-free. The authors of a study that reviewed the research on gluten and Hashimoto's thyroiditis concluded that hypothyroid patients—with or without celiac disease—do better without gluten, something many of us have been seeing clinically for years.[47]

Contrary to popular belief, you don't have to have celiac disease to react to gluten. There is another, less well-known condition called non-celiac wheat/gluten sensitivity (NCGS) that has been known to researchers since 2010.[48] Celiac disease is an autoimmune condition characterized by an inflammatory immune response to wheat, gluten, barley, and rye. The body develops antibodies against its own cells and attacks the walls of the intestines. NCGS is not an autoimmune condition, so it doesn't show the hallmarks of antibodies and tissue destruction, and it's not an allergic reaction. Instead, some people develop symptoms when they eat wheat or gluten: these can include gut symptoms (bloating, abdominal pain, etc.), but also headache or migraine, foggy mind, chronic fatigue, joint and muscle pain, tingling of the extremities, leg or arm numbness, eczema, anemia, and depression.

A 2015 randomized controlled trial has proven that NCGS is a real condition.[49] The researchers enrolled 61 participants without celiac disease or wheat allergy but with self-identified gluten intolerance. They were randomly assigned to two groups: one group was given a capsule with roughly the same amount of gluten as two slices of bread, and the other was given a placebo. After one week, they crossed over so that the placebo group was now getting the gluten capsule and the gluten-capsule group the placebo. The researchers found that intake of gluten significantly increased both gastrointestinal symptoms (bloating and abdominal pain) and other symptoms like depression, brain fog, and canker sores compared with placebo.[49] And this isn't the only trial to make this conclusion. An earlier trial of 276 patients with suspected NCGS found that their results confirmed the existence of NCGS as a distinct clinical condition.[50]

Since then, there have been numerous other studies on NCGS, and on other conditions such as autoimmune diseases, to try to understand whether NCGS is itself an autoimmune condition. People with one autoimmune condition (like celiac disease) often develop multiple autoimmune conditions (like Hashimoto's thyroiditis). One study examined the medical records of 131 patients who had been diagnosed with NCGS and 151 patients who had been diagnosed with celiac disease, to see whether they'd also had a separate autoimmune disease. Just as many patients with NCGS tested positive for an autoimmune condition as those with celiac disease (29 percent of both groups).[51] As this study just looked retrospectively at the patients' health history, the researchers also investigated another group of 142 patients who had been diagnosed with either NCGS or celiac disease but no other autoimmune conditions, and followed this group plus a control group for a period of time. They found that—perhaps unsurprisingly—people with NCGS were as likely (if not more likely) to go on to develop an autoimmune disease as were those with celiac disease.[51]

> The reason why I'm going into so much detail here is that there are many people who think that non-celiac gluten-sensitivity is a load of garbage, so I want to arm you with the studies and research that you need to back you up. But when it comes down to it, you don't need to justify your food choices to *anyone*. You do what you need to do, and if anyone asks then you can just respond with "I just don't feel like it."

I recommend that anyone with inflammatory conditions, hypothyroidism, or autoimmune diseases should remove gluten from their diet completely for two months (and better if you can make it three). Get your inflammation and thyroid levels checked before and after the two (or three) months. If your symptoms and/or lab results improve, you're better to keep on avoiding gluten. If you want to know for sure, the test I use clinically for non-celiac gluten sensitivity is one from Cyrex Laboratories (see the Resources section).

Dairy

Dairy is another food group that can be potentially inflammatory to those of you with inflammatory or autoimmune conditions. Dairy contains a protein called beta-casein. There are two types of beta-casein, A1 and A2 types, that differ very slightly in structure. However, this small difference changes the way in which the two types interact with digestive enzymes, and may make a big difference when it comes to inflammation. While the research is far from clear-cut, there are indications that milk containing A1 beta-casein is potentially quite inflammatory for some people.

One randomized controlled trial gave two groups of people either milk containing both types of beta-casein or milk containing just A2 beta-casein for 14 days.[52] At the end of the 14 days, the participants were given a break for a few weeks (a washout period) and then swapped over, so that those who were previously getting the A2 milk now received both A1 and A2 (and vice versa). The participants who drank milk containing the A1 beta were found to have significantly more gastrointestinal symptoms and higher inflammatory markers in their blood than those who drank the A2 milk.[52]

A review of 39 studies on A1 vs. A2 milk concluded that in animal studies, the research is "conclusive" that A1 promotes more inflammation and gastrointestinal issues.[53] But when it comes to human studies, the current research is only "emerging" and more work is needed. While we wait for the research to be done, it's up to you what you want to do— but if I were suffering from an inflammatory or autoimmune condition, I would think that the inconvenience of removing dairy from my diet for at least two months was worth a potential improvement in symptoms. Get your inflammation and thyroid levels checked before and after the two months. If your symptoms and/or lab tests improve, you're better off avoiding dairy.

Note for those of you with endometriosis

Endometriosis (endo) is a condition that affects about 1 in 10 women, and it's common to have both endo and PCOS. I write about how endometriosis can also affect fertility in Chapter 11, but for those of you who already know that you have endo, you might also want to remove dairy and gluten from your diet to help relieve some of the symptoms.

Endometriosis is essentially an issue with the immune system going a little haywire. So you're going to want to do everything you can to support your immune system and avoid things that could inflame it. Gluten and dairy are two such foods. Gluten can promote inflammation, even in people who don't have celiac disease, and 75 percent of women with endometriosis reported a statistically significant reduction in pain after 12 months on a gluten-free diet.[54] (This wasn't a small study either, with 207 endometriosis patients participating.) Dairy, especially conventional dairy that contains A1 beta-casein, can also promote inflammation. While there is little research currently on the effect of dairy on endometriosis symptoms, and it is still in its infancy for A2 milk in general, both human and rat studies have shown a higher level of inflammation with A1 milk products.

So even if you don't have a thyroid condition, if you have endo or suspect that you do, I recommend avoiding gluten and dairy, at least for some time to assess its effect on you. For more endometriosis-specific advice, I highly recommend Lara Briden's book *Period Repair Manual*.

RECIPES FOR REDUCING INSULIN

Blueberry Protein Pancakes

SERVES 2 | PREP TIME: 10 MINUTES

¾ cup unsweetened almond milk (or any nut milk)

2 eggs

1½ tsp vanilla extract

1¾ cups fine almond flour

¼ cup collagen or egg white protein powder (you can also use pea protein)

1 tsp baking powder

1 cup frozen blueberries

oil to fry (I use a neutral oil such as avocado oil)

coconut yogurt, to serve

fresh or defrosted berries, to serve

Pancakes are one of my favorite brunch dishes, but the standard white flour-based ones aren't great for insulin levels. These are made from almond flour instead and have some added protein from collagen protein or egg white protein powder. You can also use pea protein powder, although I don't like that as much.

Whisk together the almond milk, eggs and vanilla in a medium-sized bowl.

In another medium-sized bowl, mix together the almond flour, collagen or protein powder and baking powder.

Add the wet ingredients to the dry ingredients and mix to a smooth batter, then gently stir through the frozen blueberries.

Add about 1 tsp of oil to a pan over a medium heat. Pour about ¼ cup of batter into the pan and cook pancakes until just slightly brown on the underside and the edges are crispy enough for you to slide a spatula underneath and flip them over.

Serve with your choice of low-sugar toppings, such as a dollop of coconut yogurt and more berries.

Chocolate Thick Shake Smoothie

SERVES 1 | PREP TIME: 5 MINUTES

1 cup cubed frozen zucchini (courgette) or cauliflower (see note)

¼ cup chocolate protein from protein powder (see note)

1 Tbsp dark unsweetened cocoa powder (optional)

1 Tbsp almond butter (optional)

½–1 cup water or nut milk

Frozen zucchini (courgette) or cauliflower is the surprising winner in this recipe. Not only does it make the shake cold and deliciously thick, but it also adds a serve of vegetables and fiber to your morning to get those bowels moving! The protein powder helps to keep your blood sugar stable, and cocoa is a good source of antioxidants.

Put all of the ingredients into a blender or food processor. Use more or less water or nut milk depending on your preferred thickness. Start with a bit less, as you can always add more.

Blend until smooth.

Smoothie bowl option

Make this into a smoothie bowl by using less liquid, to make the texture thicker. Pour into a bowl and top with any combination of the following ingredients:

- Blueberries, strawberries, raspberries, cranberries
- Macadamia nuts, almonds, walnuts, pili nuts, pecans
- Cacao nibs
- Shredded/flaked/coconut chips
- Chia seeds, hemp seeds, sesame seeds, pumpkin seeds
- Peanut butter, almond butter, pecan butter, cashew butter.

Notes

- You can prepare the frozen zucchini or cauliflower the night before. Cut the zucchini into ½ in (2.5 cm) cubes, or chop the cauliflower into small florets. Blanch in boiling water for 1 minute (this isn't essential, but it makes the shake smoother). Store in the freezer in a glass dish or a bag.
- Forgotten to freeze your zucchini? Just use cubed fresh zucchini and some ice cubes.
- The protein content of different protein powders can vary a lot—check the protein content on the brand you use to work out how many scoops you'll need. I use NuZest protein powders, which translates to 4 scoops.

Strawberry Shortcake Smoothie

SERVES 1 | PREP TIME: 5 MINUTES

1 cup frozen
  strawberries
2 scoops vanilla protein
  powder
1 cup almond milk
½ cup frozen cauliflower
  florets (optional)
cold water to thin if
  needed

The wonderful combination of strawberries and vanilla makes you think you're drinking strawberry shortcake.

Place all the ingredients except water in a blender or food processor.

Blend until smooth, adding a little extra water if needed.

Note

Add some frozen zucchini (courgette) if you want an extra serving of undetectable vegetables. It will also make the smoothie colder and thicker.

Breakfast Caesar Salad

SERVES 1 | PREP: 30 MINUTES

For the salad:
3½–5 oz (100–150 g)
  skinless chicken breast
2 eggs
¼ head romaine or cos
  lettuce, chopped
handful of baby
  spinach, chopped
1 Tbsp anchovies or
  bacon bits

Optional spices for chicken:
½ Tbsp chili powder
½ Tbsp garlic powder
½ Tbsp dried oregano
salt and pepper to taste

For the Caesar dressing:
½ cup mayonnaise
2 cloves garlic, minced
2 Tbsp fresh lemon juice
2 tsp anchovy paste
1 tsp Dijon mustard
salt and pepper to taste

You might be surprised to see this in the breakfast section, but I have found Caesar salad to be one of the easiest savory options. Eggs for breakfast is something we're already used to, and the other ingredients just work as tasty added extras. You can jazz the chicken up with a bit of spice or simply leave it plain. Feel free to also add some toasted seeds or nuts for some added crunch.

Put a saucepan of water on medium heat and bring to the boil. Meanwhile, preheat the grill to 320°F (160°C), or preheat a frying pan with a little olive oil if frying.

If using the spices, place them in a cup or small bowl, and mix together. Rub the chicken with the spice mix.

Grill or fry the chicken for 5–6 minutes on each side, or until cooked through. Meanwhile, put the eggs into the pan of boiling water and cook for 5 minutes (until hard-boiled).

Whisk together all of the ingredients for the Caesar dressing until thoroughly combined.

Place the lettuce and spinach in a large serving bowl.

When the chicken and eggs are cooked, slice the chicken into strips, and cut the eggs into quarters. Add the chicken and eggs to the spinach and lettuce leaves, pour over the dressing and toss everything together gently.

Top with anchovies or bacon bits, if using.

Note

This is also one of the best breakfasts to prepare ahead of time, or make to have over a few days. Boil up the eggs, cook the chicken, whisk up the dressing, and toss the salad vegetables together, and leave everything separate in the fridge. Then each morning, it's just a two-minute job to combine it all and then sit down to this delicious bowl.

Low-sugar Brownies

MAKES 15–25 BROWNIES | PREP TIME: 17 MINUTES

1 cup fine almond flour

⅓ cup Dutch cocoa powder

1 tsp baking powder

½ tsp salt

⅓ cup melted coconut oil or butter

3 Tbsp water or additional oil

2 eggs

⅔ cup granulated erythritol or regular sugar

1 tsp pure vanilla extract

1½ cups fresh or frozen raspberries (optional)

These are incredibly delicious brownies—as good as it gets. They are dark and fudgy and super easy to make. As a general rule, the less time you cook brownies the more fudgy they will be. The longer you cook them, the more cake-like they will be. I like mine fudgy so I bake them for 15 minutes, or until the outside is cooked but the middle is still a bit wobbly. If you bake them until a skewer inserted into the center comes out clean the texture will be more cakey. The cooking time may vary depending on your oven, so the first time you make these keep checking after 15 minutes.

Preheat the oven to 350°F (180°C).

Line an 8 in x 8 in (20 cm x 20 cm) baking tin at least 2¼ in (6 cm) deep with non-stick baking paper.

Mix all the ingredients, except the raspberries, together until smooth

Pour the mixture into the prepared tin and spread out. Scatter over the raspberries if using.

Bake in the center of the oven for around 20 minutes, or until cooked on the outside but still slightly soft and fudgy in the middle. Let the brownies cool completely and they will firm up even more.

Cut into squares and enjoy. These will also keep in the fridge or in an airtight container for a week.

Bountify Bars

MAKES: 5 BARS | PREP TIME: 1 HOUR

For the coconut filling:

1 cup coconut milk

3 Tbsp coconut oil

1–3 tsp stevia or
monkfruit extract, to
taste

2¼ cups desiccated
coconut

pinch of sea salt

**For the chocolate
coating:**

3½ oz (100 g) 90 percent
dark chocolate

**If you're still struggling with a few cravings, then
these homemade Bounty-style bars should sort you
out! Bounty bars were one of my favorite treats, so
I was very keen to create a recipe that was low in
sugar but still gave me that coconutty hit.**

Place the coconut milk and coconut oil in a
medium-sized saucepan, and stir over low heat
until combined.

Add the stevia or monkfruit extract and taste for
sweetness. If you like it sweeter, add more. Add
the desiccated coconut and sea salt, and stir to
combine.

Line a deep baking tray with non-stick baking paper,
leaving it overhanging the sides a little. Scrape the
coconut mixture into the tray and press down with
the back of a spoon to about ¾ in (1.5 cm) thick.
Place in the freezer for about 1 hour until well set.

When the coconut is almost set, break the
chocolate up and place it in a heatproof bowl.
Set the bowl over a saucepan containing a little
simmering water, without allowing the bowl to
touch the water. Let sit until the chocolate has
melted, stirring occasionally until smooth. Remove
from the heat.

Remove the coconut from the freezer. Holding the
baking paper, lift out the coconut slab and place on
a chopping board. Cut into five chocolate-bar-sized
slices.

Carefully place each bar into the melted chocolate
and turn to cover evenly. Lift with a fork under the
bar, hold until the chocolate has stopped dripping,
and place on a clean sheet of baking paper laid on
a clean tray.

Place the bars back in the freezer to set. Remove
just before eating. Stored in an airtight container in
the freezer, these will keep for approx. 2 weeks.

Chocolate Coconut Ganache

SERVES 6 | PREP TIME: 40 MINUTES

3½ oz (100 g) 90 percent
dark chocolate (or
100 percent if you're
brave!)

stevia or monkfruit
extract, to taste

1 x 14 oz (400 ml) can
full-fat coconut cream,
refrigerated overnight

fresh berries, to serve

This rather decadent recipe is low in sugar, easy to make, and a great accompaniment to some fresh berries. When you're choosing your coconut milk, have a look at the ingredients on the can and go for the brand with the least additives (and certainly no added sugar). The additives, while not great for us, also prevent the coconut cream from separating—which is not what we want for this recipe. You'll need to put the can in the refrigerator the night before for best results.

Break up the chocolate and place in a heatproof bowl. Set the bowl over a saucepan with a little simmering water in the bottom, without letting the bowl touch the water. Allow to melt, stirring occasionally until smooth. If you want to make it sweeter, add the stevia or monkfruit and stir in. Remove from the heat and allow to cool a little.

Open the can of coconut cream and scoop the cream off the top into a mixing bowl. Be careful not to get too much of the watery liquid in there.

Whip the coconut cream with an electric beater (as you would with normal cream), until thickened. Add the cooled melted chocolate and fold it into the coconut cream.

Place the ganache in the refrigerator to firm up, for approx. 2 hours, then serve in small scoops with fresh berries.

This is really rich, so you don't need much.

Coconut Chickpea Curry

SERVES 4 | PREP TIME: 40 MINUTES

1 Tbsp light olive oil

1 large red onion, thinly sliced

3 cloves garlic, minced

1 in (2.5 cm) piece of fresh ginger, peeled and minced or grated

1 Tbsp garam masala

¼ tsp turmeric powder

¼ tsp ground black pepper (or ⅛ tsp freshly ground)

¼ tsp cayenne pepper (or to taste)

¼ tsp salt (or more to taste)

1½ cups diced tomatoes (or 14 oz/400 g can, drained)

1½ cups full-fat coconut milk (14 oz/400 g can)

1¾ cups cooked chickpeas (16 oz/450 g can, drained and rinsed)

2 Tbsp freshly squeezed lime or lemon juice

1 serve cauliflower rice or konjac flour rice

fresh cilantro (coriander), chopped, for serving

This curry can be made ahead and frozen, or reheated the next day. It contains loads of great veges, especially if you serve it over cauliflower rice. I like to make it for new moms to have in their freezer to heat and eat.

In a large pan, heat the light olive oil over medium-high heat. Add the red onion with a pinch of salt, and stir-fry until the onion is softened and starting to color.

Reduce the heat to medium. Add the garlic and ginger, and stir-fry for 60 seconds or until fragrant.

Stir in the garam masala, turmeric, black pepper, cayenne pepper, and salt. Cook, stirring, for 30 seconds more to toast the spices.

Add the tomatoes to the pan and stir well. Continue to cook, stirring occasionally, for 3 to 5 minutes or until the tomatoes are starting to break down and dry up a little bit. Stir in the coconut milk and chickpeas. Bring the mixture to a boil, then reduce the heat to medium-low.

Simmer uncovered for about 10 minutes, or until reduced slightly.

Stir in the fresh lime or lemon juice.

Season to taste with additional salt if you wish (about another ½ teaspoon at this point).

Spoon over cauliflower rice or konjac flour rice (you can also use black, wholegrain or basmati), and garnish with cilantro (coriander).

Fish Parcels with Cauliflower "Tabouli"

SERVES 2 | PREP TIME: 20 MINUTES

For the fish parcels:

2 x 6 oz (170 g) fillets of a firm, white-fleshed fish

zest and juice of 1 lemon

2 sprigs of mint or basil

For the cauliflower tabouli:

1 telegraph cucumber, finely diced

4 large tomatoes, diced

2 green (spring) onions, thinly sliced (or 1 small red onion, finely diced)

a handful of fresh mint, finely chopped

a handful of fresh parsley, finely chopped

1½ cups cauliflower rice (I make this using a cheese grater to grate my cauliflower)

1 tsp olive oil

For the dressing:

3 Tbsp olive oil

¼ cup lemon juice

2 cloves garlic, minced

1 tsp cumin powder

½ tsp salt

Fish parcels are by far the easiest and cleanest way to cook fish. Cooking fish in foil retains the moisture and flavor, making these parcels really delicious, too! You can reduce the quantity by half to make for 1, or save the other half for lunch the next day.

Preheat the oven to 350°F (160°C).

Cut out two pieces of foil, each big enough to hold one piece of fish with plenty of space around it. Place the fish on the foil and cover with the lemon zest and juice.

Put the herbs on the fish and roll up the foil to make a parcel. Place on a baking tray and bake for 10 minutes, or until the flesh has turned white.

While the fish is cooking, make your salad by combining the cucumber, tomatoes, onion, mint, and parsley in a large bowl.

Place the dressing ingredients in a jar and shake to combine.

Add the cauliflower rice to the rest of the salad ingredients. Pour over the dressing and toss everything together. Serve immediately with the fish on top. You can store the salad, covered, in the fridge for up to two days.

Spicy Mexican Tacos

SERVES 4 | PREP TIME: 20 MINUTES

For the non-vegetarian filling:

2 eggs

2 Tbsp Cajun seasoning

4 x 6 oz (170 g) firm white fish fillets (I use cod), sliced into four (or 2 chicken breasts, sliced into tenderloins)

olive oil, for cooking

For the black bean filling:

1 Tbsp olive oil

1 medium onion, finely diced

3 cloves garlic, minced

2 tsp Cajun seasoning

2 x 15 oz (390 g) cans black beans, drained and rinsed

½ cup vegetable stock (or water)

Avocado salsa:

1 avocado, stoned and diced

½ red onion, finely diced

1 punnet cherry tomatoes, cut into quarters

½ lemon or lime, juiced

To serve:

12 large romaine or cos lettuce leaves (for wraps)

3 cups of undressed slaw of your choice

lemon or lime juice

fresh cilantro (coriander), chopped, to garnish (optional)

This is one of my favorite recipes of all time—it's great with fresh fish, chicken, or black beans, and is a crowd-pleaser. I usually serve the tacos with a handful of sweet potato or potato wedges. Note that this is spicy, so to make a milder version use mild Cajun seasoning. I like to use broccoli slaw mix, which you should be able to find in grocery stores; it usually has broccoli, red cabbage and carrots in.

To make the non-vegetarian filling, whisk the eggs until combined. Pour about 2 tablespoons of Cajun seasoning onto a dinner plate. Dip the fish (or chicken) into the egg to coat it, then place it straight onto the Cajun seasoning to coat, then onto a separate plate. Add more Cajun seasoning as needed. Heat a little olive oil in a large frying pan over medium heat and cook the fish or chicken in batches until cooked through and lightly browned.

To make the black bean filling, heat the oil in a large skillet over a medium heat. Gently fry the onion for about 4 minutes until soft and just beginning to brown. Add the garlic and gently fry for 2 minutes, then add the Cajun seasoning and continue frying for 1 minute. Add the beans and stock. Bring to the boil, then lower the heat and simmer for about 10 minutes until the beans soften. Add extra stock or water as needed. Mash about half the bean mixture with a fork or potato masher, adding extra stock or water to achieve the desired consistency.

While the filling is cooking, make the avocado salsa by combining the avocado, red onion, and cherry tomatoes in a small bowl. Squeeze over the lemon or lime juice.

To serve, place some of the fillings down the center of a lettuce leaf. Top with avocado salsa and slaw. Drizzle with lemon or lime juice, and sprinkle with cilantro (coriander) leaves if desired.

Thai-style Salad

SERVES 2 | PREP TIME: 30 MINUTES + MARINATING TIME

10½ oz (300 g) rump or
  sirloin steak
salt to taste
1 tsp olive or avocado oil

**For the marinade/
dressing:**
¼ cup soy sauce (or
  coconut Aminos if
  gluten-free)
¼ cup light olive oil
2 Tbsp lime juice
1 Tbsp fish sauce
1 Tbsp Thai red curry
  paste
sweetener, such as
  stevia or monkfruit
  (optional)

For the salad:
½ telegraph cucumber,
  sliced into batons
½ red onion, sliced
1 medium-sized carrot,
  julienned
½ red bell pepper
  (capsicum), sliced
a handful of fresh
  cilantro (coriander),
  roughly chopped
a small handful of fresh
  mint leaves, roughly
  chopped
a handful of mixed
  greens
½ cup roasted peanuts

I love the Thai flavors of lime, cilantro (coriander), and chili, and combined with the fact that this meal is so quick to make, it's my go-to after a busy day of work. For a vegetarian version, use tofu or tempeh—just opt for one that's traditionally fermented rather than heavily processed.

In a small bowl whisk together the marinade/dressing ingredients.

Sprinkle steak with salt on both sides and place in a glass baking dish. Pour over half the marinade, reserving the other half for the salad dressing. Cover and marinate for up to 8 hours in the fridge.

Heat the olive or avocado oil in a large frying pan over a medium-high heat and cook steak for 2–3 minutes on each side, or until done to your liking. Remove steaks from pan, cover, and rest for at least 5 minutes.

While the steak is resting, combine the salad ingredients, except for the peanuts, in a large bowl. Whisk the reserved dressing and taste; to sweeten it add a sweetener of your choice, such as stevia or monkfruit.

Slice the steak at an angle across the grain. (If you've cooked the steak ahead of time, slice it just before serving.) Serve salad with sliced steak on top, drizzle over the dressing, and garnish with peanuts if desired.

Top tip

If you want to add some starchy carbohydrates to this dish, then add cubes of roasted sweet potato or serve with rice or rice noodles on the side.

SAMPLE DAY: EATING FOR INSULIN RESISTANCE

Here's how you can combine the recipes to meet the guidelines I've given you earlier in the book:

Breakfast: Chocolate Thick Shake Smoothie

The frozen zucchini (courgette) adds thickness and coolness to your smoothie with no extra taste, and is two servings of vegetables; this breakfast provides 45 g protein and very little carbohydrate.

Lunch: Leftover Spicy Mexican Tacos

Assuming that you ate Spicy Mexican Bean Tacos the night before, you could have leftovers the following day for lunch, which would give you your portion of carbohydrate and protein from the beans. The lettuce cups, slaw, and avocado salsa would give you at least 3½ serves of vegetables.

Dinner: Fish Parcels with Cauliflower "Tabouli" and Sweet Potato Wedges

The fish is your protein serve, while the cauliflower tabouli provides at least 3½ serves of vegetables. The sweet potato gives you your carbohydrate and still counts as a vegetable!

For dessert, treat yourself to two squares of 90 percent dark chocolate with a cup of herbal tea.

Total vegetable servings: 10! (See how you can easily get 10 or more servings of vegetables if you just make the main event the vegetables, and your protein and carbohydrate a "side.")

Chapter 8
Step 3—Address stress

There are a lot of lifestyle issues other than diet that contribute to your root cause. I've grouped them together as "stress" because, in their own way, they are stressors on the body that can affect both the root cause(s) of PCOS and the three fertile ingredients (see page 42 for a reminder if you need one).

When you think of stress, you probably think of sitting in traffic when you're late for a meeting, being given a client report at 4 p.m. that needs to be completed by 8 a.m., crashing your car or getting sick when you don't have insurance cover, or receiving an exorbitant energy bill in the mail. However, these are all examples of psychological stress, and there is much more to stress than this.

Stress is, essentially, when your body perceives that it cannot cope with what you're demanding of it. Thinking of it from this point of view, it could be not getting enough sleep for your insulin receptors to work properly; it could be over-exercising, or not doing enough exercise; it could be an internal infection that your body is fighting or an external source of stress like caffeine—or many of these.

Stress isn't all bad; a little can be a positive thing. There is nothing like a deadline to make us actually get the work done, and sometimes it's our best work. There is absolutely no way I would have finished this book unless I had editing and publishing deadlines! It is the same with your body—a little bit of stress can make your body adapt positively. This is how getting fitter works. If you haven't been running for a while, you'll head out your door and may be able to run only a fairly short distance before you need to stop. But if you keep running every day, by the next week you'll be able to run half a mile (about a kilometer), and in the following weeks you'll get up to 1, 2, 3 and even 5 miles. This is the result of your body adapting to the stress (running) that you're putting it under. Your body hates not being able to complete the task: "I don't want to be caught out if she makes me do that running thing again, so I'm going to grow some more red blood cells so they can carry more oxygen, and I'm going to grow some more muscle fibers so they can do more work. This way, I can run further and faster when she asks me to." This is what we know as getting fitter.

But like anything, there is a limit. If you keep pushing your body with exercise, it won't be able to adapt quickly enough. Instead of getting fitter, you'll just get more tired, sick, and injured. This is what's known as overtraining.

The same thing happens with stress from other sources—work, social, family, etc. Just like Goldilocks, we want not too little, and definitely not too much. The complex part is knowing where that line is, and it differs for each of us. Some of us can tolerate more stress than others. If you had a stressful childhood (e.g. you were a competitive athlete, there was stress at home, or you experienced an accident or illness), or you have a particular genetic makeup (specifically your COMT gene), your stress response is likely to be heightened. Your friend might be able to handle working in a corporate job while also having young children and doing five spin classes a week, but for you this is too much.

HOW STRESS AFFECTS FERTILITY AND PCOS

Stress hormones like cortisol can be a significant contributor to PCOS and reduced fertility. When you are under a lot of stress, your brain (hypothalamus and pituitary) detects this and stimulates your adrenal glands to produce stress hormones: adrenaline and cortisol. Adrenaline is known as the fight-or-flight hormone because it is produced rapidly to prepare your body for instant action if necessary. Cortisol is normally produced to help make glucose available when you exercise and to reduce inflammation, but high levels of stress can raise blood cortisol and keep it high for a prolonged period of time. The interaction between your hypothalamus, pituitary, and adrenal glands is called your HPA axis, and this is why you might read about HPA-axis dysfunction—which is a more accurate term than "adrenal fatigue" but a whole lot harder to understand.

Stress is especially important for those of you who were identified as having an "adrenal" root cause. As I described in Chapter 1, stress affects PCOS and fertility in three ways:

- It increases dehydroepiandrosterone sulfate (DHEA-S).
- It exacerbates insulin resistance.
- It reduces fertility, even in those without PCOS.

Numerous studies have demonstrated how stress affects menstrual cycles and fertility. One study looked at stress in female nurses. The nurses recorded their temperature and period/no period daily for three months, and answered questionnaires on stress. The researchers found that the more stressed nurses had longer menstrual cycles.[1] Another study investigated cycle length differences in almost 300 women with stressful jobs, compared with other women with non-stressful jobs. The results showed that those in stressful jobs were almost twice as likely to have a short cycle (less than 24 days).[2] As mentioned earlier, the Covid-19 pandemic has affected women's cycles across the world.

We are also starting to see evidence of stress affecting fertility in IVF. For example, one study followed 192 women going through IVF for a maximum of four rounds, and measured their stress hormones to see whether there was any relationship between stress and pregnancy success. Cortisol levels were found to be significantly higher in the group of women who didn't get pregnant in their second round of IVF.[3]

While this research is still in its infancy, clinically we see this happening all the time. Women who are chronically stressed either have a long cycle because their body is trying to ovulate over and over again, or a short cycle where their luteal phase is too short and the uterine lining doesn't stay intact for long enough. Many women describe how they have been trying to conceive for years (which is inherently stressful) and then decide to stop trying, or change job, or move to the country, and then suddenly get pregnant. Of course, you don't need to move to a rural backwater to get pregnant. If you're monitoring your cycle (using the guidance in Chapter 9), you'll easily be able to spot what the issue is and fix it. This may mean some lifestyle changes, but it won't necessarily mean uprooting your whole life. It might just be some of the simple changes that I outline here, like getting more sleep, changing your exercise, or reducing your coffee intake.

Research has shown that women with PCOS have a different response to stress. Firstly, women with PCOS secrete more cortisol than other women—i.e. our stress response is heightened.[4] Secondly, we also break down cortisol differently. Studies have shown that women with PCOS have increased breakdown and excretion of cortisol. This may sound great—we're getting rid of cortisol out of our body—but what actually happens is that our brain gets a bit confused. When more cortisol is excreted, the body detects the drop in cortisol levels and increases the production of the hormone ACTH (adrenocorticotropic hormone), which tells the adrenal gland to produce more cortisol. At the same time, ACTH stimulates the production of more DHEA-S.

WHAT YOU CAN DO ABOUT STRESS

I think of stress like a bucket, and we all have a slightly different size of bucket. A little bit of stress in that bucket is a good thing because it helps weigh it down so that it won't blow away in the wind. But too much stress in the bucket will make it overflow and tip over. If you're a high-achieving female in our modern world, your bucket is already going to be half-full. You then add in a stressful job, weekends where you're rushing across town from social event to social event, or an hour-long high-intensity spin class five times a week, plus a cup of coffee or two a day—and the result is an overflowing bucket.

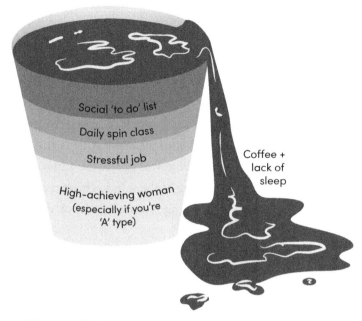

Figure 10: The stress bucket

But just as quickly as we can put stress into our bucket, we can also take it out. So let's explore some 'quick wins' when it comes to tackling stress.

- Get good sleep.
- Cut down on caffeine.
- Get the right amount of exercise.
- Avoid becoming overwhelmed.

Note: These quick wins will be unlikely to have much impact if you have some significant stressors that are filling your bucket all by themselves, such as an extremely high-pressure job, being in a bad (or worse, abusive) relationship, or serious financial stress. You're going to have to deal with these issues as well, or the measures I describe below won't help you much.

I like to think of a big issue as the "big domino." If you identify and knock out this big domino, the rest will come crashing down. However, it will likely take time to knock down that big domino. If you (say) want to change jobs, you may need to update your CV, then start looking for jobs, then go through the application and interview process if there is a desirable job out there for you. This can take six months or more.

So in the meantime, while you sort out the big domino, addressing the other quick wins is definitely going to help—and will probably make life a whole lot easier to manage while you address that big domino.

SLEEP
How lack of sleep affects you

Not only does a lack of sleep prevent us from functioning at our best, it is also a significant contributor to hormone imbalance in PCOS, via insulin resistance, inflammation, and increased stress hormones.

- **Sleep deprivation increases cortisol**—Cortisol is a long-term stress hormone, and cortisol levels are increased by sleep deprivation. The effect on cortisol levels of sleep deprivation isn't felt only the day after. Researchers found that cortisol levels were 45 percent higher two days after the sleep deprivation occurred.[5]

- **Sleep deprivation reduces insulin sensitivity**—Lack of sleep decreases your cells' sensitivity to insulin. One study showed that just one week of sleeping only five hours a night reduced insulin sensitivity by 24 percent.[6] Having decreased insulin sensitivity means that your body has to produce even more insulin to have the same effect. Sleep deprivation and PCOS are, therefore, linked due to inadequate sleep causing increased blood insulin levels, which leads to increased testosterone.

- **Sleep deprivation makes us crave sugar and other refined carbohydrates**—Not only does sleep deprivation make us less sensitive to insulin, but it also makes us crave sugar and refined carbohydrates. When your body is low on energy because it hasn't had enough sleep, it craves the next best thing: sugar! Energy drinks, chocolate bars, pastries, and pizza—we've all reached for one (or all!) of these when we're sleep-deprived.

Eating foods that are high in sugar may provide a much-needed spike in energy by increasing your blood sugar levels, but it also causes your insulin levels to rise. Do this repeatedly, and you're at risk of developing insulin resistance. If you already have insulin resistance, then eating high-sugar foods will only make your situation worse. Either way, you're increasing the likelihood of your body overproducing testosterone. As I mentioned earlier, sleep deprivation not only impairs our ability to make complex decisions, it also activates the part of the brain associated with desire and cravings.

- **Sleep deprivation makes us inflamed**—Chronic inflammation is one of the biggest causes of insulin resistance and a leading cause of PCOS. Scientists now think that inflammation and insulin resistance go hand in hand. Studies have shown that 10 nights of sleeping for only four hours caused a fivefold increase in inflammatory markers.[7] The inflammation leads to insulin resistance, which leads to PCOS symptoms. Yet another way that sleep deprivation and PCOS have a relationship.

How much sleep is enough

There is no "one amount fits all" solution when it comes to sleep. What is considered an adequate amount of sleep is unique to every individual. Adequate sleep means that you're waking up feeling refreshed, preferably before your alarm. For me, this means between eight and nine hours of sleep, but seven might be enough for you.

A good way to discover how much sleep you need is to find out how many hours of sleep you need before you wake up without an alarm. For a week, set your alarm to give yourself nine hours of time to sleep, and see how long you actually sleep. Is it seven, eight, nine hours—are you still only waking when your alarm goes off? Once you've found your natural number of sleep hours, aim to get that amount of sleep each night. Sleep is one of the priorities in my *PCOS Protocol* program; I hear so many stories of how focusing on sleep is a real game-changer.

CASE STUDY

Marie didn't think that she had an issue with sleep, but she reviewed my sleep module and purchased earplugs and an eye mask as I recommended. Within three days, she was saying how it used to take her two-plus hours to get to sleep because her partner snored so loudly, and now it was only taking her 10 minutes! She'd thought that seven hours of sleep was enough for her, but in fact it was nowhere near enough. Plus, who wants to lie in bed tossing and turning for two hours?

Tools for getting good sleep

What if you always go to bed early but find you just can't sleep? I know what it's like to be absolutely exhausted but unable to sleep. You may have been feeling tired all afternoon, but as soon as your head hits the pillow . . . *Woah.* Suddenly your mind wants all of the answers to life's great questions:

- "What should we have for dinner tomorrow?"
- "Did I actually book that Airbnb for next week, or just mindlessly scroll through the photos?"
- "What did my boss mean in that meeting this morning?"
- "How does the internet actually work?"

I'm sure you've all experienced this at some point. Your body is tired but your mind is wired! Or there is something else that is stopping you from getting to sleep (like a snoring partner).

Get regular

One of the best ways to train your body to sleep well is to go to bed and get up at more or less the same time every day, even on weekends and days off. This regular cycle will make you feel better and help your body get back into rhythm.

Keep your bed for sleep

Do you use your bed to watch television, pay the bills, or read emails that you couldn't deal with at work? Don't! You want your body to associate bed with sleep, so don't use it for anything else (apart from sex) or you won't learn this connection, and consequently you'll be tired but wired.

Use a blue-light blocker

The blue light emitted from screens affects your circadian rhythm. Your circadian rhythm is your body's natural sleep and wake cycle which responds to darkness and light in your environment. Your body's master clock in the hypothalamus of the brain controls the production of melatonin, a hormone that makes you sleepy. It receives information about incoming light from the optic nerves in your eyes. When there is less light—like at night—the hypothalamus tells the brain to make more melatonin, so you get drowsy. But blue light from devices sends the opposite signal. It tells your brain that it's daytime, and studies have shown that this results in a significant reduction in melatonin production.[8]

The best practice is to turn off all screens two hours before bedtime. However, I know this isn't always possible; if you really need to do some life admin in the evenings, make sure you reduce the blue light coming from your device. Newer Apple devices have this available as a setting, so just make sure it's turned on; for other devices, you can download apps that do the same thing (see the Resources section). I also like to use blue-light blocking glasses from about midday to reduce the impact of blue light.

Make your bedroom properly dark

When it comes to your bedroom, definitely turn those phones to night mode before you go to sleep—or even better, get them out of your room entirely and make the room properly dark with blackout curtains to help your melatonin production. If you can't do this, get an eye mask to block out any additional light. You'll be amazed at how much better you sleep.

Meditate 10 minutes before bed

Do you lie in bed at night thinking of all the things that you didn't do that day, or perhaps going over a passive-aggressive conversation you had with a colleague earlier, or thinking that you must remember to take the steak out of the freezer for dinner tomorrow night? One of the best ways to stop all these thoughts swirling around your brain is to meditate for 10 minutes before bed. This takes your mind out of thinking about the past or future and gets you focused on the present moment of sleeping. There are apps or podcasts that can help (see the Resources section)

Keep a pen and paper beside your bed

Sometimes you really do need to remember to get the steak out of the freezer—and who am I to stop you from meal prepping? But instead of lying there thinking "must not forget to take the steak out," over and over again, just write it down, then get it out of your mind and get to sleep. This can also work well if you're worrying about something—write it all down on a piece of paper to get it out of your head.

CAFFEINE

The second easy win when it comes to reducing stress is cutting out caffeine. Caffeine (in the form of tea or coffee) has become central to many cultures, and to the belief that it helps us function during the workday. The average American coffee drinker drinks more than three cups of coffee a day,[9] and when asked about what drinks they had consumed the previous day, 62 percent had drunk coffee, more than any other drink apart from bottled water.

Back in 2011, I couldn't process my thoughts to write a coherent email unless I'd had a double shot of coffee as soon as I got to the office, and then again three hours later. Every morning I'd wake up feeling like I'd been hit by a bus, with my brain foggy and slow, feeling like every thought had to push through a muddy swamp just to get out. It was awful. I felt like my intelligence was receding, and my ability to quickly pick up new tasks and concepts, which I'd once prided myself on, was vanishing. Then come evening I'd get my second wind, and by night I'd be tired but wired.

After doing some research, I realized that my caffeine intake might not be helping me and decided to stop drinking coffee completely. For over a week, I had terrible headaches. But after three weeks, I started to notice some improvements. I was waking up and feeling brighter and more alert. My sharpness started to return and, interestingly, my face became a lot less puffy.

How caffeine affects you

Caffeine stimulates your adrenal glands to produce more stress hormones. Studies have shown that even low doses of caffeine (one cup a day) activates the adrenals to produce more stress hormones.[10] What if you're drinking more than that? Well, the more caffeine you drink, the higher your stress hormones stay for longer.[10]

Caffeine actually works by blocking a receptor (or lock on the door to a cell). In this case, the lock is for adenosine—a super-important neurotransmitter, but one that also makes us feel drowsy. This is why caffeine improves our reaction time, concentration, and motor control.[11] The problem is that for every action in the body, there is a reaction. We can't just block adenosine from working without having some downstream consequences, just like we can't block our body from ovulating with hormonal contraception without consequences.

There is a second complication when it comes to caffeine, and that is your individual ability to metabolize it (break it down). Like your hormones, caffeine needs to be broken down by your liver so that you can excrete it in your urine. The longer that caffeine is in your body, the more of an effect it's going to have on you. But the ability to break caffeine down isn't the same for everyone. It's controlled by your genes (and also by medication). The genes CYP1A2 and HLA control caffeine metabolism, and variations in these genes control whether you're going to be a fast or a slow metabolizer of caffeine. This means how quickly your

DRINK	AMOUNT OF CAFFEINE
Coffee (Starbucks Venti)	475 mg
Coffee (double-shot espresso)	180–250 mg
Black tea	46 mg
Green tea	40 mg
Instant coffee	26 mg
Dark chocolate (1½ oz/42 g)	20 mg
Decaffeinated coffee	9 mg

Figure 11: Amount of caffeine in different drinks

body can break it down and get it out of your body. A fast metabolizer of caffeine can have a cup of coffee right before bed and have no issues sleeping, whereas a slow metabolizer will feel more dramatic effects that last longer. Instead of just feeling more alert, a slow metabolizer might feel jittery or even nauseous. About 50 percent of the population are slow metabolizers of caffeine.[12]

And that's not all. When slow metabolizers consume caffeine, it increases their fasting blood glucose.[13] If your insulin already isn't functioning correctly, this will exacerbate it. Caffeine consumption has also been associated with a higher risk of heart disease and hypertension (high blood pressure).[14, 15]

A third complication with caffeine is how it affects and is affected by any medication you're taking. If you're taking hormonal birth control (HBC), you're less able to metabolize caffeine. One study found that oral contraceptives almost doubled the time it takes to metabolize caffeine (10 hours vs. six hours).[16] So if you're genetically a slow metabolizer of caffeine *and* you're on HBC, you've got a double whammy and have caffeine floating around in your body for much longer.

As you can see from Figure 11, your favorite Starbucks Venti and double-shot espresso are by far the worst culprits when it comes to caffeine. Black and green tea have about a quarter of the caffeine that espresso does, so are a better choice, but if you're like my grandmother and drink 13 cups a day, you're going to get about the same as three cups of espresso.

Reducing your consumption

For the next two months, try reducing your caffeine to the equivalent of one cup of green or black tea a day. This could mean four decaffeinated coffees. If you want to have green or black tea, try to have it first thing in the morning so that your body has more time to break it down and it is less likely to affect your sleep and circadian rhythm.

To help you cut down or quit caffeine, follow these steps:

1. Don't go cold-turkey—you'll likely suffer some pretty severe headaches. Instead, wean yourself off it. Reduce your caffeine intake by half for the first week (i.e. if you have two cups a day, reduce that to one—you can make the second one decaf if you like). The next week, reduce by half again, i.e. half a cup or a single shot, then a quarter cup.

2. You don't have to give up coffee, just *caffeine*. I love the taste of coffee, so I drink decaf. Try to find one where the caffeine has been removed using water rather than chemicals.

3. Reduce down to the equivalent of 1 cup of tea per day for at least a month (preferably two), and see how it affects you. Does it make you feel better in the morning? Do you wake up feeling more refreshed, or does it makes no difference? If you're feeling better, you're likely to be better staying off caffeine. (And if you need to see what your genetics say to take it seriously, get a genetic test done.)

EXERCISE

Too much high-intensity exercise can also be a significant source of stress in your life. Exercise is critical for optimal health, and especially for PCOS. But there is definitely such a thing as too much. I'm going to break this section into two components: the effect of too much exercise on our stress hormones, and the optimal exercise, especially for insulin resistance.

The effect of too much exercise

We've all heard that exercise is great, and that as a population we need to exercise more—but what about when exercise is too much? Please don't take this out of context: if you're not exercising currently, then exercise is *not* going to be bad for you. In this section I'm talking to those of you who I used to be—those of you doing marathons, ultramarathons, six days a week cross-fit, or two hours of HIIT (high-intensity interval training) gym classes a day. If this doesn't apply to you, please skip ahead to read about what the best exercise for PCOS is.

- **Too much high-intensity exercise increases cortisol**—Studies have shown that exercise increases both cortisol and ACTH by 40 percent at 60 percent of maximal oxygen uptake and by an average of 83 percent at 80 percent of maximal oxygen uptake.[17] To put this in context, many women would be exercising at 80 percent in a spin class or a high-intensity aerobics class. And these changes don't just occur during the exercise but can last for hours afterward. As you now know, when cortisol increases, so does DHEA-S (your adrenal androgen hormone). When your eggs are exposed to overly high levels of androgens, this will affect their quality and affect your fertility.

- **Too much exercise makes us more insulin-resistant**—Cortisol is elevated when you are under chronic stress, and also during endurance exercise and for many hours afterward.[18] When cortisol is raised, our body reacts by dumping glucose into the bloodstream, preparing for the muscles to use it, either for exercise or to react to a perceived threat. In our modern-day corporate world, we're going from our morning gym class to sitting all day—so that glucose in the blood doesn't get used. Combine this with a morning coffee and a high-pressure job, which both increase cortisol, and we are literally soaking in a day-long bath of cortisol.

  For the 80 percent of women with PCOS who have insulin resistance,[19] this is a recipe for disaster. The cortisol is continually pumping glucose into the blood, but the muscles aren't doing any work, so they're not using it. The body doesn't like glucose just sitting in the blood, so it raises the glucose-storing hormone, insulin, to store the glucose for later use. However, if you have insulin resistance, this process doesn't work properly.

Why doing more exercise to lose weight is the wrong approach

As I explained in Chapter 3:

- Weight loss is not the most important thing for fertility— improving your root cause is.

- Calories are only part of the equation when it comes to weight loss; insulin and hormones are other very important factors.

But also, when it comes to endurance and high-intensity workouts, the caloric burn is not all it's cracked up to be. We've grown up with the "calorie equation" encouraging us to exercise more to "burn" calories. So we think that more must be better, and therefore an hour-long gym class is the way to go. Studies have proven this to be wrong. Under the umbrella of the Cochrane collaboration (a major and respected research analysis group), researchers conducted a review of 43 studies, each between three and 12 months long, involving exercise sessions lasting on average 45 minutes, three to five times a week. This means that the participants were exercising on average for 69 hours during the duration of the studies. The average weight loss was found to be just 2.2 lb (1 kg)— for 69 hours of working out.[20] Disappointing or what?

Other research has shown that when we burn calories exercising, our body drives us to make them up again by eating. While we might not think that we do this enough to override all of the calories we burn, we actually do. Studies have shown that we really believe we've earned those extra treats. One study compared two groups of women: one that had exercised for 50 minutes at a relatively high intensity, and one that did no exercise. The exercise group not only ate more, but they also preferred higher-fat, sweet food.[21] Moreover, the researchers hypothesized that this was completely involuntary. When we've been working hard, we are apparently predisposed to crave that candy bar instead of reaching for a can of tuna or a handful of carrots.

Don't get me wrong: exercise is beneficial for PCOS, and you can still exercise—you just might need to change the type and amount of exercise you're doing. From my own experience, I know just how hard this can be. I love working out, especially running and cross-fit. I love the competitiveness, the endorphin rush, and pushing my body to the edge. So learning to stop overworking myself was really, really hard, and to be honest with you I still battle with this. The "go hard or go home" high-achieving mentality is so deeply rooted that it takes some time to override. However, I realized after years of trying to lose weight and improve my PCOS symptoms that doing more exercise and eating less wasn't working for me. I needed to actually look at and follow what the scientific research was recommending. So if you find it hard to back off, then I empathize with you. But what I want you to ask yourself is: How long have I been doing this, and is it working for me? Is my body working the way that it should? If not, then something needs to change.

How much exercise to do

The international evidence-based guidelines for PCOS recommend a minimum of 150 minutes a week of moderate-intensity physical activity, or 75 minutes a week of vigorous-intensity exercise, or an equivalent combination of both, including muscle-strengthening activities on two non-consecutive days a week.[22] What does this look like? It could be two or three 20-minute strength sessions a week, plus walking briskly for 15 minutes each way to and from your car every day. Or it may be more for you.

I don't want you to be scared of exercise—I just want you to check in with yourself to see whether you might be overdoing it. Ask yourself these questions:

1. How do I feel after exercise? Am I exhausted, or do I feel more energized?
   It's normal to feel tired after a tough workout, but you should recover within about 10 to 15 minutes. If you're still tired after an hour, you might be pushing a bit much.

2. How quickly can I get to sleep at night?
   If the answer is it takes more than 20 minutes, then your stress
   hormones might be struggling a little and exercise could be playing
   a role there.

3. Do I sleep through the night? How do I feel when I wake up in the
   morning?
   If you don't sleep through the night, and you wake up feeling like
   you've been hit by a bus, your stress hormones could be causing this.

The best types of exercise for PCOS

When it comes to exercise, the most important thing is that you enjoy
it. Here I'll talk about a couple of things that are particularly good for
PCOS.

Strength training and HIIT

When it comes to improving insulin resistance, the best type of exercise
is strength training. Strength training helps to improve your muscles'
sensitivity to insulin.

If you don't have high DHEA-S or any symptoms of high stress (i.e.
you don't have adrenal PCOS), one to two HIIT sessions per week might
also be great for you. HIIT means lifting heavy things and sprinting,
but for short periods, with rests in between and for a maximum of 20
minutes. Studies have shown that short HIIT not only improves insulin
sensitivity during the exercise, but also up to one to three days afterward.[23]

But what about cardio exercise?

Endurance exercise has often been promoted as the king of
cardiovascular health (building the heart, lungs, and vascular
system to protect us from heart attacks, strokes, etc.). However,
studies have proved HIIT to be just as effective in improving
cardiovascular health, and, better yet, to be more effective in
improving almost every other health marker. One study that
compared sprinting on a bike for a maximum of 20 minutes
(HIIT) vs. steady-state cycling for 40 minutes (cardio) found that

while both exercises increased cardiovascular fitness, only those in the HIIT group:

- significantly decreased weight
- significantly decreased fat mass
- lost a significant amount of fat around their stomach and legs
- significantly improved their insulin sensitivity
- significantly improved their sensitivity to leptin (satiety hormone).[24]

And, by the way, this had nothing to do with calories burned during exercise, as both groups ate the same number of calories. I'm not saying that endurance exercise is bad, just that other forms of exercise can be better.

Walking and standing as much as possible

Alongside strength training and/or HIIT, you should be trying to do as much low-intensity physical activity as possible. Studies have shown that low-intensity activity such as walking or slow cycling actually decreases cortisol levels and helps to further reduce inflammation and insulin resistance.[17] Low-intensity activities have also been shown to reduce ACTH.[17] ACTH stimulates your body to produce more androgens ("male" hormones). These hormones are responsible for some symptoms of PCOS, such as acne and unwanted hair growth or loss, so less of them is much better for you.

A good way to build low-intensity exercise into your day is actively commuting to work, going for a walk at lunchtime and during breaks, meeting friends for a walk instead of a coffee, and taking up an active hobby like hiking or surfing.

In the corporate world, we sit a lot. Unfortunately, standing meetings have never really taken off; you just end up being the weirdo, always trying to push the idea of these meetings or lurking in the back corner of the room while everyone else is sitting. But you are in control of what you do at your desk, so if you haven't got a standing desk, get one of the inexpensive devices that convert a sitting desk into a standing one.

FEELING OVERWHELMED

Last but not least, when it comes to stress, we need to manage feeling overwhelmed. This can manifest in many different ways. It can come from putting far more on your to-do list than you could ever hope to achieve, or setting such high expectations that you could never meet them. It can arise from working full-time or more, or trying to be a good friend, granddaughter, daughter, sister, or partner but feeling like you are failing at all of these. You might end up having something on every night of the week, and have every weekend either away or full of commitments. You then collapse in a crumpled heap on the couch on Sunday evening, only to have to gear up to do it all over again in a few short hours.

Feeling overwhelmed might also come from worrying about things that you have very little control over—politics, climate change, what other people think of you, what might happen in 20 years if you make a wrong decision, and of course your health and fertility.

And, of course, there's the "mental load" I mentioned in Chapter 2 (see page 35) that women in particular take on. The mental load is the total sum of the responsibilities you take on to manage "the remembering of things."

- Remembering to buy toilet paper or take the bins out.
- Remembering to make a cake for your mother-in-law's birthday.
- Remembering to book that hotel for your holiday or to book travel insurance.
- Remembering to pay the water bill.

All of these contribute to feeling overwhelmed. It is something we have probably all felt at one point in time. You'll know what it feels like for you; for me, my chest feels tight, my mind is buzzing with running through all the things I need to do. I jump from task to task, trying to get more done but actually achieving less as the feeling of tightness builds up in me. This feeling comes from the adrenaline and cortisol rising in the body, and, of course, alongside cortisol comes DHEA-S, and insulin gets affected. So to improve fertility, we need to get a handle on feeling overwhelmed and get those cortisol levels down.

Here are a few key things that you can do to reduce the feeling of being overwhelmed in as little as a few days.

De-commit

Write a list of all your commitments, then go through the list to decide what is essential and what is not. Be ruthless—decide what is *absolutely essential* vs. what is optional. I'll give you a heads-up here—probably work, sleep, eating, exercising, and spending time with your partner and caring for family members are the absolutely essential ones. Everything else is optional.

Now, looking at the optional commitments, circle the two that give you a tight feeling in your chest if you just think about them. Those are the two you need to extract yourself from first. Maybe it's your work's social club, or maybe it's being the person in your household who is responsible for the bills. Whatever it is for you, I want you to sit down and think about how you can extract yourself.

This may feel challenging to begin with because you'll feel like you're letting people down; your mind will probably start racing into the territory of "what will they think of me." But once you do this, you'll realize that it is actually possible to hand over the baton to someone else, or put those bills onto auto payment, and free up some time for yourself.

Next, you need to find ways to set clear boundaries with your time so that you don't fill up every possible space. If you find it hard to say no to new commitments, there are ways to say no without having to say "No." Here are some ideas:

- "That won't work for me."
- "Maybe another time."
- "I'll have to pass."
- "I can't, but thanks for the offer."
- "Sorry, I can't this time."
- "My calendar is full."
- "I wish I could, but I won't be able to make this one."
- "I'm afraid I can't."

Reduce your mental load

There isn't a "right" way to reduce your mental load and share the burden of household tasks more evenly. But after doing much research, I like Julia Pelly's approach: specialize, don't delegate. Delegating means that you still have to remember to ask someone else to do it, which means that you bear the brunt of the mental load of "remembering everything."[25]

Pelly advocates for specializing rather than delegating or sharing the same tasks. You each have tasks that you take full responsibility for. For example, Pelly says that her husband takes full responsibility for unloading the dishwasher, vacuuming, and taking out the trash. She doesn't do those tasks, and nor does she take on any of the associated mental work: remembering to buy trash bags and detergent, emptying the vacuum filter, etc. Similarly, her husband doesn't clean the bathrooms, wash the windows, or pay a single bill. She says: "By specializing, instead of both trying to half do everything, we've found balance in the ways we distribute the work of our family."[25]

Initially it can be very hard to let go of some of the control, even to your partner, but then you remember "Oh yeah, that's right, they are perfectly capable adults who manage to hold down responsibilities in their day jobs, so they can manage to remember to get dishwashing powder."

Start with noting everything down. It's easy to remember what you do in a day, but not what you and your partner do over a week or month. Take an hour to sit down and write out a list of what your house needs on a daily, weekly, and monthly basis, and then divide up the tasks based on your skills and preferences.

Worry less about what you have little control over

This last one is slightly trickier because worry of this sort can border on anxiety. But as a general rule, if you're feeling anxious, some mindfulness, meditation, or simply deep breathing can be incredibly effective (see the Resources section for the meditation apps I recommend). Several studies have found meditation to be effective at reducing symptoms of anxiety and depression, even when compared with a control group who were practicing relaxation techniques.[26] Additionally, meditating will probably make you much more productive. One study showed that meditating for just 10 minutes per day can improve focus and help the brain become more efficient at processing conflicting stimuli.[27]

Another action to take, which I found incredibly helpful for myself, was to stop following the news and anyone who wasn't a close friend or family member on social media. It's well known that people only portray the glossy parts of life on social media, which can leave us feeling inadequate and rather overwhelmed with all the things that we feel we need to do to be adequate: we must have a thigh gap but also love our bodies for what they are; we must have the latest fashion but it must be made from recycled ocean plastic that's been hand-stitched by people as a Trade Aid project; we must have #couplegoals but also be super down-to-earth; and we also need to be ticking off the big life goals like buying a house, getting engaged, having the perfect Instagrammable wedding, having a baby (that one is a real knife in the guts). In my experience, if "influencers" are not in your face every day on social media, they are not going to be contributing to you feeling overwhelmed.

Similarly, our news media has become full of clickbait headlines and catastrophes. I found that reducing my news consumption significantly improved my feelings of being overwhelmed, because I had no control over most of what was concerning me. Yes, there seem to be wildfires burning out of control everywhere; yes, the world's leaders can't agree on how to tackle climate change; and yes, there's been another mass shooting. Can I, at this very minute, do anything about it? No.

You don't have to hide under a rock. Spend 30 minutes a week catching up on the major news from a neutral news source, and the rest of the time you don't need to be overwhelmed.

Chapter 9
Step 4—Chart your cycles and time sex accordingly

Charting your cycles is an extremely important component of getting pregnant. You can get pregnant in the few days leading up to ovulation. It doesn't matter whether your cycle is 25, 36, or 48 days long: you can conceive if you can just identify your "fertile window."

Many of the women I worked with earlier in my career got their periods back, but still couldn't conceive, despite their blood tests showing that everything was normal. I was stumped.

Then I heard an interview with Dr. Kerry Hampton, a researcher at Monash University in Melbourne, Australia. Kerry studies women's understanding of their menstrual cycles and whether they can accurately identify the fertile window within which they can conceive. In one of her studies, Kerry found that over 80 percent of women going through IVF were not able to accurately identify their fertile window.[1] That means that over 80 percent of people going through IVF potentially didn't need to do so; they might just need to know how to time sex correctly. This study is not the only one to report this; the findings have been replicated in large studies in both India and New Zealand.[2,3]

The interview was an eye-opener. I knew this could well be the reason why most of the women I was working with weren't getting pregnant. It inspired me to become qualified to teach natural fertility education so that I could teach women how to identify their fertile window.

CASE STUDY

Amy hadn't had a period for about two years, and she and her husband had been trying to conceive without success. We discovered that her insulin wasn't working properly, and she was also chronically stressed from over-exercising to try to manage her weight, and from working a busy corporate job. Amy focused on changing her breakfast to stabilize her blood sugar and reduce her sugar cravings, switching to more strength and calming exercises to reduce her stress hormones and improve her insulin, and taking vitamin and mineral supplements to improve her insulin sensitivity.

Amy's body responded at lightning speed, and she got her period back in the first month. She was extremely excited (naturally) and was gearing up to get pregnant within a month or so. But two months went by and nothing . . . We jumped on one of my live Q&A sessions and did some problem analysis.

Me: "Have you been figuring out when you're actually fertile by taking your temperature and noting your cervical fluid?"

Amy: "I don't know how to do that, but I've been using the ovulation test kit."

Me: "Aha! That's where this is going wrong then."

I suggested to Amy that she start taking her temperature every morning and taking note of her cervical fluid characteristics (i.e. charting her cycle). After doing this for just one month, she could see when she was fertile, and the next month she and her partner got the timing right. Boom! Pregnant!

Detecting those few fertile days isn't hard once you know how to do it, but it just isn't taught, despite the research proving that this is a huge contributing factor to the "infertility crisis" we're going through.

It is likely that no one from your medical team has actually sat down with you to check the first, very basic fertile ingredient: whether one of your eggs is meeting the sperm, i.e. whether you're timing sex correctly. The medical advice is usually to take a scattergun approach and have sex every second or third day, which is not only impractical but also has no scientific backing.[4] In terms of fertility, there is no benefit to you of having sex after you've ovulated. If you're using this approach, you don't know when you're ovulating, so you're likely stressing every night of the month because you think it could be the make or break of whether you get pregnant or not.

In addition, the scattergun approach won't pick up a luteal phase deficiency or when your luteal phase (the days after ovulation) is too short to allow implantation (more on that below). Nor will ovulation predictor kits or apps. The scattergun approach is also not practical for most couples, who have already been trying for many months or even years. It can put a huge strain on an already (fertility-related) emotionally strained relationship. The scattergun approach also doesn't work where one or both of you frequently travel for work.

CASE STUDY

Ciara's partner is in the military and often lives two and a half hours away while on base. As Ciara explained to me, they could travel to meet each other for a conjugal visit, but doing a five-hour commute every second day of her cycle was ridiculous. Especially when she and her partner had already been trying for a baby for six years!

Through my *Eggducated* program, Ciara learned to use her basal body temperature and cervical fluid characteristics to identify exactly when she was fertile to time sex correctly to get pregnant. She told me that doing the program gave her such peace of mind through knowing when it was important to travel and when it wasn't. It was worth every penny she spent doing the course and all the time she spent learning to chart her cycles.

See the Resources section for a link to my interview with Ciara.

Identifying your fertile window gives you a much better chance of becoming pregnant. In a 2017 study, women who were on the waiting list for fertility treatment were offered training on how to identify their fertile window (using the same method that I will be teaching you in this chapter). Training was given to 187 women who had been trying to conceive for one to two years, and the women were then followed for eight months. Within that eight months, 56 percent of the women conceived naturally. This is quite an incredible result. It shows that more than half the women who were about to embark on invasive and expensive treatment with risks for both their health and that of their baby did not need it. All that these women needed was information on how to chart their cycles and time sex correctly.[5]

THE IMPORTANCE OF FERTILITY AWARENESS

The fertility awareness method (FAM) is a technique that helps you determine which days of your cycle are fertile or infertile. There is no single universal fertility-awareness-based method, but the one I teach is the symptom-thermal method, which involves tracking your two main fertile signs: cervical fluid (symptom) and basal body temperature (BBT; thermal). Cervical fluid (CF), otherwise known as cervical mucus, is released by your cervix when you're leading up to ovulation to help transport the sperm up to your fallopian tubes. It's pretty amazing what our cervical fluid can do. If you look at it under a microscope, you can actually see how it changes during your cycle. When your body is nowhere near ovulation, the cervix releases sticky fluid (you might notice that in your underwear) which has a crystalline structure to make it impenetrable to sperm; it's saying: "No entry, we're not ready for you yet." In the lead-up to ovulation, this changes to a wet/slippery fluid with channels that act as a vortex to suck sperm up into your cervix. In fact, without the structure of this cervical fluid, the sperm wouldn't reach your fallopian tubes just by swimming, as they only live for a fairly short time. So this characteristic of CF is a *really* accurate indicator that you're fertile.[6]

Your BBT is your temperature first thing in the morning, and it's a very accurate indicator that you've ovulated. The surge in LH that stimulates ovulation also results in a rise in BBT by 0.5 to 1°F (0.2 to 0.6°C).[7] This higher body temperature is maintained during the luteal phase due to the rise in progesterone during this phase.[8]

The beauty of using FAM if you have PCOS is that you don't have to be getting a regular period. You can still use it even if your cycle is 35, 40, or even 50 days. In fact, you don't even have to have a period.

CASE STUDY

Rebecca hadn't had a period for years before she got pregnant. She was diagnosed with PCOS at 19 and didn't think too much of it. She stopped HBC when she was 30, expecting to get pregnant immediately. Instead, all of her PCOS symptoms came back, and they got progressively worse over six months. Night sweats, missing periods, acne, facial hair, polycystic ovaries, and fatigue.

Her primary care and obstetric/gynecologic physicians were in disagreement regarding her PCOS diagnosis, and neither offered any help other than clomifene for infertility. Feeling frustrated, Rebecca started doing her own research and found my *PCOS Protocol* program. Through this she learned that her insulin wasn't functioning properly, and she was an absolute star in implementing all the steps to improve it. Her energy returned like a bolt of lightning, and her night sweats disappeared after just two weeks. After six weeks, her acne had disappeared, and she lost 15 lb (6.8 kg). Rebecca jumped on one of the Q&A calls with me, and we got into problem-solving mode.

Again, I realized that one of the missing pieces was fertility awareness. Rebecca didn't see much point in doing FAM as she wasn't actually getting a cycle. I explained that she had to ovulate to get a period (as a period is usually a result of ovulation if you haven't become pregnant). So Rebecca started learning about BBT and cervical mucus, and just a few months later, she got a positive pregnancy test. The first time ovulating in years and she got pregnant. *That* is the beauty of fertility awareness.

Understanding the fertile window

The fertile window is the period of time around ovulation when you can actually conceive. Contrary to popular belief, you don't conceive after you ovulate (i.e. after the temperature rise). You need to have sperm in your fallopian tubes waiting for you to release the egg—not the other way around. If you want to get pregnant, you can't wait until you ovulate and then have sex.

This means that you need to know when you're leading up to ovulation so that you can time sex accordingly, and this is what your CF indicates. The length of the fertile window differs between couples. It's dependent on how many days you release slippery CF, and on how long your partner's sperm can survive. Many women start releasing slippery CF five days before ovulation. Sperm can live, on average, three to five days (some "marathon" sperm can last up to eight days), so if you have sex five days before ovulation and your partner's sperm lasts only three days, then you won't conceive. For some women their fertile window is much shorter, at only one to two days before they ovulate.

A large study that analyzed 7017 cycles from 881 women found that sex in the earlier part of the fertile window, and especially the two days before ovulation, gave the best chance of conception.[7] These findings have been supported by two studies that show that conception is very unlikely if intercourse doesn't happen in the five days before ovulation.[9, 10]

You may get advice from your doctor or online to have sex between Days 10 and 17 of your cycle. However, one study that followed 221 women for three to four months found that only 30 percent of women have their fertile window between these days.[11] The guidelines of

Days 10 to 17 being your "primetime" are based on the assumption that you ovulate 14 days before you get your period. But this study showed that this wasn't the case at all. Only 10 percent of the women who had a 28-day cycle got their period 14 days after ovulation, and the range was actually 7 to 19 days! For those of us with PCOS and more-irregular cycles, this variability is even greater.[11]

Karen (who you met in Chapter 5, page 83) went through my *Eggducated* program, and her story is a really great example of why the advice you're getting from your doctor might not be accurate when it comes to timing sex correctly. The reason is simply that they haven't had proper training in this area, and for good reason: they have to know so much about so many different illnesses and medical complications that their advice can only be quite general in this specialist area. But you're in the right place now to get good advice.

Ovulation and periods

But I'm getting my period, so I'm ovulating, right? Not necessarily. You can be getting a period without ovulating. While it's not common to get a period *every* month without ovulating, it *is* common for at least some of your cycles to be anovulatory.

During the first half of your cycle your estrogen levels steadily increase, causing your body to build up your uterine lining (called the endometrium) so that a fertilized egg can implant in it. In a normal ovulatory cycle, after an egg is released from the ovary, the remains of the follicle that was housing the egg stay behind; this is called the corpus luteum. For the rest of your cycle, until you get your period, the corpus luteum produces progesterone, and estrogen levels drop; this period in between ovulation and the end of your cycle is known as the luteal phase. The reduced estrogen levels slow the development of the endometrium, but progesterone provides it with structural support until conception or the next cycle. If conception doesn't occur, the corpus luteum stops producing progesterone about 12 to 16 days after ovulation. This signals to your body that conception did not occur, and the endometrium is shed—meaning you get your period (this is also known as progesterone withdrawal bleeding).

If no egg is released from the ovary, there is no corpus luteum, meaning your body won't produce progesterone. Without progesterone, estrogen is unable to support the growing endometrium on its own. Eventually the uterine lining is shed, and you get what seems to be your period. But because ovulation did not occur, this type of anovulatory bleeding is not a true period; it is known instead as "estrogen breakthrough bleeding."

Professor Jerrilyn Prior, an endocrinologist and an advocate for why women actually need to ovulate for health, not just for fertility, has looked at the cycles of 3,163 women and found that in approximately one out of every three cycles, we don't ovulate, even when these look like perfectly normal cycles.[12] This makes complete sense from an evolutionary point of view. I grew up on a farm, and we always had chickens to give us a supply of eggs. It was quite normal, especially over the winter, for those chickens to "go off the lay"—to not produce any eggs—for a couple of months. So why would we expect our body to produce an egg every month, for up to 40 or 50 years?

When you don't ovulate, it's common to have a slightly off-looking period. Rather than at least two days of bright red flow, it's likely short, light, spotty, or reddish/brown. However, Professor Prior's research has shown that it's just as common to have a completely normal-looking period but no ovulation.[12]

The beauty of learning fertility awareness and how to track your cycle is that you'll know exactly whether you've ovulated or not.

Other techniques and their pitfalls
Can't I just use one of those apps?

Apps can be a great way of recording and keeping track of your BBT and cervical fluid, but they can't accurately tell you when your fertile window is by themselves, especially if you're only recording the days of your period!

There are many different apps on the market, so I'll break this down into two categories because not all apps are made equal. There are the apps that count days, and those that record temperature.

First, let's look at the apps that just count days. These record your period and try to predict your fertile window. This is called the rhythm method. Let's think about this for a second: You already know that ovulation can be delayed by many things, such as stress, your diet over the past three months, whether that egg has grown properly, and just having PCOS and what can often be very irregular cycles. So how can a computer algorithm possibly be able to interpret all this information and adjust accordingly? Of course it can't, and that's why the rhythm method is not very helpful for getting pregnant. (It is also only about 60 percent effective for those using it as contraception, i.e. an excellent path to an unplanned pregnancy.)

The second group of apps get you to record your temperature and then interpret when you ovulated. Temperature is a really helpful tool when it comes to fertility, but it's only useful for confirming that you have ovulated. After you have ovulated, your body produces progesterone, which increases your metabolic rate and causes a rise in temperature. While this is great for confirming that you did indeed ovulate, it doesn't help you time sex correctly. It takes a couple of days for your temperature to rise after you've ovulated, so by the time you've seen the temperature increase, it's too late.

Even the smartest algorithm in the world can't predict the fertile window from month to month. A recent study, in 2018, compared many of the apps currently on the market, including six calendar-based apps (Clue, Flo, Maya, Menstruationskalender Pro, Period Tracker Deluxe, and WomanLog) and also temperature apps (Ovy and Natural Cycles), and found that due to variations in the menstrual cycle from month to month there is no way that the fertile window can be predicted; instead, you need to be tracking your own signs from month to month.[13] The researchers concluded that apps based just on data from previous cycles are not able to indicate the most fertile days.

You need to know when you are leading up to ovulation (your fertile window), and you can only know that by checking your cervical fluid.

Can't I just use an ovulation predictor stick/test kit?

I often see women in PCOS online groups and forums showing positive results from their ovulation test kits, and I want to scream "It's not accurate! Don't plan your life around that stick!"

Ovulation predictor kits work by measuring the LH levels in your urine. In Chapter 1, I explained that LH's job is to shoot up and release the egg into the fallopian tube so that it's ready to meet any awaiting sperm (see page 28). But in PCOS our LH levels are actually too high,[14] and this increased LH can not only disrupt the delicate ratio between LH and FSH but can also lead to false-positive results on these ovulation test kits. The result is that you could see the positive result and think "Whoop! Time to get to bed." You proceed to have sex for a couple of days and then not worry about it because you think you've already nailed it; when in actual fact, it is likely to have been a false-positive and you actually ovulate two weeks later.

Clearblue is the market leader in LH ovulation predictor kits, and their own literature is clear on this: "Certain medical conditions and medications can adversely affect the performance of the Clearblue Fertility Monitor. If you have menopausal symptoms, **polycystic ovarian syndrome** [my emphasis], impaired liver or kidney function, or if you are pregnant or have recently been pregnant (even if not carried to full term), you may get misleading results."[15]

The second reason why ovulation test kits are not useful in PCOS is that they don't tell you anything about the length of your luteal phase—the third fertile ingredient: the nest staying intact long enough to keep the fertilized egg safe. Your luteal phase has to last at least 11 days, or the egg won't have enough time to burrow into your uterine lining and signal to your body that you're pregnant. If you're just tracking ovulation on a test kit, you won't get any of this information.

HOW TO CHART YOUR CYCLES

Charting is the single most important thing you can start doing today to help you conceive, so I've created a step-by-step guide on how to do this. These instructions are taken from my *Eggducated* course, so for more interactive elements you might like to join that course.

Step 1: Chart your basal body temperature (BBT)

The first step is to start recording your temperature, as body temperature confirms that you have ovulated. The LH surge that stimulates ovulation causes your BBT to rise a little, and this higher body temperature is maintained during the luteal phase by the progesterone being released by your corpus luteum.[6] As progesterone rises, your metabolic rate also increases and this increases your temperature. It's a bit like a hen sitting on eggs that have been fertilized. Your body is doing the same—it's increasing the temperature to incubate your eggs. But just like a hen doesn't sit on the eggs before she lays them, your temperature doesn't increase until you've released an egg (ovulated). Interestingly, this is also why you get really hungry and often crave a bit of chocolate before you get your period. Your metabolic rate has increased (in some cases burning up to 300 kcal more a day), so your body is craving a bit more food to make up for that.

Here is how to measure your BBT.

1. Get an oral digital thermometer. You'll likely find one at your local drugstore. There are loads of different options on the market, with all kinds of extra features, like syncing to your phone app and a backlight so that you can read it in the dark. But my advice is to just buy a basic one, and upgrade later if you want to.

2. Measure your temperature orally (in the mouth, under the tongue), *as soon as you wake up*. As my lecturer in natural fertility told me, "It doesn't need to be anywhere more exotic; just the mouth." The important part is that it needs to be as soon as you wake up. This means no getting out of bed to make a cup of tea or go to the toilet, no fooling around in bed, and no getting up to retrieve your thermometer from where you left it on the windowsill yesterday. To be accurate, your temperature needs to measured before *any* activity. And it needs to be done at the same time (within the hour) every morning.

3. Leave your thermometer in place for 10 minutes before pushing

the button. If you put the thermometer in your mouth and push the button, it will beep after about 12 seconds. However, this often isn't long enough to get an accurate reading; you might find that you get a reading of 79.5°F (36.4°C), and then put it back into your mouth only to find it's gone to 79.9°F (36.6°C). Keeping it in for 10 minutes helps your thermometer to warm up and gives a more accurate reading once you do press the button.

3. Record your BBT! This can be in an app or on a PDF printout (I've created you one that you can download from my website; see the Resources section)—just make sure you note it down immediately before you forget. Sometimes paper can be easier to start with because you can see the temperature rise more easily when you're drawing your graph. Apps are also very convenient, though, so use what suits you.

4. Start now! Don't wait for your next period to start, just start measuring your temperature tomorrow morning. The more data you have, the more quickly you can start to recognize your temperature rise pattern.

Also, note the following guidelines:

- You need to have slept for about four to six hours before taking your temperature—it doesn't matter whether you're on night shift or you're jetlagged. If you haven't, that's okay—take your BBT anyway, but note down that you've had limited sleep so you can discard this temperature later if it falls outside your usual pattern.

- Take your temperature at approximately the same time every morning, within an hour of when you usually wake up. If most days you get up at (say) 6 a.m., but don't wake up until 7 a.m. on the weekend, that's fine. But if you sleep in on a Saturday until 9 a.m., your temperature will probably be higher. Again, make sure that you note down in your app or on your printout that this temperature could be inaccurate and might need to be disregarded.

- Get your partner involved—they can help monitor your

temperature, whereas they can't monitor the sensation of your cervical fluid. Sometimes it can feel like you're the one doing all the work when it comes to finding the fertile window and timing sex correctly, so if you share the responsibility then it doesn't become another burden to you and your partner doesn't feel isolated.

Step 2: Chart your cervical fluid

The next step is to record your CF. You're probably wondering what I'm talking about; although you've probably noticed your CF change before, you just didn't know its significance. It is a feeling of wetness in your underwear that might make you think you've wet your pants. Or when you've gone to the bathroom, you've wiped and it's been so slippery you've almost hit the bathroom wall. That is cervical fluid, not discharge, and it's your body getting ready for you to ovulate.

If you've been on HBC you might not have felt this for a while because HBC stops ovulation. If this is you, then think back to when you were younger (before going on HBC). We produce a lot more CF when we're in our teens and twenties, so you might remember the feeling from then.

When you're not ovulating, your CF is thick and impenetrable and stops sperm getting up into your cervix when you're not fertile, and this will result in you feeling quite dry. During this time, you cannot conceive. As your body prepares to ovulate, your CF changes, and you will be able to feel it. What it feels like is a wet/moist or slippery sensation in your vulva (vaginal "lips") or when you wipe with toilet paper.

The reason why this change in the CF is so important is that it now acts like a jet-pack for sperm, to move them up into your cervix so that one can get in there and fertilize your egg. Slippery cervical fluid is incredible! When you look at it under a microscope, you can see that there are channels in it, and these are what suck the sperm up. Without it, the sperm literally wouldn't survive long enough to reach your fallopian tube.

Another important function of CF is that it actually filters out the suboptimal sperm we don't want. If the sperm isn't quite right—maybe the head's a bit pointy, it's got a stumpy tail, or maybe a growth out the side—our CF will filter it out so that the good guys get through and fertilize the egg.

Cervical fluid can be hard to assess, so I have two techniques for you.

The "sensation" method

1. Stand up and walk around, so that your vulva (vaginal lips) slide across each other.

2. Now bring your attention to your vulva. Does it feel completely dry there? Or does it feel moist or wet? Is your vulva maybe sticking or catching as you walk (dry), or is it gliding across itself (moist or wet)?

On your app or printout, note down the characteristics of your CF—see Figure 12.

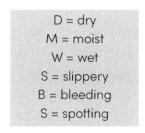

D = dry
M = moist
W = wet
S = slippery
B = bleeding
S = spotting

Figure 12: How to record your cervical fluid

You'll probably second-guess yourself here, so don't think about it too much; just record in your app or on your printout what you think, and repeat the exercise tomorrow. You might think that you don't feel anything, and this is probably because you're in your dry period. So record it as dry, and move on. Of course, if you have your period you won't be able to tell the difference between cervical fluid and blood, so just write down B for bleeding or S for spotting.

Set yourself an alarm on your phone to remind yourself to do this every day. I recommend doing it multiple times a day, especially sometime in the morning, e.g. when you're walking around in your underwear getting ready for work, or on your way to work.

Don't worry if you think you won't be able to feel your cervical fluid;

most people feel this way, but when they start bringing their attention to it, they actually do. So just give it a go.

The toilet paper method

If you're not getting the whole "sensation" thing, then try focusing on what it feels like when you wipe with toilet paper.

1. Every time you go to the bathroom, check your CF. Before you pee or poo, get some toilet paper, fold it flat and wipe your vulva from front to back. Pay close attention to how it feels at the perineum (the smooth piece of skin between your vulva and anus).

2. What do you notice? Does it glide, does it feel wet, or does it tug?

3. Look at the toilet paper—can you see mucus that you can actually pick up and stretch between your fingers? This is slippery CF, which means you're leading up to ovulation.

Record it on your app or printout—see Figure 12. Note that this method only works if you're recording it so that you can look at your pattern. Do this again every time you go to the bathroom.

When you feel or notice the wet/ slippery cervical fluid, you're fertile!

Don't worry about waiting until you have a full cycle charted, if you feel or notice the wet or slippery cervical mucus, you're fertile. So if you want to get pregnant, you need to be having sex now!

Can't I just use temperature to tell me when I'm going to ovulate? Do I have to use the cervical fluid as well?

Oral temperature can only confirm that ovulation has occurred. We cannot use it to indicate when ovulation is going to happen.

As I mentioned earlier, your body releases the egg and then increases the temperature to incubate it. So it can only tell you when you've already ovulated, not when you're leading up to ovulation. You might read online that you get a dip in temperature right before ovulation that can signal the fertile window. However, oral temperature measurements aren't sensitive enough to pick this up, and in all my years of measuring my temperature I've never seen this in my own charts.

Step 3: Interpret your temperature chart

Once you have a full cycle charted, including your period, look back about 11 to 16 days before your period and see whether there is any change in temperature. It's important to wait and chart all the way through to your period for this first chart, because your temperature can fluctuate during your cycle, especially if your body is trying to ovulate more than once during the cycle, which is very common in PCOS.

1. Start by looking for three temperatures that are at least 0.3°F (0.1°C) but more likely 0.5 to 1°F (0.2 to 0.6°C) higher than the six temperatures that immediately precede it. A simple way to remember this is *three over six*. Three temperatures higher than six lower ones. If you have this pattern, then those three temperatures are your ovulation temperature spike. Congratulations—you ovulated!

   In Figure 13 below, which is one of my personal charts, I've marked the three higher and the six lower temperatures. Mine are

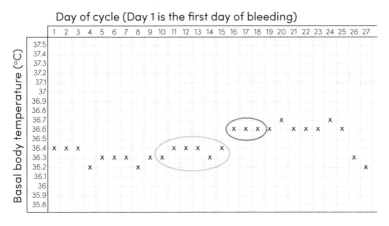

Figure 13: The "three over six" rule—three higher temperatures following six lower ones = ovulation

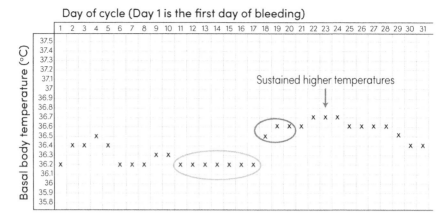

Figure 14: Sustained temperature rise between ovulation and start of period

done using °C, but the process is exactly the same for °F.

2. Now check: Is that higher temperature sustained for most of the remainder of your cycle, almost until you get your period? It's normal for your temperature to drop before you get your period because your progesterone also drops, which reduces your BBT. But until then, it should generally stay high. Figure 14 is for a slightly longer cycle, but you can clearly see the sustained temperature rise until two days before the period starts. Note that in all of these charts, Day 1 is the first day of bleeding so that you are making sure you chart a complete cycle.

You will see the same pattern—a rise in temperature that is sustained until your period starts—even if your cycle is 40, 50, or even 90 days long. The chart for a 47-day cycle is shown in Figure 15.

What about missing temperatures? It's okay to have a missed temperature (one you forgot to take), as long as there's only one missing from the six lows. If you miss one day, then you can put an approximate temperature in there with confidence, but if there are a lot of gaps then it's hard to see when there was a temperature rise. So try not to miss taking too many temperatures!

Step 4: Now bring it all together with cervical fluid

How do you bring this all together? You look at both CF and BBT, and

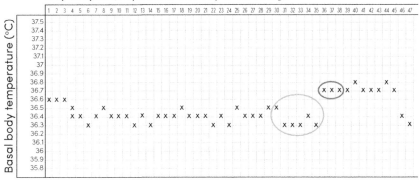

Day of cycle (Day 1 is the first day of bleeding)

Figure 15: BBT pattern in a longer cycle

can see when you've ovulated and what it felt like before you ovulated (your fertile window).

Once you have a full cycle of CF and BBT charted, all the way through to your period, look back about 11 to 16 days and see whether you noticed any change in your CF around that time. Were there any days around then that you marked moist or wet? How does this compare to the timing of your temperature rise? Was there any wet or slippery CF just before or around the time your temperature rose? If there was, BOOM! That was the fertile CF that was going to help propel sperm up through your cervix to meet your egg.

In Figure 16, you can see that my wet/slippery CF (the fertile stuff) on Days 13 to 15 immediately preceded my temperature rise on Day 16. Days 13 to 15 (see the gray shading) were therefore my fertile window, the days when I could have potentially conceived.

Think back to those days when you had the fertile CF . . . What did it look like? What did it feel like? Was it wet? Was it just moister? Was it slippery? Did you notice the toilet paper slipping? Now you know what it feels like to have that cervical fluid before you ovulate. Going forward over the next month, that's the feeling you need to look out for. Whenever you notice that cervical fluid, head to the bedroom because that's when you're fertile and want to be having sex.

If you didn't, that's okay, just try the cycle again. If you saw the temperature rise, you will know that you ovulated.

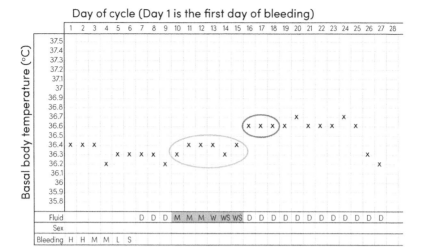

Figure 16: Bringing CF and BBT together to show the fertile window

Note that you can have more than one bout of fertile CF per cycle, meaning that your body has tried to ovulate more than once (see Figure 17). This is really common in PCOS, but you won't know at the time whether you're going to ovulate or it will be a missed attempt. All you need to remember is: If the fertile cervical fluid is there, it's time to have sex.

Additional guidance

1. When looking at your charts, you might notice that you had some fertile CF present but there was no change in temperature. Or maybe you had repeated patches of wet/slippery cervical fluid over a couple of weeks before the temperature rise. This is your body trying to ovulate, and it's very normal in PCOS. This is why we use both the CF characteristics and your BBT, as cervical fluid alone can be misleading in PCOS.

2. You won't know whether the fertile CF will be followed by ovulation until after the ovulation has occurred and the temperature rise has occurred. You just have to presume that every time you notice that wet cervical fluid, that that is fertile time.

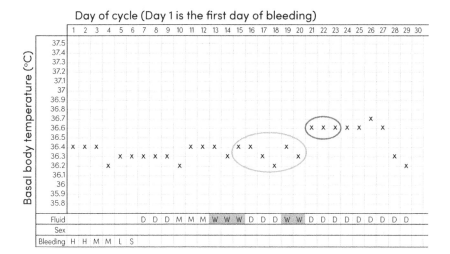

Figure 17: Cycle showing two bouts of fertile cervical fluid in one cycle

Note that on Figures 16–19 I've included days of bleeding (your period). H = heavy bleeding; M = medium bleeding; L = light bleeding; S = spotting.

Step 5: Keep going!

If you're looking at your chart and thinking "Hold on, we got everything right! I felt the cervical fluid, we had sex, I can then see that my temperature rose so I know I ovulated. So why aren't we pregnant?", don't worry—this is completely normal. Even if you time everything perfectly, you've still only got a 10 to 30 percent chance of getting pregnant. Put another way, you need up to 10 perfectly timed cycles to have a 100 percent chance of conceiving.[9] So please don't get discouraged, and do keep going.

There may be many reasons why you don't conceive even though everything seemed to go perfectly: Maybe the egg didn't move down the fallopian tube far enough, or maybe your body determined that this particular egg wasn't great quality or the sperm weren't quite right. These are all great survival mechanisms to make sure we're not conceiving when there is an underlying issue. You need to think about getting pregnant as a six- to 12-month process, and that every cycle is one step closer to increasing your probability. Of course you'll hear stories about women who've conceived on their first try, but there are just as many stories about women who've taken three, six, 12 or more cycles to conceive.

Step 6: Check your luteal phase

Another really important part of charting your cycle is to make sure that your "nest" (uterine lining) is staying intact long enough for your egg to be able to burrow into it. If it isn't, you could be doing everything else right—ovulating, and timing sex correctly—and yet still not conceive because your egg doesn't have enough time to get down the fallopian tubes to your uterus before your uterine lining breaks down.

This is your luteal phase: the number of days between your first temperature rise and the day before your period starts. **Your luteal phase must be longer than 11 days for you to be able to conceive.** Anything shorter than 11 days is called a luteal phase deficiency.

You can have a 28- to 33-day cycle that seems completely normal, but when you look more closely you see that the first half of the cycle is 23 days long and the second half only 10 days. This is really common in PCOS, and can be one of the main reasons why you're not getting pregnant. Your body has attempted to ovulate many times. If this is the case, you often get a short luteal phase afterward. But it's also very common in the normal female population. A study done by Professor Jerrilyn Prior followed the cycles of 66 women for a year, and found that over 25 percent of the cycles had a short luteal phase.[16]

How to check your luteal phase

On your chart, find the first day of your temperature rise. Count that day, plus the number of days between that day and the last day before your period started. For example, say your last day of fertile cervical fluid was on Day 19, and you saw your temperature rise on Day 20, and then you got your period on Day 28. Counting from Day 20 (inclusive) to Day 27 is only eight days, so your luteal phase is much too short to conceive.

Figure 18 shows an example of this, where the luteal phase is only nine days. The first day of the temperature rise is Day 21, and counting this and through to Day 29—the end of the cycle—gives the nine days.

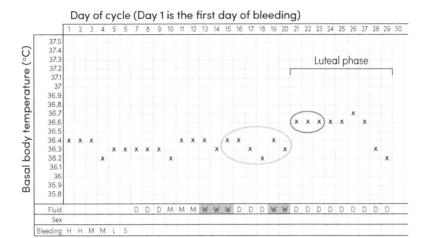

Figure 18: Short luteal phase

How to make your luteal phase longer

A short luteal phase is caused by too little progesterone, which is generally a manifestation of your root cause, i.e. your insulin,[17] adrenals (stress), etc.

If your insulin is high, your egg might be of a poor size or poor quality; or your LH might be too high and the egg can't be released. The result will be that your body attempts to ovulate two, three, four, or more times before it's successful. High insulin significantly reduces your progesterone.[17] Even if this doesn't cause multiple attempts at ovulation, it is still likely to be responsible for your short luteal phase.[18] Research has shown that your luteal phase can be increased by improving your insulin sensitivity.[17]

The same goes for stress. I've seen many charts for women who have been under significant stress during their cycle, which has resulted in delayed ovulation and a subsequent short luteal phase. These are all the things that we cover off in my *PCOS Protocol* program, so if you need more help, join us there.

CASE STUDY

When I first met Hannah, her cycles were months apart. We identified that her insulin was high, and she implemented lots of changes to bring that down. After a few months, her cycles

---

regulated to every 33 days like clockwork.

After deciding to try for a baby, Hannah joined my *Eggducated* program to learn how to chart her cycles. While these looked "normal," her body was actually trying to ovulate three times during the cycle—as shown by the wet/slippery (WS) cervical fluid (shaded in Figure 19). When she did actually ovulate (shown by the three shaded days following the six shaded days), we could see that her luteal phase (Days 25–33) was only nine days and therefore too short. She knew from the *PCOS Protocol* what to do, so doubled down on her lifestyle changes. Her short luteal phase continued in March, but by June she was pregnant.

If you've addressed your underlying root cause and your luteal phase is still too short, then you might need some further support. Some research has suggested that the cells of some women with PCOS might not be able to produce enough progesterone after ovulation. If you do have a short luteal phase, please visit your doctor or fertility specialist and ask to have your progesterone tested in the middle of your luteal phase. They might tell you that this is "Day 21," but because you're monitoring your cycles you will know what day it actually is. If your blood tests show that your progesterone is lower than the normal range on the lab report, you might want to look at using some micronized progesterone (bio-

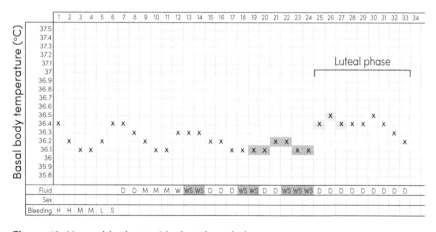

Figure 19: Hannah's chart with short luteal phase

identical progesterone) during the second half of your cycle to help. The brand name for this in the US is Prometrium, and in New Zealand it's Utrogestran. The synthetic progestin Provera won't work in the same way.

As your doctor might not have been trained in the use of micronized progesterone to support the luteal phase, Dr. Prior and the team at the Centre for Menstrual Cycle and Ovulation Research have developed some guidelines that you can print off and take to your doctor to help them understand how to use this (see the Resources section for the link).

Please read about reducing miscarriage risk in Chapter 12, as a short luteal phase may be a sign of too little progesterone.

Chapter 10
Step 5—Get your nutrients and herbs

One of the most common questions I am asked is: "What are the best supplements for PCOS?" My response is always the same frustrating answer: "It depends."

What supplements might help you is very dependent on a number of factors:

- What's driving your PCOS root cause?
- Do you have suboptimal levels of vitamins and minerals, or a full-blown deficiency?
- Are you trying to conceive?

You can end up wasting a lot of money on supplements that you don't need or that might be doing more harm than good.

The herb vitex is a great example of this. Vitex is often praised by women for helping to get their period back. This may be true for some women, but first you need to understand how vitex works. It has been shown to increase LH, which can be very helpful for some women who aren't ovulating because their LH is too low. But as you've already learnt,

LH is too high in most women with PCOS so if you have high LH and that's stopping you ovulating, you may be making it worse by taking vitex.

Chantelle was diagnosed with PCOS at 19 years old when, after years of irregular periods and acne, she consulted a gynecologist.

"The diagnosis scared me! I remember getting the ultrasound because the insensitive lab technician blurted out 'WOW' while examining and measuring my ovaries. When I tackled him about his response, he only responded with the question 'Have you ever had children?' When I said no, he just shook his head and told me to get dressed. I cried uncontrollably when I got home, not understanding the meaning of it all.

"When I went back to my gynecologist, she explained that I had PCOS. I was lean, so the advice wasn't to lose weight. I was just put on birth control for the acne, and to give me a monthly bleed. I wasn't given any other information. As the years passed, I developed IBS and eczema, and had thinning hair. My anxiety levels were high!"

After no periods, Chantelle and her husband managed to conceive with clomifene. They were excited, but the pregnancy was difficult, and Chantelle was constantly ill. Her blood pressure skyrocketed, and she had a lot of spotting and had to go on bedrest 16 weeks into her pregnancy. After they had their miracle son at 30 weeks, Chantelle was "assaulted" with acne and weight gain and had consistent stomach pains and IBS. She was also constantly tired, stressed, and anxious.

"My days were spent at the gynecologist and the gastroenterologist to get to the root cause of my issues, but they offered no solutions besides birth control and antacids."

Chantelle went on a "relentless search for answers online," and spent a small fortune on every supplement that anyone, anywhere, said could "help" PCOS. But her symptoms just didn't improve, and some got even worse. This is the problem with blindly buying supplements, especially herbs—if you don't know what they do, you could be making things worse.

When Chantelle came to see me, I could see that her insulin wasn't working optimally, and nor were her stress hormones. We focused on her diet and stress management and a few *targeted* supplements for her insulin and stress hormones. Within a few months she saw real results:

"Everything has been reversed! I no longer have acne or eczema, I get my period EVERY month, my hair has stopped falling out. My IBS and pain are no more. My palpitations are gone, I am no longer anxious, and my waist measurement is down 10 inches [25 cm]—all of this in four months! I love the energy I now have!"

See the Resources section for a link to Chantelle's podcast.

In PCOS, there are three types of nutrients and herbs that can be helpful:

- Those that address your root cause
- Prenatal vitamins
- Androgen (testosterone) blockers—these don't fix the root cause, but they are a great Band-Aid for helping improve the quality of your egg (as well as hair growth, hair loss, and acne) while you address the root cause.

There is no single "list of nutrients for PCOS" to take, but I can give you some guidelines based on the various root causes, and also give you some guidance on what you should be focusing on prenatally. But first, let's have a look at what we mean by "supplements."

WHAT SUPPLEMENTS ARE

When I say supplements, I mean vitamins, minerals, herbs, antioxidants, polyphenols, and amino acids. Some of these are essential components in your body, and others cause a favorable reaction in your body.

Vitamins and minerals

Vitamins and minerals are naturally occurring substances, such as vitamins A, B, E, C, and D, along with selenium, zinc, copper, magnesium, and iron. Vitamins and minerals are critical for your body to work properly. They are co-factors in every system in your body, meaning that they assist the normal biological processes. If you don't have enough vitamins and minerals, your body will just shut down or slow the affected systems. This is why the availability of vitamins and minerals is called a rate-limiting factor. Most vitamins and minerals are called "essential," meaning that our body can't make them and we have to get them from our food (or supplements).

What vitamins and minerals do

Imagine that your body is a factory making toy cars. The factory normally produces 100 cars an hour, but this is dependent on how many car parts the factory has. If the factory only has enough wheels for 40 cars per hour, it will only be able to produce 40 cars per hour. You cannot produce a car without wheels; this is a rate-limiting factor. In your body, this might show up as processes not able to work as efficiently; for example, if you don't have enough vitamin B_6, your liver won't be able to clear as many toxins per hour. In the case of growing a baby, you might not have enough vitamins and minerals to grow the tissue correctly. The formation of the neural tube (the tube from which your brain, spinal cord, and the entire nervous system grow) in babies is dependent on how much folate, vitamin B_{12}, and choline you have. If you're trying to conceive, you will have no doubt heard that you need to take folic acid (actually folate, but we'll talk about that later) to help the neural tube grow properly. The reason for this is that if you don't have enough folate, your body can't properly code the genes (DNA and RNA) to make the neural tube.

Herbs

Herbs, on the other hand, are not natural inhabitants of our body. Instead, we use them because they make our body change or adapt in a certain way. Herbs have been used in medicine for centuries, especially in traditional Chinese medicine (TCM), and through modern research we can now see why. It has now been shown that herbs like berberine can make your body more sensitive to insulin.[1]

Phytophenols and antioxidants

These compounds occur naturally in the food we eat, but are extracted and used in much higher quantities than you would find in food. One example is resveratrol (a phytophenol), which is a compound found in red wine. Studies have shown that it improves insulin sensitivity,[2] but the amount you need for this is the equivalent of 300 glasses of red wine a day! I'll let you put two and two together about why it needs to be extracted.

Antioxidants are molecules that help counteract oxidative stress in your body. Oxidative stress occurs when you have more free-radicals than your body's natural antioxidant defenses can cope with.[3] Some good examples of antioxidants are *N*-acetylcysteine, glutathione, and vitamin C.

Effects on PCOS

Herbs, polyphenols, and antioxidants aren't essential, but there have been a lot of studies showing that they can help improve some of the root causes of PCOS.

For example, the herb berberine has been shown to very helpful in improving insulin sensitivity.[1] Imagine that you have 1,000 insulin receptors (locks) along your thigh muscle. Insulin's job is to bundle up the glucose when you eat, herd it to your muscle, and use its key to open up the lock and let it into your muscles. The more receptors you have, the more glucose your body can process. But what happens in PCOS is that a few of those locks become clogged up, and insulin can't fit the key in any longer. So instead of having 1,000 locks we now have only 500. Insulin is trying to do the same job but with only half the number of locks, so it takes twice as long. In the meantime, your body is getting panicky that it's taking so long, so it's excreting more and more insulin to try to speed things up. Berberine appears to come in and "clean out" the lock, helping to get it functioning properly again. This makes you more sensitive to insulin, as more insulin receptors are available and it takes less time to get the glucose into your cells. However, you can't use herbs all the time—your body becomes less sensitive to them over time.

THE BEST SOURCES

When it comes to vitamins and minerals, you want to try to get as much as possible from your diet. There is a special benefit to getting vitamins and minerals from real food that you don't get when these have been extracted from the natural sources. There are a few reasons:

- Nutrients affect each other's absorption. You may have heard that iron and vitamin C have a special relationship. If you take iron with vitamin C, the iron will be absorbed more easily. Similarly, vitamins A and D, copper and zinc, and manganese and iron have similar relationships. These interdependent nutrients tend to appear together in foods, but not necessarily in isolated supplements.

- The way the nutrients have been produced also changes the effect of the nutrient. Trans fats produced in cows are beneficial to health, whereas trans fats artificially produced in the processing of your average cookie are harmful.

Researchers have also shown that in most cases, wholefoods are more effective than supplements. For example:

- People eating broccoli, cauliflower, cabbage, and kale had fewer free-radicals in their bodies compared with those taking the same amount of nutrients in a supplement.[4]

- Eating whole tomatoes is much better for cardiovascular health than taking a supplement of lycopene, the nutrient responsible for this health benefit.[5]

So, on the whole, you should be trying to get as many nutrients as possible from real food, and then "supplementing" the essential nutrients that you absolutely can't get from your diet, or when your nutrient needs exceed what you can reasonably get from your diet, i.e. when you're growing a baby. Other situations where you may need supplements is if you are vegetarian or vegan, or have allergies and intolerances, or are a picky eater and don't want to eat a variety of real food. If, for example, you live far from the equator, it's impossible to get all the vitamin D you need without supplementing. If you live in New Zealand (where I'm from), our soil is deficient in selenium, and this has been associated with higher rates of depressive symptoms in young people.[6] In these cases, yes, you're going to want to take a supplement to boost your food intake.

What I'm *not* okay with is eating a poor diet and then taking a multivitamin to make up for this! Actually, I'm not a fan of most multivitamins—they can do more harm than good, as they often contain fewer of the things you actually need and too much of what you don't. What I'll be doing in this chapter is telling you where you can get the nutrients you need from your diet, and then how to top up if necessary, from supplements, in the correct quantities.

In this book, I am using the term "supplements" to cover vitamins, minerals, herbs, polyphenols, and antioxidants because there isn't another term that fits. Just remember that this doesn't mean that they have to come from pills. It's food first, always.

WHAT ADVICE DO I NEED?

In Chapter 2, I explained that there are different root causes for PCOS, of which the main ones are insulin, thyroid, stress, hormones, and inflammation. As there are many possible root causes, there isn't a single "set" of supplements that suits everyone, so here are some things to watch out for:

- You might be deficient in a vitamin and mineral that I don't mention, and if that's the case you're going to need that, too.

- There are also reasons why a supplement might not work for you. Herbs can interact with one another and with medications, and can have a different effect on some people.

- Vitamins and minerals can be toxic at high levels. Be careful with the vitamins that are stored in your fat tissue (vitamins A, D, E, and K)—your body can't just pee these out if you have too much. Instead, they build up in your fat tissue and can become toxic. Similarly, minerals like selenium can be toxic at high levels.

I always recommend working with a functional nutritionist, naturopath, naturopathic doctor, or someone with a lot of experience in this area to draw up your own personal supplement list. Such people have the knowledge and training to make sure that none of the supplements will interact with one another, and can check your levels using the proper tests and reference ranges to make sure that these are optimal rather than just being "not deficient."

Not being deficient and having optimal levels are not the same thing, but many doctors will just use the laboratory reference ranges to make sure you're not deficient. These laboratory reference ranges are generally based on what's common for the population currently—the range of results that are found in 95 percent of people generally.

Do you see the issue here? A laboratory reference range doesn't specify how much of the nutrient you need to function properly (remember the rate-limiting toy car example above), but instead what level is commonly found in the population. This relies on most of the population actually having optimal levels. But we know that this is not the case. We know that vitamin and mineral levels in the soil and in our food have been declining over the past century due to practices like not rotating crops, genetic modifications, and artificial ripening.[7] If our food has fewer nutrients, it makes sense that we have fewer nutrients, too.

> In the following sections, I've included optimal ranges for most nutrients. It's important to note that the units not only vary between nutrients but also differ between countries. Commonwealth countries tend to use one set of units, and the US a different set—just like the units we use for temperature, distance, etc., are different. You don't need to understand what each unit means in order to understand what your levels are

telling you, but you do need to make sure that you're comparing your result with the correct optimal range.

TREAT YOUR ROOT CAUSE

Supplements can be really helpful for improving your symptoms, but you need to use the ones that are important for your root cause.

Insulin root cause

Insulin requires a lot of vitamins and minerals to function properly; these are known as co-factors, which help the insulin "key" to fit into the receptor "lock." If your insulin isn't working optimally, we aim to improve your lock's sensitivity to the key, so that it opens more quickly. This will stop your body from overproducing insulin. Here I have included nutrients that are essential for your insulin to work properly, and the supplements that have most research evidence regarding improving insulin sensitivity.

> In many cases, I compare the supplements to metformin (Glucophage) to demonstrate differences in effectiveness. This does not mean that you should stop taking metformin. If you've been prescribed this, you should always inform your doctor about what else you're taking. Do also make sure that you discuss with your doctor the research on the potential negative effects of metformin (see page 74), especially on the baby.

Inositol

When it comes to improving insulin, first up is inositol. This is a naturally occurring compound in the body that is an essential co-factor for the insulin lock-and-key reaction.[8] Researchers have proposed that inositol deficiency could directly cause insulin resistance.[8]

There are two forms: myo-inositol and D-chiro-inositol, both naturally occurring. The research shows that supplementation with just myo-inositol is effective, while the combination of myo-inositol and D-chiro-inositol is possibly more effective.[9, 10]

A systematic review of the trials on inositol in PCOS found that it can help improve ovulation rates and fertility.[11] Clinical trials have shown that in PCOS, myo-inositol combined with D-chiro-inositol improves weight loss, ovulation, and pregnancy more than metformin.[9] They've also shown that combined D-chiro- and myo-inositol improves insulin resistance and reduces testosterone,[10] and that the combined supplement reduces the risk of metabolic disease in women with PCOS who are overweight, compared with myo-inositol supplementation alone.[12]

> **Sources:** Inositol is found in small amounts of grains, fruit, and legumes, but to get the quantities you need, you'll also need to supplement.

B vitamins

B vitamins, especially B_{12} and folate (B_9), are very important for allowing your insulin receptor to work properly, and for a large number of other processes including hormone production, DNA and RNA synthesis, and nerve conduction. Studies have shown that the lower your B_{12} and folate, the more likely you are to have insulin resistance and weight gain,[13] and that treatment with vitamin B_{12} and folate improves insulin resistance and decreases inflammation.[14]

Unfortunately, the most common drug used for PCOS and insulin resistance, metformin, strips the body of essential nutrients, especially vitamin B_{12}.[15] It has been reported that an average of 6–30 percent of women could be deficient in vitamin B_{12} due to metformin use.[16, 17]

The optimal level is under debate. It is well established in the scientific literature that people with vitamin B_{12} levels between 200 pg/mL and 350 pg/mL—levels considered "normal" in the US—have clear vitamin deficiency symptoms.[18]

> **Optimal range:** 332–1,475 pmol/L or 450–2,000 pg/mL
>
> **Sources:** Beef, liver, chicken, fish and seafood, dairy products, eggs

Vitamin D

Vitamin D, or the sunshine vitamin, is essential for many of our body systems, but especially for insulin. It's been shown to be low in most women with PCOS, and especially in those with insulin resistance. In fact, 67 to 85 percent of women with PCOS are deficient in vitamin D, and low levels of 25-hydroxyvitamin D (the active metabolite of the vitamin) have been found to be significantly correlated with PCOS and insulin resistance.[19-21] Vitamin D is stored in your fat tissue, so if you have a higher body fat percentage your body might not be able to use your vitamin D as easily, as it's bound up within your fat tissue.[22]

Supplementation with vitamin D has also been shown to lower anti-Müllerian hormone levels (which are high in PCOS) in women with PCOS who were deficient in the vitamin.[23] One study of over 1,000 women with PCOS found that women who were deficient in vitamin D when starting fertility treatments were 40 percent less likely to have a live birth compared with those who had good levels of vitamin D.[24] Reviews of research on PCOS and vitamin D supplementation concluded that vitamin D improves insulin resistance[25] and could help improve fertility by improving ovulation rates.[26]

If you get a vitamin D test (which I highly recommend, at least every six months), your doctor will be looking to see whether you are deficient. But as I've explained earlier, I don't just want to see that you're not deficient—I want you to have optimal levels. So when you get your tests back, check your level against the optimal range given below.

> **Optimal range for 25-hydroxyvitamin D:** 35–60 ng/dL or 87–150 nmol/L[27]
>
> **Sources:** Sunshine, oily fish (salmon, tuna, mackerel, etc.), fortified eggs, dairy products, mushrooms that have been left on the windowsill to absorb vitamin D from the sun

Vitamin D is a fat-soluble vitamin that can increase to toxic levels in the blood. I recommend that you always get your levels tested before supplementing with high amounts. Ask for a 25-hydroxyvitamin D test.

Berberine

Berberine is a herb that has been used in TCM for centuries to treat type 2 diabetes. Clinical trials have found that berberine reduces blood glucose compared with metformin in people with type 2 diabetes.[1] It has also been shown to reduce bodyweight and cause a significant improvement in glucose tolerance without altering food intake in diabetic mice.[28] As high insulin pushes your LH too high and stops you ovulating, making your body more sensitive to insulin is critical.

> **Important:** Don't use berberine if you're also using metformin, as they both can have an unwanted effect on the gut. Like all herbs, berberine is best used for a time and then stopped. Otherwise, you can become desensitized to it.
>
> **Sources:** No food sources, just a supplement

N-acetylcysteine

N-acetylcysteine (NAC) has antioxidant effects and is a precursor of the amino acid cysteine, which the body needs for hormone health, especially insulin. In clinical trials, NAC has shown significant improvement in pregnancy and ovulation rates for women with PCOS.[29] Additionally, a study of 100 women with PCOS found that NAC treatment had significant effects on:

- lowering insulin and increasing weight loss (similar to the effect of metformin)
- decreasing facial and body hair
- decreasing free testosterone
- improving ovulation (i.e. egg quality and egg release).[30]

  Sources: Cysteine comes from food sources high in protein such as meat, fish, poultry, and legumes, but you'll need an NAC supplement, too.

Chromium

Chromium is a mineral that is essential for insulin sensitivity. While it's found in many foods, like meat and potatoes, supplementing with chromium picolinate is very effective in helping to improve insulin sensitivity (comparable with metformin). Clinical trials have shown that chromium picolinate decreased fasting blood sugar and insulin levels and increased insulin sensitivity in women with PCOS who were resistant to clomifene (discussed on page 71); this was comparable with the effect of metformin.[31] Chromium supplementation has also shown beneficial effects by decreasing BMI, fasting insulin and free testosterone, and improving blood glucose control.[32, 33]

Sources: Broccoli, liver, potatoes, grains, seafood

Magnesium

Magnesium is an essential nutrient. It's the fourth most abundant mineral in our body, and helps more than 600 enzymes in the body to work properly.[34] One of the most important roles of magnesium is to make our insulin receptors work properly.[35] It's now thought that magnesium deficiency could be one of the predisposing factors for developing insulin resistance.[36] Clinical trials have shown that supplementation with magnesium improves insulin sensitivity and metabolic control in people with type 2 diabetes who have decreased serum magnesium levels.[37, 38]

The standard diet in the US contains only about 50 percent of the recommended dietary allowance (RDA) of magnesium, and up to three-quarters of the population is likely not getting enough magnesium in their diet.[39, 40]

Sources: Leafy greens, figs, avocados, nuts and seeds, legumes

Probiotics

Probiotics are the "good" bacteria that we often try to "plant" in our gut. Our gut has been shown to contribute up to 70 percent of our immune system,[41] and our gut bacteria can affect our body's ability to regulate insulin and blood sugar.[42] This might be why the research shows that people with insulin resistance have very different gut bacteria than those without insulin resistance.[43] Research has shown that people with type 2 diabetes and women with PCOS have altered gut bacteria.[44] While there is limited research on probiotics and insulin, studies in mice indicate that probiotics improve insulin sensitivity.[45] It is a good idea to take a good-quality probiotic containing different strains to help promote more growth of the "good bacteria."

> **Sources:** Fermented food and drinks: kombucha, kefir, sauerkraut, kimchi, etc.

Prebiotics

Prebiotics are food for your probiotics and gut bacteria. If you think of your gut bacteria as a garden, then the probiotics are the seeds you plant, and the prebiotics are the fertilizer. There is no point in planting the new seeds (probiotics) if we then don't feed them.

> **Sources:** Fiber from vegetables, whole grains, fruit, seeds and nuts; or extracted, e.g. inulin powder, beta-glucan, oligofructose, psyllium husk

Adrenal (stress hormones) root cause

This section is directed at those of you with stress as a component of your PCOS. If you don't have any issues with your stress hormones, you don't need to read this, but the other sections in the chapter may be relevant.

Rhodiola, schisandra, and holy basil

Rhodiola, schisandra, and holy basil are all adaptogenic herbs, which means that they help the body to adapt to stress and therefore reduce the amount of damage that stress causes. There is a significant body of evidence showing the efficacy of rhodiola, and also many positive studies for schisandra and holy basil. These herbs are often found together in stress-specific herbal remedies.

One clinical trial showed that rhodiola (*Rhodiola rosea*) significantly reduced self-reported anxiety, stress, anger, confusion, and depression, with significant improvements in total mood after just 14 days.[46] Rhodiola has also been shown to reduce fatigue while improving mood and cognition in those feeling stressed or anxious,[47] and to markedly decrease the stress-induced elevation of stress hormones.[48]

> **Sources:** No food sources; obtained from the herb or a supplement

Magnesium

Think of magnesium as your stress shield. When we're stressed, the magnesium that's normally locked in our cells actually moves into our blood and organs to protect them from the damage caused by high levels of stress hormones.[49] This is likely why a review of the studies on magnesium found that magnesium supplementation can help reduce feelings of stress and even anxiety.[50]

Over time, however, that shield becomes weaker as our magnesium levels get depleted.[49] As I mentioned above, the standard American diet (and I would extrapolate that to "standard Western diet") is woefully inadequate when it comes to magnesium content.[39, 40] This is a good reason to make a very conscious effort to eat more of the magnesium-containing foods listed below or consider supplementing with magnesium if you have adrenal PCOS.

> **Sources:** Leafy greens, figs, avocados, nuts and seeds, legumes

Inositol

Inositol is a powerful insulin sensitizer. The reason I include it here is that high stress causes the body to dump sugar into the bloodstream. Therefore, there is often some blood sugar dysregulation associated with HPA-axis dysfunction in "adrenal" PCOS.

Regarding fertility, as I mentioned earlier in the chapter, a combination of the two naturally occurring forms of inositol, myo-inositol and D-chiro-inositol, showed significantly better results in terms of weight reduction, resumption of spontaneous ovulation, and spontaneous pregnancy than metformin in women with PCOS.[9]

> **Sources:** Small amounts in grains, fruit, and legumes, but to get the quantities you need, you'll also need to supplement

Omega-3 fats

Omega-3s are a type of fatty acid that our body can't make—we must get these from our diet, and they have a big impact on how our brain and body respond to stress. Low intake of omega-3 fats is associated with higher levels of cortisol[51] and inflammation; whereas research has shown that if we get good amounts of omega-3 fats, our body doesn't produce as much cortisol and adrenaline (epinephrine) when we're faced with the same stressors.[52]

> **Sources:** Oily fish (salmon, tuna, mackerel, etc., preferably wild-caught); if you can't get three to four servings of oily fish per week, cod liver oil or fish oil supplements might be necessary

B vitamins, especially pantetheine (B$_5$)

Vitamin B$_5$ (pantetheine) plays a part in producing sex and stress-related hormones in the adrenal glands (among other things, like converting food into energy). B$_5$ helps make cortisol and is also needed to support the normal functioning of our adrenal glands.[53] This is why pantetheine helps to reduce the damaging effects of stress.[54]

If you've been on metformin, you may have lower levels of B vitamins, especially B$_{12}$ and folate, as metformin leaches both of them from the body.

> **Sources of vitamin B$_5$:** Shiitake mushrooms, salmon, avocados, chicken breast, beef, pork, sunflower seeds, whole milk

N-acetylcysteine

N-acetylcysteine (NAC) is a precursor to cysteine, one of the amino acids needed to produce glutathione, which is a powerful antioxidant. An antioxidant's job is to mop up the free-radicals that can cause oxidative damage in your body. Glutathione is called the "mother of all antioxidants" because it does many more times the work of other antioxidants like vitamin C.

Chronic stress contributes to a huge amount of oxidative damage in the body. In animal studies, NAC has been shown to reverse anxiety and oxidative damage caused by stress.[55] Additionally, NAC has been found to improve pregnancy rates in those who have previously suffered from infertility.[56]

> **Sources:** Cysteine comes from food sources high in protein, such as meat, fish, poultry, and legumes, but you'll also need a supplement.

Inflammation/thyroid root cause

This section is directed at those of you with thyroid issues or an inflammatory condition as a component of your PCOS. These issues may occur as well as insulin and adrenal issues, so you may need to read those sections as well. But if you just have hypothyroidism and/or another inflammatory condition, follow these guidelines.

Magnesium

Magnesium is an essential mineral in the body. As well as being important for insulin resistance and the stress response, it also has a powerful anti-inflammatory effect.

Inflammation is a cornerstone of hypothyroidism. Clinical trials have shown that too low a magnesium intake (less than 250 mg/day) and low magnesium levels in the blood (0.75 mmol/l or less) have both been associated with high levels of C-reactive protein (CRP), which is a marker of inflammation.[57] Another recent study found that a combination of zinc and magnesium significantly reduced CRP levels in women with PCOS.[58] Considering that 50 percent or more of the US population doesn't get enough magnesium from their food,[59] this is a good reason to supplement with magnesium if you have inflammatory or thyroid PCOS.

Sources: Leafy greens, figs, avocados, nuts and seeds, and legumes

N-acetylcysteine

N-acetylcysteine is a precursor to the amino acid cysteine, which is an important component in the body's production of glutathione—which is fondly known as the master antioxidant because of the powerful effect it has. An antioxidant mops up free-radicals in the body, preventing them from causing oxidative damage and creating inflammation. Inflammation also depletes glutathione levels, which creates a vicious cycle. Studies have shown that reduced glutathione levels lead to increased levels of inflammation.[60]

Oxidative stress and inflammation have also been found to contribute to infertility by making the environment in the uterus "uninhabitable."

NAC has been shown to offer protection for the ovaries and uterus from oxidative damage.[61] In this way, NAC can help fertility.

Antioxidants are also very important for egg quality. In studies on IVF retrieval, researchers have found that the level of antioxidants in the fluid around the eggs influences the quality of those eggs and, therefore, how many eggs can be retrieved.[62] The study authors concluded that a focus on increasing antioxidants three months before egg retrieval could increase the number of quality eggs retrieved.[62]

> **Sources:** Cysteine comes from food sources high in protein, such as meat, fish, poultry, and legumes, but you'll need an NAC supplement, too.

Curcumin

Curcumin is a naturally occurring chemical extracted from the roots of the turmeric plant. You might have heard that turmeric is anti-inflammatory; while that's true, it's not potent enough to have much of an effect when inflammation is already quite high—turmeric only contains a few percent of curcumin. Curcumin extract is far more potent. It has been widely studied and shown to have a powerful anti-inflammatory effect. In animal studies of PCOS, researchers found that curcumin significantly reduces the inflammatory marker CRP.[63] A meta-analysis (a review of a large number of studies) showed that supplementation with curcumin can reduce CRP levels, but this depends on the bioavailability of the supplement (meaning how well it is absorbed by the body).[64]

> **Sources:** Turmeric, but it's not potent enough so you will need a supplement

Vitamin D

Inflammation and vitamin D deficiency is a vicious cycle: vitamin D deficiency is associated with high levels of inflammation,[65] and inflammation stops our body from being able to use vitamin D.[66] Vitamin D is also crucial for good thyroid function.[67]

Vitamin D is a natural antibiotic that assists white blood cells to clear up infections. It does this by stimulating immune cells. This doesn't happen well in our gut, but works really well in our skin with UV rays as the catalyst. Low levels of vitamin D are a risk factor for hypothyroidism, especially Hashimoto's hypothyroidism.[67]

Vitamin D_3, which is made in our skin when exposed to sunlight, has been shown to restore vitamin D levels more effectively than vitamin D_2, the form that is produced by plants.

> **Optimal level:** 35–60 ng/dL or 87–150 nmol/L
>
> **Sources:** Sunshine, fatty fish (salmon, tuna, mackerel, etc.), fortified eggs, dairy products

Vitamin D, which is a fat-soluble vitamin, can reach toxic levels in the body, so it's important to get tested before supplementing. Ask for a 25-hydroxyvitamin D test.

Probiotics

Too many bad bacteria in the gut can lead to the release of compounds called lipopolysaccharides, which can then cause inflammation. Supplementing with probiotics ("good" bacteria) helps improve the balance between good and bad bacteria in your gut. This is one way that probiotics help to reduce inflammation. It has also been found that probiotics might actually activate our T regulatory cells, which help control the immune response and inflammation.[68]

> **Sources:** Fermented food and drinks: kombucha, kefir, sauerkraut, kimchi, etc.

Special considerations for thyroid conditions

The following are some additional nutrients that you might want to consider if you have a thyroid condition.

Selenium

Selenium is an important mineral and antioxidant. It is required to convert the thyroid hormone thyroxine (T_4) to the active form, triiodothyronine (T_3), and therefore is essential for metabolism in the body. Selenium also works in synergy with iodine (see below), so you need optimal amounts of both for your thyroid to work properly.

Thyroid hormones can stimulate the production of free-radicals and lead to oxidative stress, which is where selenium's antioxidant powers come in, to neutralize this. Not having enough selenium will lead to inflammation and can trigger an autoimmune response. This is why selenium is so important in Hashimoto's thyroiditis, an autoimmune condition; several studies have shown that selenium decreases the levels of thyroid antibodies (TGAbs and TPO antibodies; see pages 115–116).[69] Note that the maximum safe level of selenium is 400 microg/day.[70]

Sources: Brazil nuts, meat, fish, grains

Iodine

Iodine is also critical for thyroid function. Your thyroid uses iodine to make your T_4 (thyroxine), and iodine deficiency causes hypothyroidism. You need to make sure that you have a good iodine intake if you have hypothyroidism, but make sure that your selenium intake is also optimal (see above). If you have Hashimoto's thyroiditis and your selenium levels are low, high doses of iodine may actually exacerbate your symptoms.[71] Iodine is also essential for pregnancy, so it should be in your prenatal supplement, but if you have hypothyroidism you'll likely need more than what is usually prescribed. I recommend getting a hair iodine test if you have hypothyroidism—spot urinary iodine testing isn't particularly accurate for long-term iodine status; for this, get the hair iodine test.

Sources: Iodized salt, kelp, seaweed

Iron

Iron is essential for thyroid function. The TPO enzyme that converts the inactive thyroid hormone T_4 to the active form T_3 needs iron to work.[72] If you don't have enough iron, this conversion won't work properly. I strongly recommend you get the iron you need from your food, especially animal products (the iron in these is more easily absorbed than that of plant sources).[73] Supplements aren't particularly well absorbed and can often leave you nauseous and constipated (what a combo!).[74] If you do have to take a supplement, go for iron bisglycinate (instead of the more popular ferrous fumigate or ferrous sulfate)—it has fewer side-effects and is better absorbed.[74]

If your iron levels are still not rising even after you have increased your food sources and supplements, talk to your doctor about an intramuscular iron injection. Many don't like doing these, but they are an option if all else fails.

> **Optimal levels:** Serum iron: 15.22–23.77 µmol/L or 40–135 µg/dL
> Ferritin: 30–100 ng/mL
> Transferrin saturation: 17–45%
>
> **Sources:** Red meat, dark poultry meat, liver or desiccated liver capsules; tofu, lentils, tomato sauce, spinach, other leafy greens. (Additionally, cook food in a cast-iron pan to absorb some iron from the pan.)

PRENATAL NUTRIENTS

In addition to treating your root cause, there are certain vitamins and minerals that are important for your baby. Growing a human baby is an (almost) superhuman feat. In a recent human endurance study, the authors concluded that "In pushing the boundaries of human endurance, extreme athletes and pregnant women are unmatched." [75] As well as needing more calories from food during pregnancy, you also need more vitamins and minerals to help grow everything from those tiny perfect fingernails to the beautiful lungs you may come to have stern words with.

In the nicest way possible, a baby is the cutest but also the largest parasite that could enter your body. A parasite is an organism that lives in or on another species (its host) and benefits by deriving nutrients at the other's expense; in other words, it will prioritize its needs over the host—you. Simply put, if you only have seven units of iron when you get pregnant and the baby needs six units, it will take that, and you will be left with one unit and anemia. If you've ever been anemic, you'll know that you feel like a piece of trash that's been run over by 15 buses and a mobility scooter. Now imagine being anemic, *and* having a crying infant, *and* getting a maximum four hours' sleep a night for three months. Not pretty.

The aim of prenatal nutrition should not be just to prevent the baby from defects and prevent you from severe deficiency. It has to make sure that you have a pregnancy where you're not lying on the floor of the kitchen eating pickles straight from the jar because you don't have the energy to haul yourself up and get a fork. You want to ensure that your stores of nutrients are good before getting pregnant, and that you can maintain those levels as best as you can both during and after pregnancy.

The good news is that many of the foods that contain lots of the nutrients you need for pregnancy are also great for PCOS. Nutrients like iron, folate, choline, and vitamin B_{12} come from real, not manufactured, foods. So if you prioritize getting a wide variety of food from real food sources, you'll get a good portion of the nutrients from your diet.

What and how much you need

Believe it or not, we still don't exactly know what goes on in fetal development, including which vitamins and minerals are essential and, specifically, the quantities that are needed. The current recommended dietary allowances (RDAs) for nutrients in pregnancy[76] are just best guesses. Most have been calculated based on data from men, and then an estimated amount to account for fetal growth and development. As well as being only a guess, this doesn't account for the changes in pregnancy that affect the absorption or excretion of a vitamin or mineral.[76] In addition, these RDA levels are set just to prevent severe deficiency—not to ensure that you have optimal levels.

New research indicates that you do need a lot more than the current RDAs for many vitamins. For example, research into vitamin B_6 levels in the umbilical cord in pregnant women found that 56 percent of the women had suboptimal levels even though they were meeting the recommended intake.[77]

Sources of prenatal nutrients

As we've already discussed, I'm a true advocate of getting nutrients from food wherever possible. However, pregnancy is one of those times when most women struggle to get most of their needs from diet alone, even if they're eating a nutrient-dense diet. Intakes of vitamin D, calcium, vitamin E, folate, iron, zinc, and magnesium have all been found to be lower than recommended in pregnant women.[78, 79] BUT, as I outlined above, nutrients are likely best absorbed in their wholefood form, so focus on eating real, nutrient-dense diet, and use a supplement as it's intended—as a *supplement*.

Going into all the research on what to eat during pregnancy is outside the scope of this book, so instead I really recommend that you get a copy of Lily Nichols' book *Real Food for Pregnancy*.

Choosing prenatal supplements

Choosing what supplements to take when you're pregnant is both important and hard! Most of the commonly available commercial nutrient combinations don't have enough of the right kinds of nutrients based on the new research. Going into every nutrient and the research behind how much you would need would take up a whole chapter on its own, so below I will just focus on a few nutrients that I see are missing entirely, or in the incorrect form, or are commonly deficient in common formulas.

I can sense you tearing your hair out, screaming "Just tell me what to take!" And I get that—but manufacturers are constantly changing their formulas, and better ones are being developed all the time. For that reason, I've provided a list of the most up-to-date recommendations on my website (see the Resources section).

Folate, vitamin B$_9$ (not folic acid)

You will likely have been told that you need folic acid for pregnancy to help reduce the chance of a neural tube defect like spina bifida. What your body actually needs is folate, which is the naturally occurring form of folic acid. Folate is found naturally in various foods, while folic acid is manufactured and is what you'll find in most dietary supplements and fortified foods (it's a lot cheaper than natural folate supplements).

The body should be able to convert folic acid to folate, but a genetic defect in a gene called the MTHFR gene stops many people from being able to do this. This defect is very common, affecting approximately one in four people seriously and nearly one in two people mildly.[80] I go into more detail about this in Chapter 11 as a potential factor to look into further if you continue to have trouble conceiving (see page 278).

Briefly, your body has to go through a three-step process to convert folic acid and food folate into L-5-methyltetrahydrofolate (L-5-MTHF)—the active form your body can use. One of the steps relies on you having enough vitamin B_6, and the next step requires an enzyme called MTHFR (methyltetrahydrofolate reductase), which is produced with the help of the MTHFR gene. If there is a problem with your MTHFR gene, you won't have enough MTHFR enzyme to produce the L-5-MTHF (the bioactive form of folate) you need.

So, supplementing with L-5-MTHF is a better alternative than supplementing with folic acid.[81] Pregnant women supplementing with L-5-MTHF have been shown to have higher red blood cell folate levels than when supplementing with folic acid.[82]

> **Sources:** Liver, legumes, leafy greens, avocados, yeast extract, eggs, nuts and seeds
>
> **Optimal intake during pregnancy:** 600 microg/day

Choline

Choline is similar to the B vitamins and is an essential nutrient. However, it is frequently forgotten about, even though choline is just as important as folate (see above) in preventing neural tube defects and improving brain development. A survey of American diets found that 94 percent of women do not get the current recommended intake of choline.[83] In addition, this current level looks to be far too low for optimal pregnancy. A recent clinical trial found that a choline intake of double the current recommended level resulted in less pre-eclampsia (high blood pressure in pregnancy, which is already higher in PCOS) and babies that had better cognitive function.[84]

Sources: Liver, eggs, and cauliflower in much smaller amounts

Optimal intake during pregnancy: 930 mg/day[84]

Vitamin B$_{12}$

Another of the essential B vitamins in pregnancy, vitamin B$_{12}$, is only found in high amounts in animal products—so if you're vegetarian or vegan, you're likely going to have insufficient intake. Additionally, if you've been on metformin, you'll likely have low levels as metformin is known to leach B$_{12}$ from your body. Recent research shows that *triple* the current RDA of B$_{12}$ is actually the optimal level for pregnant women.[85]

Sources: Beef, liver, chicken, fish and seafood, dairy products, eggs

Optimal intake during pregnancy: 8.6 microg/day[85]

Vitamin D

We've already talked about vitamin D (see pages 241 and 249), but as well as being essential for your insulin and thyroid, it's also essential for growing a healthy baby. Your requirements for vitamin D increase during pregnancy because your vitamin D is needed to grow the baby's bones and teeth. If you don't have enough vitamin D, it's more likely that your child will be born with a lower bone mass,[86] and this can influence their bone mass later in life[87] and may predispose them to fractures or osteoporosis.

How much vitamin D is enough during pregnancy? One well-designed study measured the levels of vitamin D in 450 pregnant women who were given either the RDA amount of vitamin D (400 IU) or a much higher dose of either 2,000 IU or 4,000 IU.[88] The results showed that only 50 percent of the women who received the 400 IU dose had sufficiently high levels of vitamin D, and only 39.7 percent of their babies had adequate levels. Not only were the higher doses safe throughout the pregnancies, but they were far more effective, both in helping the women to achieve optimal vitamin D levels and in helping the babies be born with adequate levels—70.8 percent of the women taking 2,000 IU and 58.2 percent of their babies had sufficient levels of vitamin D, while 82.0 percent of women taking 4,000 IU and 78.6 percent of their babies had sufficient levels.[88]

As you can see, it took almost 10 times the RDA for many of the women participating in this study to achieve optimal levels of vitamin D. Given that up to 85 percent of women with PCOS are deficient in vitamin D,[19] we are arguably a group that's at even greater risk of severe deficiency and need to make sure that we get adequate amounts of vitamin D.

Remember to ask for a 25-hydroxyvitamin D test, and ask for the actual results—don't just accept being told they are "normal."

> **Optimal range during pregnancy:** 35–60 ng/dL or 87–150 nmol/L[89]
>
> **Sources:** Sunshine, fatty fish (salmon, tuna, mackerel, etc.), fortified eggs, dairy products

Vitamin K$_2$

Vitamin K$_2$ works hand-in-hand with vitamin D to keep the calcium in your bones rather than in your soft tissue, like your arteries and other blood vessels. This helps to create your baby's skeleton and teeth, and, of course, keep your bones healthy, too. It's found in fatty animal foods, and the only vegetarian source that has high quantities is a fermented soybean product called nattō; unfortunately, the form in nattō may not be able to cross the placental barrier,[90] so if you are vegetarian or vegan you will want to supplement with Vitamin K$_2$.

> **Sources:** Fatty animal foods, including full-fat dairy, eggs, and liver; or supplements if necessary
>
> **Recommended intake during pregnancy:** There is no RDA for vitamin K$_2$ alone; just be aware that if you aren't eating any animal products, you are likely deficient.

Iodine

Iodine is an essential nutrient that is often deficient in women, and is linked to cognitive development in children. During pregnancy, iodine requirements increase by 50 percent, partly due to your increased needs and partly due to the baby's.[91] The requirement increases even more during breastfeeding. If you aren't consciously making an effort to consume iodine-rich foods, then you're more than likely not getting enough. In the UK, 73 percent of pregnant women were found to have deficient iodine levels.[92] Alarmingly, just over half of the prenatal vitamin formulas on the US market neglect to include iodine,[93] even when it's known that most pregnant and lactating women in the U.S. are consuming iodine below the recommended daily intake.[94]

> **Sources:** Iodized salt, kelp, seaweed
>
> **Recommended intake:** 220 microg/day for pregnant women, and 290 microg/day for breastfeeding women[95]

Iron

Iron is a mineral that we need to make red blood cells. As you're growing a *lot* of new red blood cells during pregnancy to make both the baby and the placenta, your iron requirements are about 1.5 times higher than normally.[96] I strongly recommend you get your iron from your food; animal products in particular contain a form of iron that is two to four times better absorbed than that from plant sources.[73] Supplements aren't particularly well absorbed and can leave you nauseous and constipated.[74] Your doctor should monitor your iron levels during pregnancy; if you do have to take a supplement, ask for iron bisglycinate (instead of the more popular ferrous fumigate or ferrous sulfate) as this has fewer side-effects and is better absorbed.[75]

> **Sources:** Red meat, dark meat on poultry, liver or desiccated liver capsules; tofu, lentils, tomato sauce, spinach, other leafy greens. (Additionally, I recommend cooking food in a cast-iron pan to absorb some iron from the pan.)
>
> **Optimal levels:** Serum iron: 15.22–23.77 μmol/L, or 40–135 μg/dL
> Ferritin: 30–100 ng/mL
> Transferrin saturation: 17–45%
>
> **Recommended intake during pregnancy:** 25 mg/day

ANTI-ANDROGENS

High levels of androgens (testosterone, DHEA-S, and androstenedione) contribute to your egg not developing properly, as well as to acne, hair loss, and hair growth. They are always stimulated by your root cause, so you need to address this, too. But in the meantime, an anti-androgen is something you can take that blocks androgens from working. While it can be very helpful in PCOS, research studies are few and far between for women.

Options for anti-androgens
Black cohosh

Black cohosh (*Cimicifuga racimosa*) is a herb that's beginning to be studied more and more in PCOS and fertility studies. Black cohosh may improve fertility in PCOS by thickening the endometrial lining,[97-99] increasing estrogen and decreasing luteinizing hormone (LH).[99, 100]

One study compared the rates of conception among women using clomifene or black cohosh for three months, and found that more women got pregnant using black cohosh (14 percent) than clomifene (8 percent);[101] however, this was not a statistically significant difference, possibly due to the small size of the group studied. What *was* statistically significant was that black cohosh was more effective than clomifene at lowering LH and improving the LH to FSH ratio,[101] which we've already learned is critical in helping many women with PCOS to conceive.

Another study, involving almost 200 women with PCOS, added black cohosh to clomifene cycles to see whether it improved their pregnancy rate. The researchers found that the group that were given the black cohosh in combination with the clomifene had about a 50 percent higher pregnancy rate compared with the group just given clomifene.[99] Similar results have been found in other trials of black cohosh with clomifene, and women given black cohosh had quicker development of follicles and a thicker endometrial lining.[102, 103]

Important: Please treat black cohosh like a prescription drug, i.e. only use it under the supervision of a trained practitioner.

Spearmint tea

Spearmint and peppermint teas are great anti-androgenic herbs, and we can use the whole plant in a drink rather than extracting the components into supplements. The anti-androgenic properties were discovered when men from a region in Turkey (where spearmint and peppermint are commonly used in tea) started complaining of low libido. As testosterone is what drives libido, researchers started looking for what could be blocking the testosterone, and thus the effects of spearmint and peppermint tea were discovered.[104]

There has been only a small number of studies on the use of these herbs in PCOS, but they have been positive. However, so far they have only tested spearmint tea rather than the more commonly consumed peppermint tea. One study got women to drink two cups of spearmint tea a day for 30 days; after this time, their testosterone levels had significantly reduced and their LH and FSH levels had improved; in addition, their facial and body hair growth had also noticeably reduced.[105]

Peony and licorice

Peony and licorice are both androgen-blocking herbs. One study showed that licorice reduced testosterone by 40 percent over just two menstrual cycles.[106] In Chinese medicine, licorice is frequently used in combination with peony. Peony and licorice work by converting testosterone into estrogen, instead of DHT (the potent form that causes all the hair growth, hair loss, acne, etc.).[107] The combination was shown (in large doses) to significantly decrease testosterone by up to 35 percent in just four weeks, and also significantly improve pregnancy rates.[107]

Important: Please treat these herbs like prescription drugs, i.e. only use them under the supervision of a trained practitioner.

> **Caution:** If your root cause is adrenal, I would not recommend licorice for you as it is quite stimulating for the adrenal glands. It also raises blood pressure in some susceptible people, so always consult someone experienced with its use.

TROUBLE-
SHOOTING

Chapter 11
Still not pregnant?

If you've followed all the guidelines in this book for at least six months, and are still not ovulating or still not pregnant, it might be time to seek some medical assistance or to look a bit deeper at what else could be going on. But before heading off to investigate anything else, you need to check that you've got the fundamentals right. I know there is a lot to take in, so I've created a decision tree for you to check off all the important branches.

In the rest of this chapter we'll look at some of the common factors that can affect fertility. Note that this is not a comprehensive look at every possible thing that could be affecting your fertility, but it is a good starting point. These are the issues that I'll be covering:

- Male factor infertility—Chapter 6 gives guidelines for optimal sperm, but what can you do if there is more of a problem?
- Do you have an STI or candida infection?
- Could it be endometriosis?
- Do you have one of the big PCOS mimickers rather than actual PCOS?
- Could it be another immune or autoimmune issue (including celiac disease)?
- Do you have an MTHFR genetic mutation?

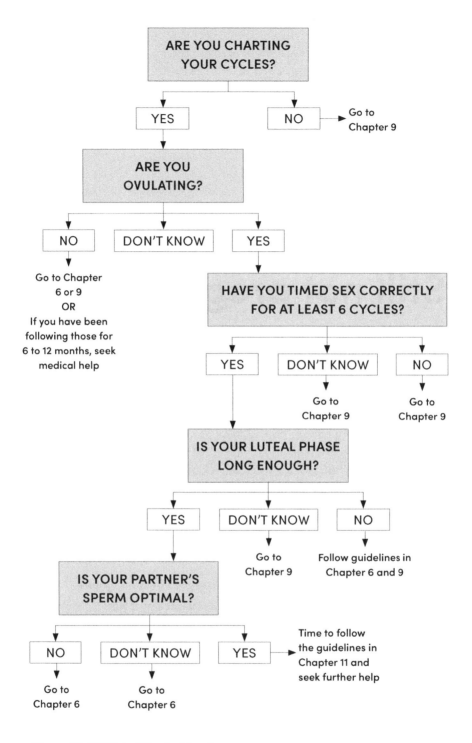

Figure 20: PCOS fertility decision tree

MALE FACTOR INFERTILITY

As I mentioned in Chapter 6, almost 50 percent of all cases of infertility may be down to male factor infertility, and there are lifestyle changes your partner can make to improve the quality of his sperm. However, if your partner's sperm morphology (the way the sperm look) is less than 10 percent normal, or you've had poor results with IVF fertilization, or have had recurrent miscarriages, you might want to also look at a sperm DNA fragmentation test. This takes a closer look at DNA damage in sperm that conventional tests don't detect. The results will be presented as a DNA Fragmentation Index (DFI) score:

15 percent or less DFI = excellent to good sperm DNA integrity

15–25 percent DFI = good to fair sperm DNA integrity

25–50 percent DFI = fair to poor sperm DNA integrity

50 percent or higher DFI = very poor sperm DNA integrity

One of the most common causes of DNA fragmentation is oxidative stress. As I discussed in Chapter 6, this can affect sperm count, motility, and morphology. In addition to the causes of suboptimal sperm I outlined in Chapter 6, some additional factors could be:

- varicocele (enlargement of one of the veins in the scrotum—the bag that holds the testicles)
- chronic disease
- infection
- enlarged prostate (prostatitis).

I recommend seeking medical advice to rule out any of the above factors.

Giving sperm some help—DIY insemination

If you've found that your partner's sperm isn't optimal, then as well as following the guidelines in Chapter 6 to help improve sperm quality, you can also give the sperm a bit of a help to reach your cervix. Don't worry—DIY insemination is not as barbaric as it might sound; your partner is going nowhere near your vagina with his cordless drill! DIY insemination just gives an extra head-start for those sperm that might not be the strongest of swimmers. Instead of ejaculating inside you, your partner ejaculates into a cervical cap, and you then insert this into your vagina to cover your cervix.

Rather than having to paddle like a bat out of hell to get up through your vagina just to reach your cervix, the semen have been dropped off at the front door, as it were, and only have to swim a short way. This simple trick also extends the time that the sperm are exposed to your cervical fluid close to your cervix, which makes it more likely that they'll get sucked into the vortexes created by the channels in the fluid (see Chapter 9, page 220). Those sperm can just kick back and glide straight up your cervix.

Many women try to get the same effect by lying on their backs, sometimes with their legs in the air. But this doesn't work—even if you're on your back with your legs in the air, your cervix is still higher than your vagina. So if the sperm are not strong swimmers, the effect of gravity is still going to be working against them. Standing on your head or indulging in a bit of acro-yoga might work, but that's way more effort than using a cervical cap.

I also want to be clear: This is no "turkey-baster" insemination. A turkey baster will just shoot the sperm up near your cervix in exactly the same way ejaculation does. But then gravity will hold, and the sperm will slide back away from your cervix. With the cervical cap method, your cervix will literally be bathing in the sperm for six hours, giving them the best possible chance of getting caught in a cervical fluid riptide.

This method has been around since the 1970s, and has been well studied. One study involving over 60 couples who'd been trying to conceive for up to 11 years found some amazing results.[1] The women used the cervical cap method alongside charting their cycle and timing sex for when they were fertile (see Chapter 9). They were told to use the cap one to three times in each cycle for at least six cycles. After an average of just three to four cycles, 53 percent of the women successfully conceived, and the miscarriage rate was no higher than what would normally be expected.[1] Another study found that 44 percent of couples conceived after using the cervical cap method for at least six months.[2]

Here's how to do the cervical cap method (three steps).

Step 1—Chart your cycles and find your fertile window

As I explained in Chapter 9, you are only fertile when you have fertile cervical fluid present; the challenge lies in finding these days (your fertile window), especially if your cycle is still a bit irregular. Use the fertility awareness method (FAM) that I've outlined in Chapter 9. This combines your cervical fluid characteristics and your basal body temperature to determine when you are leading up to ovulation and when you have ovulated.

Step 2—Get a cervical cap and learn how to insert it properly

The best type of cervical cap is a little silicone cup shaped like a sailor's cap (somewhat fitting for those swimmers!) with a loop to help you remove it easily. It is usually used for contraception, to stop sperm entering your cervix, but we're using it for the opposite reason. They are smaller and fit more tightly onto your cervix than a diaphragm. The brand name in some parts of the world is a FemCap—and no, your moon cup or another type of menstrual cup won't do the job. A menstrual cup sits much lower down in your vagina and doesn't go anywhere near your cervix.

To insert the cervical cap, squat all the way down like a frog, or put one leg up on the toilet like you're going to insert a tampon. Reach up and feel your cervix to see where you're aiming for. The cervix will feel a bit like the tip of your nose, and it moves around depending on where you are in your cycle.

Squeeze the top rim of the cervical cap so that it flattens it out—but be careful not to squeeze any sperm out at each end—and hold it in your dominant hand. With your free hand, separate the lips of your vagina (your vulva), insert the cap, and push it all the way along the vagina to the end. You'll then have to maneuver it around to make sure it's up and over the cervix. Press down on it for 10 seconds to make sure it's on properly; you might feel that your cervix underneath is a little uncomfortable from the pressure—that's okay, just don't press too hard as your cervix is a sensitive wee thing. Then feel around to just check that your cervix isn't peeking around the side of your cervical cap.

Family planning centers or trained doctors and nurses can train you in how to place the cap correctly, and also make sure that it fits properly.

Step 3—Get your partner to ejaculate in the cervical cap and insert it

The ejaculation doesn't have to happen via masturbation—you can have sex as usual and have the cup handy so that he can withdraw and ejaculate into it. You decide what works for you.

Insert the cervical cap just like you've practiced, and leave it in place for at least six hours. The hardest part of the cervical cap method is inserting the cap properly so that it fits snugly around your cervix without spilling all those wee swimmers down your thigh. It's definitely possible for most women, and practice makes for less sperm lost to the shower drain. However, if you've been trying for some time and still can't get it right, a device called "The Stork," which has a cervical cap on the end of an applicator, could help. It's like inserting an applicator tampon, but further up so that you feel the pressure of it at the end of your cervix. There's a YouTube video on how it works—see the link in the Resources section.

STI OR CANDIDA INFECTION

Sexually transmitted infections (STIs) are one of the most common causes of infertility. They can be present with no symptoms for years, leaving you none the wiser that they are affecting you and/or your partner. Chlamydia and gonorrhea can both cause pelvic inflammatory disease (PID) and infertility. Chlamydia can also cause fallopian tube infection without any symptoms.[3] I would recommend that everyone gets checked for STIs before they start trying to conceive.

Candida is a yeast (*Candida albicans*) that is a natural inhabitant in your body in small amounts, but when it becomes overgrown, it causes fungal infection (candidiasis). This has been called "the most important sexually transmitted fungal infection"[4] when it comes to fertility. As you may know (see page 89), our gut bacteria (microbiome) play a huge role in our health. But you might not know that we also have a vaginal microbiome—a community of bacteria, yeasts, and fungi that live in the vagina. And this is very tightly linked to our gut microbiome, because of the proximity of the anus to the vagina, and bacteria being able to spread between the two.

We are only just starting to understand how the vaginal microbiome contributes to fertility. A 2016 study with Danish women undergoing IVF found that just 9 percent of those who had an abnormal vaginal microbiome got pregnant, versus 44 percent that had a normal vaginal microbiome.[5] While this is just a correlational study, the mechanism does make sense. If you have a lot of bad bacteria, yeasts, and fungi in your vagina (or higher), these can potentially do things like altering the pH of your vagina to make it less optimal for sperm.

One of the most common symptoms of candida infection is thrush, and another is urinary tract infections (UTIs).[6] Other signs are athlete's foot or other fungal skin infections. Thrush is one of the most common vaginal disruptions I've seen in women with PCOS. Insulin resistance causes the perfect conditions for candida to thrive in. The high levels of glucose circulating in the body due to impaired insulin feed the candida, and suppression of the immune system (also due to insulin resistance) allows them to breed without opposition.[7] We also know that in PCOS the gut microbiome is not as good as it should be (this has even been suggested as a "root cause" for PCOS on its own).[8]

Men as well as women can be affected by candida. Candida causes semen candidiasis, which affects sperm motility (swimming ability).[9] So both you and your partner need to be checked for candida overgrowth, especially if either of you has ever had thrush, UTIs, or fungal nail or skin infections. The test that I would recommend for this is a comprehensive stool (poo) analysis by a functional medicine practitioner.

ENDOMETRIOSIS

Endometriosis can be a significant factor when it comes to fertility, and you likely won't know that you have it.

Tara had come off hormonal birth control to get pregnant. After a year and no success, she was diagnosed with PCOS. She was suffering from weight gain, severe sugar cravings and hangry attacks, fatigue, and missing periods.

I sent Tara for some tests, and identified that her insulin and stress hormones weren't working optimally. After addressing these problems, she had some incredible results: she lost an amazing 29 lb (13 kg) and got a regular period for the first time in 16 years. She also found that her gut health improved massively, and she was sleeping better, was no longer getting hangry attacks, and her energy improved immensely. However, even after getting her period back regularly for a few months, Tara still wasn't pregnant, and some other symptoms had appeared. Her period pain was getting worse, intercourse was painful, as was trying to pass a bowel movement. After doing some of her own research, she thought that some of her symptoms sounded an awful lot like endometriosis.

Her primary care doctor agreed that Tara had many of the symptoms of endometriosis and referred her to a gynecologist for an internal examination. This confirmed that she did indeed have endometriosis, and surgery successfully removed the associated scar tissue and lesions.

A few months post-surgery, Tara was able to become pregnant.

Unlike PCOS, endometriosis is not a hormonal condition. It's an inflammatory immune condition where a lining like your uterine lining (which you shed when you get your period) grows in other parts of your abdomen where it's not supposed to. Imagine that your immune system is like an army fighting on the front line in a war; in the case of your body, it's a war against foreign objects that need to be killed and eradicated. The job is both physically and mentally demanding, so the soldiers (your white blood cells and other immune cells) can only fight for a few weeks before they need to rest and repair. When you have a systemic immune condition like endometriosis, your immune cells have been fighting for years, if not decades, rather than just a few weeks. The result is that your poor soldiers (immune cells) are exhausted and delirious, and can no longer tell who's the enemy and who's on their side. Your immune system starts to attack your own cells, and one of the results is that uterine-like tissue grows on your ovaries and colon, and causes severe pain, scarring, and infertility.

Diagnosis

Endometriosis affects up to one in 10 women.[10] However, diagnosing endometriosis is quite tricky currently because there is no straightforward blood test (although this is very close to being available).[11] The diagnosis usually requires you to have many of the typical symptoms, and then a pelvic exam or ultrasound will be done. If your doctor can't see or feel any lesions during the exam, you may be referred for a laparoscopy. This is a surgical procedure where an incision is made near your navel (belly button) to allow a laparoscope (a camera in a long, thin tube) to be inserted to look for endometrial tissue. If endometrial tissue is found, it can often be removed there and then so you only need the one surgery.

Links to PCOS and infertility

Clinically, I see many women with PCOS who also have endometriosis, but this is probably just because they are both quite common. Like Tara in the case study opposite, symptoms of endometriosis often start to show after PCOS symptoms have begun to resolve, because endometriosis is sensitive to estrogen. If you haven't had a period in a while or have been on HBC, your estrogen levels are going to be fairly low. Then, when you get your period back or come off HBC, your estrogen will rise and endometriosis may flare up.

As endometriosis is an immune condition, it can affect both the quality of your eggs and the hospitality of your uterus. If your eggs are exposed to high levels of inflammation as they are growing, they may not be of great quality. Endometriosis also doesn't make your uterus a very hospitable place to be. Instead of it nurturing your fertilized egg, it attacks the egg before it has a chance to implant.

The other component of endometriosis that affects fertility is scar tissue. Uterine-like tissue that grows all around your pelvis can lead to scar tissue forming. When there is scar tissue in your fallopian tubes or joining your fallopian tubes to your ovaries, this makes it really hard for your egg to make its way down the fallopian tubes.

What causes endometriosis

It would be wrong to say that we know exactly what's going on with endometriosis (especially when new research is coming out as frequently as it is currently); however, what we do know is that it's a chronic inflammatory disease, and when inflammation is involved, so too is the immune system.

There is also research supporting the theory that immune dysfunction might be caused by bacteria. Women with endometriosis have a high level of Gram-negative bacteria (which are more resistant to antibodies) and the bacterial toxin LPS (lipopolysaccharide) in their pelvis, which has been shown to contribute to endometriosis.[12]

Symptoms of endometriosis

Two of the main symptoms of endometriosis are period pain and infertility, which can often be mistaken for PCOS. It's a misconception that severe period pain is a symptom of PCOS. The heavy periods that PCOS can cause do lead to a dull ache, but the pain of endometriosis is the sort of pain that makes you need to miss school, work, or social events, have vomiting or nausea, or take high-dose painkillers.

Bear in mind that endometriosis doesn't *always* cause severe period pain. I recently met a woman who had never missed a day of school in her life and had managed her pain with acetaminophen (paracetamol; often sold as Tylenol or Panadol)—and it turned out she had endometriosis. Pain is not the only way to diagnose endometriosis. Endometriosis U.K. has compiled a file of some of the main symptoms of endometriosis which you can download—you'll find the link in the Resources section of this book. If you do suspect that you have endometriosis, you can print the file off to use as a talking tool with your primary care doctor.

CONDITIONS MIMICKING PCOS—NCAH AND HYPOTHALAMIC AMENORRHEA

The advice I have offered in this book assumes that you have correctly been diagnosed with PCOS. However, this is not always the case. I've seen many women who have been diagnosed with PCOS but don't actually have PCOS. In some cases they might have fitted the PCOS diagnostic criteria; in others they have been told that they had PCOS solely on the basis of an ultrasound scan.

I explained in Chapter 1 (page 24), the Rotterdam diagnostic criteria can over-diagnose PCOS. Many women diagnosed with PCOS, actually have one of the big PCOS mimickers: non-congenital adrenal hyperplasia (NCAH) or hypothalamic amenorrhea.

Non-congenital adrenal hyperplasia (NCAH)

NCAH is a condition caused by a genetic mutation that results in your body overproducing androgens (testosterone and its relatives DHEA-S and androstenedione). Unlike PCOS, NCAH isn't limited to women, but it's less obvious in men because they already produce high amounts of androgens—so symptoms like facial and body hair are completely normal for these men.

The increased levels of testosterone in women mean that they:

- have an irregular period, or it's plain non-existent
- aren't ovulating, so the eggs or follicles stay "stuck" on the ovary and appear as "cysts."

This can result in infertility, and you might get facial hair, acne, hair loss, or other symptoms associated with high androgens. Sounds like PCOS, right? Exactly—but the difference is that the cause of the high androgen levels is entirely different. In PCOS it's a mixture of your genes interacting with the environment, whereas in NCAH it's a genetic mutation. Unsurprisingly, the treatments for the two conditions are different.

Like PCOS, NCAH is also quite common. Research shows that up to 9 percent of the women who overproduce testosterone actually have NCAH,[13] but are misdiagnosed with PCOS as it looks so similar.

Recently I saw a patient, Alicia, who wanted help with facial hair growth and hair loss. She also had a bit of weight gain and irregular periods. On the face of it, this sounded like a very normal PCOS case. During the consultation, however, I asked Alicia about what happened when she hit puberty, and something interesting came up. She explained that she got her period rather late, at 15 years old, but starting growing pubic hair really early—at about eight years old. That set alarm bells going off for me. Late-starting periods but early pubic hair is one of the key signs of NCAH.

How to differentiate NCAH from PCOS

Unfortunately, PCOS and NCAH look incredibly similar; there are also a lot of misconceptions about NCAH, which is partly to blame for the common misdiagnosis. Many doctors are under the impression that if you have NCAH, you won't have insulin resistance. However, this is not true. If you have high levels of testosterone, you're more likely to put weight on around your middle and also go on to develop insulin resistance. The results of one study showed that women with NCAH are more likely to have insulin resistance than women without NCAH, even if they have the same body weight.[14]

Another misconception is that you must be lean to have NCAH. Insulin resistance is a really common cause of weight gain, and as women with NCAH are likely to have insulin resistance, they are also likely to gain weight. In a study on NCAH and PCOS, researchers reported an average BMI of 33 in the PCOS group and 29 in the NCAH group, both of which are in the "overweight" category, bordering on obese.[15]

And finally, even if you have polycystic ovaries, this can also be caused by NCAH. Having multiple "cysts" on your ovaries doesn't necessarily mean that you have PCOS. Notice that I put cysts in quote marks—in PCOS these are not actually cysts but instead baby eggs or follicles that stayed "stuck" on your ovaries when you didn't ovulate. As many women with NCAH also don't ovulate, it's not surprising that 50 percent of them have these "cysts" on their ovaries, too.[15]

Symptoms alone cannot differentiate NCAH from PCOS; you need the correct test. The correct test to differentiate NCAH from PCOS is a 17-hydroxyprogesterone test, and then an ACTH stimulation test to confirm the diagnosis.

Hypothalamic amenorrhea

Lean women with PCOS-like symptoms are often misdiagnosed as having PCOS—particularly if they've been diagnosed by ultrasound or AMH (anti-Müllerian hormone) levels alone. Hypothalamic amenorrhea (HA) is a condition caused by your brain (hypothalamus) stopping your ovaries from ovulating. It is basically when your brain is saying "Whooooa! We're in danger; this is NOT the right time to bring a baby into the world!" and subsequently sends a message to the ovaries to stop ovulation. This danger generally arises from three issues:

- undereating, even if not underweight
- undereating carbs
- stress.

As women with HA don't ovulate, they can therefore have "cystic" ovaries and high AMH levels;[16] they can also have facial or other body hair. However, in the case of HA this is not due to high testosterone or androgen levels as is the case in PCOS. It's also very possible to switch between PCOS and HA.

CASE STUDY

Mandy was diagnosed with PCOS when she was 17. She'd had high insulin and testosterone, missing periods, acne, and "cysts" on her ovaries—a "textbook-perfect" PCOS case. However, when I saw Mandy, she was 31 and trying to conceive, and it became clear that this wasn't the case. After a brief stint of classic university overconsumption, Mandy became very image-conscious and started strict dieting and heavy exercise. She cut out all sugar and carbohydrates, eating 800 kcal a day and running twice-daily. She lost a lot of weight; her periods returned for a year, but then disappeared again. At the time I saw Mandy, she still thought she had PCOS—but her androgens were normal and her LH was extremely low. This is the opposite to what typically happens to hormones in PCOS. The missing periods and fertility challenges weren't caused by PCOS anymore; it was hypothalamic amenorrhea.

The same thing that happened to Mandy can happen if you've just come off HBC. Hormonal birth control, and anti-androgen pills like Yasmin (Yaz), artificially suppress androgens. When you come off HBC, your androgen levels will jump up, which can stop your period coming back, and you'll also probably get some acne around your chin and jawline. If you went to the doctor at this point, you'd likely be diagnosed with PCOS. However, very commonly this jump in levels is just temporary and will come down with time (you can also help it along with some specific nutritional strategies—see Chapter 10). But say that you tried the ketogenic diet at this time—while this might improve your symptoms for a while, and your insulin sensitivity might improve, if you stayed on it for longer it might turn into HA.

Test to differentiate HA from PCOS

Levels of LH and FSH are a good way to distinguish between PCOS and HA. They are best measured on Day 3 of your cycle (or any day if you have no cycle). If the ratio of LH to FSH is greater then 2 to 1, it's likely that you have PCOS. If it's not, then you may have HA. This is not a foolproof method, however; you will need the clinical guidance of a good gynecologist or endocrinologist to look at all the factors and make an informed diagnosis.

AUTOIMMUNE CONDITIONS

Autoimmune conditions are where your immune system has gone a bit haywire and started attacking your own body tissue, rather than foreign invaders. Autoimmune conditions include Hashimoto's thyroiditis (which is super-common in PCOS, and has been discussed where relevant throughout the book), celiac disease, lupus, rheumatoid arthritis, and type 1 diabetes, among others.

When you have an autoimmune condition, your body will create antibodies against your own cells and tissue. Normally, antibodies are created when you have a virus and then successfully fight it off, or when you receive a vaccine—the little bit of modified virus contained in the vaccine is enough for your body to create antibodies against it without the virus being able to invade your body. The next time your body comes into contact with that disease, it already has the ability to mobilize an army of antibodies to fight it. However, in an autoimmune condition it's not a disease from outside your body that the antibodies are fighting— it's your own tissue and cells.

Autoimmune antibodies can be present years before you actually get any symptoms, but during this time they may still affect fertility. For example, celiac disease has been linked to recurrent miscarriage, pregnancy complications, and infertility. A clinical trial in 2010 found that between 5 and 10 percent of women with recurrent miscarriages or stillbirths tested positive for one of the celiac disease antibodies, transglutaminase IgA.[17]

Autoimmune conditions can also affect male factor fertility. Anti-sperm antibodies are another form of autoimmunity, and they do what the name says: they attack sperm by either attaching to the tail of the sperm to stop it swimming so fast, or blocking it from penetrating the egg. These antibodies can be present in either you or your partner, and you'll need your doctor to test for them. Around 5 percent of subfertile women and 10 percent of men have these antibodies in their bloodstreams.[18]

If you have a family member with any autoimmune condition, but particularly those listed above, get your antibodies tested, as genetics plays a major role in whether you are likely to have one of these conditions, too. In my *PCOS Protocol* program we cover these tests in more detail.

GENETIC MUTATION IN THE MTHFR GENE

As we covered in Chapter 10 (page 235), you need folate for the neural tube (spine and brain) of your baby to form properly. Your ability to use folate can be affected by genetic mutation in a particular gene, the MTHFR gene. A mutation in the MTHFR gene is a very common genetic defect—it affects approximately one in four people seriously, and nearly one in two people mildly.

At this point I want to explain what a genetic mutation (or coding error) is and why it's not the end of the world. You may remember from biology that to make a new cell the existing cell divides in two. Before it does this, it copies (duplicates) its DNA so that after division each of the new cells will have a full copy of the original cell's DNA.

During the DNA copying process, small coding errors are sometimes made. These are called "single nucleotide polymorphisms," or SNPs (pronounced "snips"), and are just like a typo in the DNA. These "typos" mean that the DNA that makes up the MTHFR gene will be very slightly different in different people. A lot of the time this doesn't matter, but particular variants of the MTHFR gene will mean that you don't make enough methylated folate and will need some help with this.

If your body has a mutation in the MTHFR gene, you will produce less MTHFR enzyme, and therefore less methylated (active) folate. How much this affects you will depend on what MTHFR gene variant you have. People with the variant of MTHFR called C667T were found to have a 40 to 60 percent decreased ability to produce methylated folate.[19]

Preventing neural tube defects in developing babies is not the only job that L-5-MTHF does. It's a critical factor in neurotransmitter production, DNA regulation, immunity, and the cardiovascular system, and it also affects hormone levels and oxidative damage. This is really important for getting pregnant.

The main roles that the MTHFR mutation plays in fertility are that it decreases our ability to reduce oxidative damage (detoxify) and increases homocysteine levels. Elevated homocysteine isn't a good thing—it's been cited as a factor contributing to recurrent pregnancy loss, pre-eclampsia, infertility, Down syndrome, and other serious concerns surrounding pregnancy.[20, 21]

Note: The MTHFR mutation is not the *only* thing that causes high homocysteine (other factors include low vitamin B_{12} and vitamin B_6), but it's a pretty common cause.[22]

Given the grave consequences of a poorly functioning MTHFR gene, if you are trying to conceive and it isn't happening for you, then you should seriously consider screening for the MTHFR genetic defect. Remember that if you do have it, it's not the end of the world—you just likely need the proper food and nutrients to help you with the folate pathway (i.e. lots of leafy greens for folate, and a methylated folate supplement— *not* folic acid).

Chapter 12
Reducing your risks during pregnancy

Pregnancy puts a lot of strain on the body—and as I've said previously, a recent study showed that pregnancy pushes the body so far to the limit that it is only matched by elite-level sport.[1] This is even more so for women with PCOS. Pregnancy complication rates are much higher in PCOS—but from my experience, they don't have to be. I've found that the pregnancy complications that often come with PCOS have little to do with the actual PCOS, but instead are due to the root cause, especially when this is insulin or a genetic condition like an MTHFR genetic defect.

In this chapter, we'll look at the three most common pregnancy complications in PCOS:

- gestational diabetes
- miscarriage
- pre-eclampsia and late preterm delivery.

I will take you through why they are common in PCOS and what you can do about them.

GESTATIONAL DIABETES

Gestational diabetes is similar to type 2 diabetes (non-insulin-dependent diabetes) that develops during pregnancy. Many hormonal changes happen during pregnancy, and one of them[15] is to make you more insulin-resistant to help you deliver nutrients to your growing baby.[2] The insulin resistance is caused by hormones produced by the placenta, so it gets more exaggerated the further through the pregnancy you are.

In most women, the body just compensates by producing more insulin, and so their blood glucose stays normal.[3] But for many women with PCOS, who already have (in most cases undiagnosed) insulin resistance, their body has already been overproducing insulin for many years. So when pregnancy comes along, their body can no longer produce enough insulin to keep up, and their blood glucose rises. This results in gestational diabetes.

Gestational diabetes exposes babies to higher levels of insulin in the uterus, which can damage their metabolism. This is why babies born to mothers with gestational diabetes are often larger than average, have higher body fat as babies,[4] are more likely to be born preterm,[5] and are at greater risk of cardiac disorders.[6]

About 20 to 50 percent of women with PCOS will develop gestational diabetes (compared with about 10 percent of the "normal" population), but it doesn't have to be this way.[7, 8] Studies have repeatedly shown that if you make your body more sensitive to insulin, you can reverse insulin resistance, pre-diabetes, and even diabetes.[9] And the best time to do that is before getting pregnant. This is why I'm so passionate about addressing the root cause first, or at least at the same time as fertility treatments.

The best way to improve insulin sensitivity is to follow my Steps 1 to 5 to address insulin resistance (see Chapters 6 to 10). Especially, take note of the supplement inositol (see Chapter 10, page 240) because research has shown that it can reduce the risk of developing gestational diabetes.[7]

If just improving insulin sensitivity doesn't work and you need more help, studies have also shown that metformin[10] helps to reduce the risk of developing gestational diabetes. Although my preferred method is always to improve insulin sensitivity before getting pregnant (because of the potential risks that I explained in Chapter 5), if you're unable to do that, then managing your blood glucose with diet and/or metformin or inositol is the way to go if you do develop gestational diabetes.

If you do develop gestational diabetes, I can recommend the book: *Real Food for Gestational Diabetes* by Lily Nichols. She gives you all the evidenced-based advice for a healthy pregnancy with gestational diabetes.

MISCARRIAGE

We've all heard of miscarriages, but what are they? A miscarriage is pregnancy loss before the twentieth week, but most miscarriages happen before 10 to 12 weeks of pregnancy. Many miscarriages occur in the first few weeks before you even know you are pregnant.

Miscarriage doesn't look the same for all women. The earliest bleeding can vary from a brownish discharge to clear fluid with a pink tinge. Bleeding can often start with this spotting and then move to a heavier flow, which can start suddenly and come as a shock. Usually, the heavier bleeding lasts one to two days.

If the miscarriage is before four to five weeks of pregnancy, it may just look like a heavy menstrual period with no clots. But if it happens after six weeks, clots are more likely, and there may be an identifiable fetus and placenta, which may be greyish in color. I'm telling you this to prepare you, because if you're not expecting it, then it can be very traumatic. Miscarriage is an incredibly tough experience, but the more you know, the better prepared you can be.

Some studies show that miscarriage is more common in women with PCOS than those without PCOS. For example, one large Australian study showed that the miscarriage rate in women with PCOS was 20 percent compared with 15 percent in those without PCOS;[11] another study found a miscarriage rate of up to 40 percent in women with PCOS.[12] A study on women going through IVF found that the miscarriage rate for women with PCOS was twice as high as for women without PCOS.[13] But *please* don't let these figures scare you—I've seen that addressing the root cause of your PCOS can reduce the risk of miscarriage dramatically.

Causes of miscarriage

Many things can cause a miscarriage. Some of these are actually protective. For example, we know that when a fertilized egg has an abnormal number of chromosomes, your body will often choose to miscarry instead of carrying a child to term that might not survive for very long. These abnormal numbers of chromosomes occur at random, so you can't either prevent it or cause it to happen. Other factors leading to miscarriage can include certain illnesses, a very serious infection, or a major injury; being over 30 years of age also increases your risk of miscarriage.[14] Again, these are causes that you can't really prevent.

However, other causes *are* preventable. As a miscarriage is often devastating emotionally, you want to reduce your risk as much as possible. In PCOS, the things that can increase your risk of miscarriage are the same things that are contributing to your PCOS symptoms: your "root cause(s)". As you now know, each root cause has adverse effects on your "fertile ingredients," especially in the case of insulin.

High insulin leads to low progesterone

We know that insulin plays a major role in miscarriage.[15] As we've already discussed, if your body is overproducing insulin, this will affect all of your fertile ingredients (see page 39–40). High levels of insulin lead to low progesterone levels,[16] and this increases the risk of miscarriage because progesterone keeps your "nest" (uterine lining) in place. If your uterine lining falls away, the fertilized egg or fetus will be lost (miscarried) along with it.

The importance of progesterone for maintaining pregnancy in the first trimester (the first three months of pregnancy) was first recognized in the 1970s. The corpus luteum (the follicle the egg develops in and leaves behind after ovulation) provides all the progesterone to the fetus until the eighth to twelfth week of pregnancy,[17] after which the fetus can produce its own.[18] The pioneering researchers back in the 1970s demonstrated that if the corpus luteum was removed before seven weeks of pregnancy, it always resulted in a miscarriage.[19]

Low progesterone is very treatable, but unfortunately many women go undiagnosed because the standard laboratory reference ranges are too low. The optimal level of progesterone for preventing miscarriage is actually 25 ng/mL, which is *much* higher than the lowest end of the current reference range, which is 11.2 ng/mL.[20] One study investigated what would happen to miscarriage rates if women took natural progesterone supplements to increase their progesterone to above the 25 ng/mL level. The researchers measured the progesterone of 182 women seen in fertility clinics every two to six weeks, and the women who had levels below 25 ng/mL were given natural progesterone supplements to improve their levels. The results showed that only 12 percent of women with progesterone levels below 25 ng/dL threshold carried a baby to term, as opposed to 72 percent of those who were over the threshold![20] The effect of supplementing with progesterone was even more dramatic for women over 35 years old—none of the older women with low progesterone levels carried a baby to term, but 58 percent of those with higher progesterone levels did.[20]

High insulin leads to high LH

The second way that insulin can contribute to miscarriage is by raising the level of LH. In Chapter 2 (page 40), I talked about how insulin drives up LH, upsetting the ratio of LH to FSH and stopping you ovulating. Well, it turns out that if your body isn't ovulating properly, this may also affect your ability to carry a baby to term—high levels of LH are linked with high miscarriage rates. In one study of women with PCOS, the researchers found that women with lower LH levels were more likely to conceive and also less likely to miscarry.[21]

> Findings like these for LH are precisely why I'm so vocal about treating the root cause *first*—or, at the very least, alongside a medication that helps improve your fertility. As I explained in Chapter 4, the problem with the current medical model regarding fertility and PCOS is that it focuses just on treating the symptoms, not the root cause. And the root cause, if untreated, has a massive knock-on effect.

Reducing the risk of miscarriage
Address insulin and progesterone levels

To reduce the risk of miscarriage, we need to fix the root cause of your PCOS. If your insulin sensitivity improves, then your LH levels reduce, and your progesterone levels increase, and you are more likely to carry to term.

One clinical trial showed that improving insulin sensitivity decreased miscarriage rates from 40 percent to 8 percent.[12] This improvement was even more pronounced for women who had a history of miscarriages, where the rate fell from 50 percent to 11 percent.[12] Note that in this study the researchers used metformin, but as you now know (see Chapters 7 and 8, in particular), this isn't the only way to improve insulin sensitivity, and metformin has its own risks (see Chapter 5).

> Just another note—as I mentioned in Chapter 3, many doctors will tell you to lose weight "to reduce your risk." What they actually mean is "to improve your insulin," as improving your insulin will help you lose weight. It was originally thought that obesity was what caused miscarriage. However, a study that looked into this found that obesity was linked to increased miscarriage rates, *but* this was associated with insulin, and insulin was an *independent* risk factor for miscarriage.[15] In other words, you could be lean, but if you also had high insulin levels, then you were still at higher risk of miscarriage.[15]

Additionally, when you do get pregnant, have your progesterone tested a few times during the first trimester. If your progesterone level is below 25 ng/mL, get your doctor or naturopathic practitioner to prescribe some micronized (natural) progesterone supplements to bring the levels up. I do not recommend using synthetic progestins, because these don't have the same effect as micronized (natural) progesterone.

Address hypothyroidism
As we discussed in Chapter 2 and Chapter 6, your thyroid plays a major

role in you getting pregnant. But it also plays a role in whether you can stay pregnant, even if you're not clinically hypothyroid (have too little thyroid hormone). For many years, researchers have been reporting that women with thyroid levels that are not outside the reference range but are on the low side (subclinical hypothyroidism), are at greater risk of miscarriage.[22] In a systematic review of the research, it was found that women with subclinical hypothyroidism have higher miscarriage rates than women with normal thyroid levels.[22]

Thyroid hormones are crucial for the normal development of your baby's brain and nervous system. During the first trimester, your baby depends on you to supply thyroid hormone through the placenta. At around 12 weeks, your baby's thyroid starts to work on its own, but it doesn't make enough thyroid hormone until 18 to 20 weeks of pregnancy.[23] This is why hypothyroidism can increase your risk of miscarriage.

Hypothyroidism is defined as having high thyroid-stimulating hormone (TSH) and low thyroid hormone levels.[24] Most of the time, your doctor will only check your TSH levels. TSH is produced by the pituitary gland in your brain (not by your thyroid). When your brain detects that your thyroid levels are low, it tells your pituitary to pump out more TSH, which then stimulates your thyroid to produce more hormones. The reason behind checking your TSH levels is that the higher these are, the lower your thyroid hormone levels are meant to be. But it doesn't always work quite this way; I've seen many cases where TSH looks normal but the actual thyroid hormones that do the work, T_4 and T_3, are low.

One study looked at women with either really low thyroid hormone levels (overt hypothyroidism) or with borderline levels (subclinical hypothyroidism, meaning low levels that are still just within the reference range).[25] When left untreated, 60 percent of the hypothyroid women and 71 percent of the subclinical women miscarried. However, if they were adequately treated with thyroid hormone replacement (the study used levothyroxine), 100 percent of the overtly hypothyroid women and 90.5 percent of the subclinical women carried pregnancies to term.[25]

In 2009, the American Thyroid Association (ATA) formed a task force to put together guidelines for the management of thyroid conditions in pregnancy. This task force consisted of international experts in the field of thyroid disease and pregnancy, and included representatives from the ATA, the Asia and Oceania Thyroid Association, the Latin American Thyroid Society, the American College of Obstetricians and Gynecologists, and the Midwives Alliance of North America. They reviewed all the evidence and put together a recommendation that TSH levels should be maintained at between 0.2 and 2.5 mU/L in the first trimester of pregnancy, and between 0.3 and 3 mU/L in the remaining trimesters.[26]

Check your thyroid antibodies

Low levels of thyroid hormone (see above) are not the only issue—the presence of thyroid antibodies is also a factor. There have been many studies over the past two decades that show that women with high levels of thyroid antibodies have a higher risk of miscarriage, even if their other thyroid levels are completely fine.[27] This is really important to know, as a quarter of women with PCOS have thyroid antibodies or subclinical hypothyroidism,[28] and most often your doctor will test only TSH, as mentioned above—so they may completely miss that your body is producing thyroid antibodies.

If any of your family has a thyroid condition (and it's especially common in females—up to five times higher in women of childbearing age than in men), get a full thyroid panel tested every six months.[29]

In the first stage of Hashimoto's thyroiditis, your thyroid hormone levels will be normal but your thyroid antibodies will be high. Studies have shown that this is enough to cause a three-fold increase in miscarriage and pregnancy complications.[30] This occurs because high thyroid antibodies are the first warning sign—your thyroid hormone levels will already be declining but are not yet out of the reference range. However, when you become pregnant, your body's demand for thyroid hormone skyrockets, and if your thyroid is already struggling then it will really struggle to keep up with the new demand.

One study involved 1,500 pregnant women in Pakistan, who had their thyroid antibodies and thyroid hormone levels measured throughout their pregnancy. Women with high thyroid antibodies but normal thyroid hormone levels had a miscarriage rate of 36 percent, compared with only 1.8 percent for those that had no thyroid antibodies.[31] In addition, 27 percent of women with high antibodies had a preterm birth compared with just 8 percent of women with normal thyroid antibody levels.[31] Note that all of these women had normal TSH and thyroid hormone levels—it was just their thyroid antibodies that were high!

As this was only a correlational study, it was not able to prove that it was the antibodies that caused the high rates. So, a group of Italian researchers sought to check the theory out. They recruited a group of 948 women from southern Italy who were in their first trimester of pregnancy, and measured their thyroid levels and their thyroid antibody levels. The 115 women who had high thyroid antibodies were allocated two groups; one group received thyroid hormone replacement drugs (levothyroxine) and the other group, along with the 869 women who didn't have thyroid antibodies (the control group), did not receive anything. The rate of miscarriage in the women with high levels of antibodies who didn't receive the treatment was significantly higher, 14 percent, compared with only 3.5 percent in the levothyroxine group and 2.4 percent in the control group.[32]

It is especially important to get your thyroid antibodies checked if you've had recurrent miscarriages (i.e. three or more). Many studies have shown that women with recurrent miscarriages tend to have higher thyroid antibody levels.[27] Of course this isn't the only reason for recurrent miscarriages, but it's a good thing to check.

Check for the MTHFR genetic mutation

Another factor that can increase the risk of miscarriage in PCOS is a mutation in one of your genes, the MTHFR gene. As we discussed in Chapter 11 (page 278), a defect with your MTHFR gene can affect your ability to get pregnant—and it may also cause miscarriage, especially recurrent miscarriages.[33] If you have inherited the MTHFR genetic mutation from both your parents, studies have shown that you could be three times more likely to miscarry compared with women with a normally functioning gene.[34]

As we also learned in Chapter 11, the MTHFR genetic mutation can result in high levels of homocysteine in your body. Homocysteine is an amino acid that we naturally produce to help our body use B vitamins. However, if you have the MTHFR C677T mutation, your body can't produce an enzyme that breaks down homocysteine;[35] it accumulates in your body and you develop homocysteinemia (high homocysteine levels). This causes your body to develop tiny blood clots, which stop oxygen and nutrients from being able to reach the placenta and subsequently the fetus. The result is that the fetus essentially starves and is miscarried.

A good analogy for this is a blockage in the exhaust pipe of your car. When you drive, the engine converts petrol to energy, but there are byproducts of that conversion. The purpose of your car's exhaust is to get rid of these byproducts out of the car, as they'll affect the car's ability to run. If the pipe is blocked and the exhaust gases can't get out, there will be no room for fresh air to get into the combustion chambers—the engine won't be able to run, and the car will stall.

Your ability to produce the MTHFR enzyme that breaks down homocysteine is reduced by about 35 percent if you've inherited the genetic mutation from one parent (heterozygous), or by about 70 percent if you've inherited the mutation from both your parents (homozygous).[35] While there is no conclusive "proof" that an MTHFR genetic mutation causes miscarriages, it's been described as a "strong risk factor" for recurrent miscarriage,[36] and there is a plausible mechanism as small blood clots have regularly been found in women with a history of recurrent miscarriages.[37] And, interestingly, it's not just your genetics that matter—it's also your partner's. A study has shown that MTHFR mutations on the male side are also associated with a higher risk of recurrent miscarriage.[36]

But remember, having this genetic mutation doesn't mean the end for you—there are treatments available. If you have had recurrent miscarriages, the first step is to get a genetic test for both you *and* your partner to see if you do have one or more copies of the MTHFR genetic mutation, and also get your blood homocysteine levels tested.

PRE-ECLAMPSIA AND LATE PRETERM DELIVERY

Pre-eclampsia and late preterm delivery are also potential pregnancy complications in PCOS. Pre-eclampsia is a disorder that causes high blood pressure and large amounts of protein in the urine, and is the most common medical complication in pregnancy. It can lead to eclampsia (seizures), which is a major cause of death in both mothers and babies during pregnancy—eclampsia can also affect the placenta, resulting in a lack of oxygen and nutrients for the baby, which can impair fetal growth and/or result in stillbirth.

Pre-eclampsia can more commonly occur in late preterm birth. Late preterm birth is defined as birth between 34 and 37 weeks of pregnancy, and commonly causes issues. Many people, even medical professionals, believe that 37 weeks is "almost term," so it's fine, but the research shows that this is not the case. Babies born between 34 and 37 weeks (rather than 39 to 40 weeks, which is when most women go into labor) are up to six times more likely to die at birth or as an infant than are full-term babies.[38] They are also far more likely to get jaundice (yellowing of the skin), which is caused by high levels of bilirubin and can cause brain injury, and are also more likely to suffer developmental issues later in life.[38] Babies born before 37 weeks are three times more likely to be diagnosed with cerebral palsy, and are also more likely to have mental retardation and schizophrenia.[38] They have been shown to have worse school performances than their full-term counterparts in every aspect.[38] I am outlining all of this not to scare you, but simply to highlight that fact that there are risks even with later preterm births, which is why it's a good idea to reduce your risk if possible.

Women with PCOS have a 2.7 times higher chance of developing pre-eclampsia and a 1.5 times greater risk of having a preterm baby, compared with women without PCOS.[39] However, it's not just "PCOS" that increases our risk—it's having high levels of androgens (testosterone, DHEA-S, etc.).[40] When researchers looked into what was going on, they found that just having PCOS puts women at no greater risk, but having high androgen levels does.[40]

As you've learned in earlier chapters, we can lower our androgen levels if we address the root cause—whether that's insulin or high-stress hormones, or something else. In so many cases, including my own, I've seen that when we address the root cause, we can easily bring down our androgen levels. In 2013 my testosterone was well over the high end of the normal range, whereas in 2018 it had significantly reduced to the low end of the normal range. I achieved this just by making my body more sensitive to insulin—eating food that suited my insulin, changing my exercise, bringing down my stress levels (by doing less extreme endurance training and just chilling out), and getting the vitamins and minerals my body needed. So focus on your "root cause" and the steps outlined in Chapters 6 to 10 for at least six months.

Chapter 13
Protecting your fertility

If you're not looking to conceive now but would like to in the future, then this book is perfect for you too (and massive kudos to you for thinking about this now and giving yourself time to prepare). With fertility and the art of getting pregnant it can feel like you can't do anything until you actually start trying, but this is absolutely not true. You can start preparing your body for fertility years ahead of actually wanting to become pregnant, and I would actually recommend that you do this. If you have PCOS, it can sometimes take that long to get your cycles normal, especially if you've been on hormonal birth control (HBC). Similarly, if your partner's sperm is suboptimal, it could take up to two years to resolve that.

In this chapter, we're going to cover everything you need to know to give your body the best chance of conceiving naturally in the future. (Your partner's sperm is covered in Chapter 6.) But as you'll also learn, getting all this sorted now isn't just important for fertility—it's actually important for your optimal health now and in the future.

START PROTECTING YOUR FERTILITY EARLY ON
Understand your "root cause(s)"

The most important first step is to investigate your personal PCOS root cause(s). Do this as early as possible! This isn't just about fertility, or your acne, weight gain, hair growth, hair loss, or other symptoms. It is also about you being in optimal health, rather than just "getting by."

It can take many months to understand what's going on with your body and then implement the correct lifestyle changes to address it. So the earlier you get onto it, the more years you'll have of fertility and (hopefully) reduced PCOS symptoms. In my experience, it realistically takes most women at least three months, if not six months, to see any changes in symptoms. And most women will need to keep up with those lifestyle changes for most of their life. So, instead of thinking that you're going to do a 12-week "diet," think about it as a lifestyle change.

Go back to Chapter 6 and implement the steps to understand your root causes. Then move on to Chapters 7, 8 and 10 and implement the appropriate lifestyle changes for you.

CASE STUDY

Alana is a great example of someone who was proactive in protecting her future fertility. Alana was what the medical world might call a "classic" PCOS case. She had a long family history of insulin resistance and diabetes, and had always struggled with her weight. This started when she was a child, and her weight steadily increased by about 6 to 9 lb (3 to 4 kg) every year. Her periods were also extremely irregular, and she was diagnosed with PCOS and insulin resistance when she was in her teens. Like me, Alana was told that she would probably have trouble conceiving.

She was advised to lose weight if she wanted to improve her symptoms. In her twenties, Alana lost around 45 lb (20 kg) but still felt heavy, sluggish, and out of sorts. As a midwife and nutritionist, she was well aware of what PCOS was and how to live a "healthy" life. She joined my *PCOS Protocol* program and learned about the specifics of what she needed to do to really improve her insulin—

not just her nutrition, but also how to manage her sleep and stress, her exercise, and the vitamins and minerals that her insulin receptors needed to work properly.

Alana lost 15 lb (7 kg), her cycles regulated to 30 to 36 days, and through using fertility awareness she could see that she was now ovulating every month (for one of the first times in her life). Her skin cleared up, her hair stopped falling out, her hirsutism disappeared, and her bloating ceased. Again, like many other women I've seen, her weight was the last thing to change—proving yet again that we need to improve the insulin before the weight moves.

After 12 weeks of using the *PCOS Protocol*, Alana got married, and a few months later she and her partner decided to start trying for a family. They conceived in the first month of trying and now have a healthy baby boy.

Just this result is incredible on its own, and shows that it is possible to go from not ovulating for years to ovulating every month and conceiving on the first try. But additionally, Alana was able to see that her insulin levels and Hb1Ac were now in the normal range, showing that she had reversed her insulin resistance. This was huge for Alana, as she is a midwife with a special interest in the first 1,000 days of a baby's life—which includes the time when the egg is developing. Alana was motivated to try to break her family's cycle of type 2 diabetes by reducing her insulin and giving her baby the best chance of normal metabolism. This is why it's great if you can start preparing for fertility before you want to start trying.

Come off hormonal birth control

My recommendation is to come off HBC 18 to 24 months before you want to become pregnant. This will allow you to uncover any issues that might not have been there prior to you going on HBC, and will also allow your body to start ovulating again on its own.

I'm sure you've heard countless stories of women coming off HBC and getting pregnant the very next month. But for every one of those, I hear an equal number of opposite accounts, with periods taking months, if not years, to regulate after stopping oral contraception.

Many women, even those without PCOS, may experience an 18- to 24-month delay in their cycles returning naturally after coming off HBC. In one study, researchers compared the cycles of 175 women who'd been on the combined contraceptive pill with 284 women who'd never taken the pill at all. They found that the women who had been on the combined pill experienced more irregular cycles for several months after coming off HBC, and it took an average of nine to 12 cycles before they normalized.[1] This is nine to 12 cycles—not months; those cycles could have been 60 days or longer.

If you have PCOS and irregular cycles, you are almost certainly going to experience a delay in your cycles regulating, given what we know about HBC reducing insulin sensitivity. Research shows that if you were put on HBC to "regulate your cycles," you may have an even greater delay. In a study of 63 women whose cycles didn't return after coming off HBC, researchers found that 40 of the women had had irregular cycles before going on HBC. The researchers concluded that: "Combined estrogen–progestin contraceptives should be used with caution in women with irregular menstruation."[2]

Given this, I strongly recommend that you come off HBC at least 18 months to two years before you really want to conceive if you can. I give give some non-hormonal methods of contraception on the next page.

Get your partner to have his sperm checked

Lastly, if you have a partner, encourage him to get his sperm checked 18 to 24 months out from wanting to conceive. As I explained in Chapter 6 (see page 117), a review of all the research on fertility found that 40 to 50 percent of all infertility is caused by male factor infertility.[3] Just like it can take some time to address any issues with your ovulation, it can take some time to get sperm quality levels up to optimum. So it's best practice to do that now while you've got some time to prepare. Follow the guidelines in Chapter 6 to understand what optimal sperm quality is and how to achieve (or at least improve) it.

NON-HORMONAL METHODS OF CONTRACEPTION

So, what do you use for contraception instead of HBC? Contraception is a very personal choice, and this is where you need to decide what works for you. That might even mean that you choose not to take the above advice to come off HBC. And that's okay—you need to do what's right for you. You may be in a situation where you absolutely cannot become pregnant in the 18 to 24 months prior to wanting to conceive, and in that case you may want a form of birth control that allows for virtually no human error.

However, in my experience of working with women from a natural fertility perspective, there are many non-hormonal options available which can be both really well liked and incredibly effective when you have learned to use them correctly. It all comes down to you, your appetite for an unplanned pregnancy, and your willingness to learn new techniques for contraception so that you can use them properly.

Here I will discuss the copper coil, the symptom–thermal fertility awareness method, and barrier methods of contraception.

Copper coil

The copper coil is a non-hormonal IUD (intrauterine device)—it's inserted into your uterus. It doesn't have any hormones, so it doesn't stop you from ovulating. Instead, it works by damaging sperm and disrupting their motility so that they are not able to join with an egg. The way it does this is by actually cutting off the tails of the sperm[4]—how fascinating is that?

This is a completely reversible form of contraception; and because it doesn't stop ovulation, your periods continue as usual and you can conceive immediately after it's removed.[5] It's got one of the highest satisfaction ratings of any birth control method,[6] and I know countless women who've used the copper IUD for years without any issues. It's also incredibly effective, with just a 0.1 to 0.4 percent failure rate with perfect use.[7]

However, it's not without faults. In some cases it can increase bleeding and cramps;[8] and many women, including myself, have found that it increases anxiety levels. As someone who'd never suffered from anxiety before, I had no idea what was going on with my body. On an evening out in London in 2016, I suddenly felt an extremely tight sensation in my chest, my breathing got shallow and rapid, and my heart was racing. After this happened a few more times, my doctor told me they were panic attacks. We put this down to starting a new business and all the stress and financial pressure of that, and of living in a country that wasn't my home, away from family. While I agreed that this was probably part of the puzzle, it still didn't quite add up. I had been under a lot of stress before, as an élite athlete and doing my honors thesis, and had not reacted in this way. The only thing that had really changed in the past six months was that I'd had a copper IUD inserted. I googled "copper IUD and anxiety"— and saw thousands of stories from other women with similar symptoms: panic attacks, anxiety, depression, chronic fatigue, and hair loss. For most women, including myself, the symptoms disappeared when the IUD was removed.

Not all women react badly to the copper IUD, and this is likely due to individual variation. While there is no proof that the copper IUD can cause the symptoms I've described above, that may just be because, to date, there are no published studies that have looked into a possible connection. But there is a very plausible mechanism. Copper works in combination with zinc in your body in a ratio that your body normally keeps tightly controlled at 1:1. Multiple studies have reported increased blood copper levels and lower zinc levels in people suffering from anxiety,[9, 10] and the copper IUD is known to increase copper levels after three months of women having had the copper IUD inserted.[11]

Additionally, copper can kill bacteria and fungus, and it works well in humid environments. If there is an infection or inflammation in your body, your body will draw more copper from the IUD to fight the infection, which can create an imbalance in minerals and cause symptoms of copper toxicity. Safety information for the copper IUD Paragard states "Do not use Paragard if you have a pelvic infection, or get infections easily."[12]

In addition, excess estrogen can also cause copper retention, and women with PCOS often have high levels of estrogen. But even without an infection or estrogen excess, the copper content in the IUD may cause issues depending on how much zinc you have. Excess copper in your body can cause issues with your thyroid in particular, so you need to be aware of this if you have a thyroid condition.

Given all this information, it's very plausible that the connection between the copper IUD and anxiety isn't just "women crying wolf." However, the issues certainly don't happen to all women—the majority find that it works really well for them. So try the copper IUD for yourself, consider taking some extra zinc, and be alert for symptoms indicating that there is a problem. If you do get these symptoms, you can always have the IUD removed.

Fertility awareness method (FAM)

Before you roll your eyes, hear me out. FAM is completely misunderstood, and is widely believed to be unreliable. But if done correctly, studies have shown that it's 99.4 to 99.6 percent effective (i.e. as effective as HBC).[13] I know this because I'm a qualified teacher in fertility awareness; this means that I've done a lot more training in this area than your average doctor or even family planning practitioner.

The fertility awareness method outlined in Chapter 9 uses your cervical fluid characteristics and your basal body temperature to determine when you are fertile (only about six days in your cycle). During that fertile window, you use condoms or diaphragms during sex. Many people, even doctors, believe that FAM just means counting days to determine when you're ovulating, which is completely inaccurate—counting days is only 75 percent effective as a means of contraception, and possibly even less if you have an irregular cycle.[14]

CASE STUDY

In 2018 I met Holly while on vacation. Holly confided in me that she was really concerned about her future fertility and had gone off HBC to give her body a break. She'd been on the pill since she was 16, and had heard many horror stories of women being unable to conceive after coming off it. So instead, Holly was now using the Clue app to tell her when she was fertile. She hadn't been taking her temperature every morning—all she needed to do was put in the days of her period, and the app would tell her when she was fertile and when not.

This is what's called the "rhythm" method, where you just count days, and it is extremely unreliable. It is especially so if you have irregular periods with PCOS, as your fertile days and when you ovulate change every month. But even if you have a regular cycle, your fertile days and ovulation can still change dramatically from one month to the next. I had one client with a very regular 30-day cycle, and her day of ovulation changed from Day 14 to 22 to 19 to 17 all within the space of four months. So please don't use the rhythm method if you don't want to get pregnant. (Unfortunately, this advice was too late for Holly, and she had an unwanted pregnancy.)

Instead of the rhythm method (counting days), you need to school yourself up on the symptom–thermal method of fertility awareness (see Chapter 9). Trust me, it's not hard, though it does take a bit of practice. Research has shown that with perfect use, this method can be 97 to 99.5 percent effective in preventing pregnancy.[14] Side note: This is also very useful because by the time you want to get pregnant, you will also be very experienced in detecting your fertile window!

Good books to read are *The Fifth Vital Sign* by Lisa Hendrickson Jacks—a trained fertility awareness educator, who also hosts a very popular podcast: "Fertility Fridays" or *Taking Charge of Your Fertility* by Toni Weschler. Read these, follow the rules, work with a fertility awareness educator for a few months to help give you confidence while you use condoms, and then you'll be set for life.

Barrier methods

A barrier method is anything that puts a barrier between the sperm and your cervix. Barriers include the male and female condoms, the diaphragm, the cervical cap, and the sponge, to name the most popular.

These are less effective contraceptive methods compared with the copper coil or the symptom-thermal fertility awareness method (FAM). But remember that it doesn't have to be an either/or choice when it comes to these methods. You can easily combine FAM with using condoms or a diaphragm, and even the withdrawal method as well for further protection when you're in your "fertile phase" to increase the effectiveness of all of them.

In terms of effectiveness, the diaphragm has a 9 percent failure rate with perfect use, but a 16 percent failure rate with typical use.[15] The male condom has only a 2 percent failure rate with perfect use, but a 15 percent failure rate with typical use, and the female condom has a 5 percent and 21 percent failure rate with perfect and typical use, respectively.[15]

Understanding all the barrier methods available to you can help with getting around issues with them. For example, if you or your partner has an allergy to the latex used to make condoms, you could use a diaphragm (made from silicone) instead.

A FINAL COMMENT

If you want to protect your future fertility, my advice for you would be to allow your body to ovulate, and to learn the fertility awareness method as a method of contraception. FAM won't just help you not to conceive; it will also help you understand when you're fertile so that when you *do* want to conceive, you can. It will also allow you to check whether your luteal phase is sufficiently long, and will protect your heart, breast, and bone health.

Please don't rely on apps. Take the time to learn FAM properly, and get a fertility awareness educator to help you to make it 99 percent effective.

Final word

Your body wants to ovulate and reproduce. After survival, reproduction is the next most basic instinct, and that holds true for women with PCOS, too. Getting pregnant with PCOS is very possible. PCOS isn't a condition of infertility but subfertility—it might take you slightly longer to fall pregnant than someone without PCOS, but it is very possible.

Research has proven that women with PCOS have no fewer children than those without PCOS.[1] And this isn't just due to the help of fertility treatments. The majority of women with PCOS will have at least one child without any fertility treatment at all.[2]

I hope that this book has inspired you to get to the root cause of your PCOS, not just for your fertility, but for your own health and wellbeing. I also hope it has demonstrated that you don't need to be pressured to be "all natural" on your fertility journey, but that you know what can cause fertility issues in women with PCOS and that medical fertility treatments aren't the only option nor the most effective for many women. In many cases, the best approach for you might be a combination of lifestyle changes and medical intervention.

You now have the knowledge to understand your own body and make informed decisions about your health and fertility. Much of this is within your control through the lifestyle changes you make, and when you understand the "root cause" for you, you can be so much more targeted with the changes you implement.

References

Introduction

1. Teede, H., Misso, M., Costello, M., et al. *International evidence-based guideline for the assessment and management of polycystic ovary syndrome.* Melbourne, VIC, Australia: Monash University, 2018.

Chapter 1

1. Revised 2003 consensus on diagnostic criteria and long-term health risks related to polycystic ovary syndrome. *Fertility and Sterility* 2004; 81(1): 19–25. doi: 10.1016/j.fertnstert.2003.10.004

2. Boyle, J. & Teede, H. J. Polycystic ovary syndrome: an update. *Australian Family Physician* 2012; 41(10): 752–6.

3. Azziz, R., Black, V., Hines, G. A., et al. Adrenal androgen excess in the polycystic ovary syndrome: sensitivity and responsivity of the hypothalamic–pituitary–adrenal axis. *Journal of Clinical Endocrinology & Metabolism* 1998; 83(7): 2317–23. doi: 10.1210/jc.83.7.2317

4. Khadilkar, S. S. Polycystic ovarian syndrome: is it time to rename PCOS to HA-PODS? *Journal of Obstetrics & Gynecology of India* 2016; 66(2): 81–7. doi: 10.1007/s13224-016-0851-9

5. Zegers-Hochschild, F., Adamson, G. D., Dyer, S., et al. The international glossary on infertility and fertility care, 2017. *Fertility and Sterility* 2017; 108(3): 393–406. doi: 10.1016/j.fertnstert.2017.06.005

6. Dumesic, D. A., Padmanabhan, V. & Abbott, D. H. Polycystic ovary syndrome and oocyte developmental competence. *Obstetrical & Gynecological Survey* 2008; 63(1): 39–48. doi: 10.1097/ogx.0b013e31815e85fc

7. Dumitrescu, R., Mehedintu, C., Briceag, I., et al. The polycystic ovary syndrome: an update on metabolic and hormonal mechanisms. *Journal of Medicine and Life* 2015; 8(2): 142–5.

Chapter 2

1. Azziz, R., Dumesic, D. A. & Goodarzi, M. O. Polycystic ovary syndrome: an ancient disorder? *Fertility and Sterility* 2011; 95(5): 1544–8. doi: 10.1016/j.fertnstert.2010.09.032

2. Charifson, M. A. & Trumble, B. C. Evolutionary origins of polycystic ovary syndrome: an environmental mismatch disorder. *Evolution, Medicine, and Public Health* 2019; (1): 50–63. doi: 10.1093/emph/eoz011

3. Vink, J. M., Sadrzadeh, S., Lambalk, C. B. & Boomsma, D. Heritability of polycystic ovary syndrome in a Dutch twin-family study. *Journal of Clinical Endocrinology & Metabolism* 2006; 91(6): 2100–4. doi: 10.1210/jc.2005-1494

4. Juul, F. & Hemmingsson, E. Trends in consumption of ultra-processed foods and obesity in Sweden between 1960 and 2010. *Public Health Nutrition* 2015; 18(17): 3096–107. doi: 10.1017/s1368980015000506

5. Conrad, D. F., Keebler, J. E. M., Depristo, M. A., et al. Variation in genome-wide mutation rates within and between human families. *Nature Genetics* 2011; 43(7): 712–4. doi: 10.1038/ng.862

6. Office for National Statistics (ONS). Women shoulder the responsibility of "unpaid work," London, UK: Office for National Statistics, 10 November 2016. https://www.ons.gov.uk/employmentandlabourmarket/peopleinwork/earningsandworkinghours/articles/womenshouldertheresponsibilityofunpaidwork/2016-11-10

7.   Berman, J. Women's unpaid work is the backbone of the American economy. *MarketWatch*, 15 April 2018. https://www.marketwatch.com/story/this-is-how-much-more-unpaid-work-women-do-than-men-2017-03-07

8.   Organisation for Economic Co-operation and Development (OECD). OECD.Stat, data extracted 3 July 2020. https://stats.oecd.org/Index.aspx?datasetcode=TIME_USE

9.   Barthelmess, E. K. & Naz, R. K. Polycystic ovary syndrome: current status and future perspective. *Frontiers in Bioscience* 2014; E6(1): 104–19. doi: 10.2741/e695

10. Stepto, N. K., Cassar, S., Joham, A. E., et al. Women with polycystic ovary syndrome have intrinsic insulin resistance on euglycaemic-hyperinsulaemic clamp. *Human Reproduction* 2013; 28(3): 777–84. doi: 10.1093/humrep/des463

11. Deswal, R., Yadav, A. & Dang, A. S. Sex hormone binding globulin—an important biomarker for predicting PCOS risk: a systematic review and meta-analysis. *Systems Biology in Reproductive Medicine* 2018; 64(1): 12–24. doi: 10.1080/19396368.2017.1410591

12. Dunaif, A. Insulin resistance and the polycystic ovary syndrome: mechanism and implications for pathogenesis. *Endocrine Reviews* 1997; 18(6): 774–800. doi: 10.1210/edrv.18.6.0318

13. Franks, S., Stark, J. & Hardy, K. Follicle dynamics and anovulation in polycystic ovary syndrome. *Human Reproduction Update* 2008; 14(4): 367–78. doi: 10.1093/humupd/dmn015

14. Berga, S. L., Guzick, D. S. & Winters, S. J. Increased luteinizing hormone and alpha-subunit secretion in women with hyperandrogenic anovulation. *Journal of Clinical Endocrinology & Metabolism* 1993; 77(4): 895–901. doi: 10.1210/jcem.77.4.7691863

15. Taylor, A. E., McCourt, B., Martin, K. A., et al. Determinants of abnormal gonadotropin secretion in clinically defined women with polycystic ovary syndrome. *Journal of Clinical Endocrinology & Metabolism* 1997; 82(7): 2248–56. doi: 10.1210/jcem.82.7.4105

16. Meenakumari, K. J., Agarwal, S., Krishna, A. & Pandey, L. K. Effects of metformin treatment on luteal phase progesterone concentration in polycystic ovary syndrome. *Brazilian Journal of Medical and Biological Research* 2004; 37(11): 1637–44. doi: 10.1590/S0100-879x2004001100007

17. Balen, A. H., Tan, S-L., Macdougall, J. & Jacobs, H. S. Miscarriage rates following in-vitro fertilization are increased in women with polycystic ovaries and reduced by pituitary desensitization with buserelin. *Human Reproduction* 1993; 8(6): 959–64. doi: 10.1093/oxfordjournals.humrep.a138174

18. Sagle, M., Bishop, K., Ridley, N., et al. Recurrent early miscarriage and polycystic ovaries. *BMJ* 1988; 297(6655): 1027–8. doi: 10.1136/bmj.297.6655.1027

19. Brown, A. E. & Walker, M. Genetics of insulin resistance and the metabolic syndrome. *Current Cardiology Reports* 2016; 18: 75. doi: 10.1007/S11886-016-0755-4

20. Hickey, T. E., Legro, R. S. & Norman, R. J. Epigenetic modification of the X chromosome influences susceptibility to polycystic ovary syndrome. *Journal of Clinical Endocrinology & Metabolism* 2006; 91(7): 2789–91. doi: 10.1210/jc.2006-0069

21. Nordström, P., Pedersen, N. L., Gustafson, Y., et al. Risks of myocardial infarction, death, and diabetes in identical twin pairs with different body mass indexes. *JAMA Internal Medicine* 2016; 176(10): 1522–9. doi: https://doi.org/10.1001/jamainternmed.2016.4104

22. Macdonald, I. A. A review of recent evidence relating to sugars, insulin resistance and diabetes. *European Journal of Nutrition* 2016; 55(Suppl 2): 17–23. doi: 10.1007/S00394-016-1340-8

23. Blotsky, A. L., Rahme, E., Dahhou, M. et al. Gestational diabetes associated with incident diabetes in childhood and youth: a retrospective cohort study. *Canadian Medical Association Journal* 2019; 191(15): E410–17. doi: 10.1503/cmaj.181001

24. Entringer, S., Wüst, S., Kumsta, R., et al. Prenatal psychosocial stress exposure is associated with insulin resistance in young adults. *American Journal of Obstetrics & Gynecology* 2008; 199(5): 498.e1–7. doi: 10.1016/j.ajog.2008.03.006

25. Wild, S., Roglic, G., Green, A., et al. Global prevalence of diabetes: estimates for the year 2000 and projections for 2030. *Diabetes Care* 2004; 27(5): 1047–53. doi: 10.2337/diacare.27.5.1047

26. Caricilli, A. M. & Saad, M. J. The role of gut microbiota on insulin resistance. *Nutrients* 2013; 5(3): 829–51. doi: 10.3390/nu5030829

27. Punjabi, N. M., Shahar, E., Redline, S., et al. Sleep-disordered breathing, glucose intolerance, and insulin resistance: The Sleep Heart Health Study. *American Journal of Epidemiology* 2004; 160(6): 521–30. doi: 10.1093/Aje/Kwh261

28. Pal, L., (Ed.). *Polycystic ovary syndrome: current and emerging concepts*. New York, NY, USA: Springer, 2014.

29. Christodoulaki, C., Trakakis, E., Pergialiotis, V., et al. Dehydroepiandrosterone-sulfate, insulin resistance and ovarian volume estimation in patients with polycystic ovarian syndrome. *Journal of Family and Reproductive Health* 2017; 11(1): 24–9.

30. Chrousos, G. P., Torpy, D. J. & Gold, P. W. Interactions between the hypothalamic-pituitary-adrenal axis and the female reproductive system: clinical implications. *Annals of Internal Medicine* 1998; 129: 229–40. doi: https://doi.org/10.7326/0003-4819-129-3-199808010-00012

31. Goodarzi, M. O., Carmina, E. & Azziz, R. DHEA, DHEA-S and PCOS. *Journal of Steroid Biochemistry and Molecular Biology* 2015; 145: 213–25. doi: 10.1016/j.jsbmb.2014.06.003

32. Lobo, R. A., Granger, L. R., Paul, W. L., et al. Psychological stress and increases in urinary norepinephrine metabolites, platelet serotonin, and adrenal androgens in women with polycystic ovary syndrome. *American Journal of Obstetrics & Gynecology* 1983; 145(4): 496–503. doi: 10.1016/0002-9378(83)90324-1

33. Cortés, M. E. & Alfaro, A. A. The effects of hormonal contraceptives on glycemic regulation. *Linacre Quarterly* 2014; 81(3): 209–18. doi: 10.1179/2050854914Y.0000000023

34. Mastorakos, G., Koliopoulos, C., Deligeoroglou, E., et al. Effects of two forms of combined oral contraceptives on carbohydrate metabolism in adolescents with polycystic ovary syndrome. *Fertility and Sterility* 2006; 85(2): 420–7. doi: 10.1016/j.fertnstert.2005.07.1306

35. Hansen, M., Miller, B. F., Holm, L., et al. Effect of administration of oral contraceptives in vivo on collagen synthesis in tendon and muscle connective tissue in young women. *Journal of Applied Physiology* 2009; 106(4): 1435–43. doi: 10.1152/japplphysiol.90933.2008

36. Balogh, A., Ditrói, F. & Lampé, L. G. LH, FSH, estradiol and progesterone levels after discontinuation of hormonal contraception. *Acta Universitatis Palackianae Olomucensis Facultatis Medicae* 1981; 101: 95–101.

37. Sinha, U., Sinharay, K., Saha, S., et al. Thyroid disorders in polycystic ovarian syndrome subjects: a tertiary hospital based cross-sectional study from Eastern India. *Indian Journal of Endocrinology & Metabolism* 2013; 17(2): 304–9. doi :10.4103/2230-8210.109714

38. Boyle, J. & Teede, H. J. Polycystic ovary syndrome: an update. *Australian Family Physician* 2012; 41(10): 752–6.

39. Weghofer, A., Himaya, E., Kushnir, V. A., et al. The impact of thyroid function and thyroid autoimmunity on embryo quality in women with low functional ovarian reserve: a case-control study. *Reproductive Biology & Endocrinology* 2015; 13: 43. doi: 10.1186/s12958-015-0041-0

40. Poppe, K. & Velkeniers, B. Female infertility and the thyroid. *Best Practice & Research. Clinical Endocrinology & Metabolism* 2004; 18(2): 153–65. doi: 10.1016/j.beem.2004.03.004

41. Thangaratinam, S., Tan, A., Knox, E., et al. Association between thyroid autoantibodies and miscarriage and preterm birth: meta-analysis of evidence. *BMJ* 2011; 342: d2616. doi: 10.1136/bmj.d2616

Chapter 3

1. Fica, S., Albu, A., Constantin, M. & Dobri, G. A. Insulin resistance and fertility in polycystic ovary syndrome. *Journal of Medicine and Life* 2008; 1(4): 415–22.
2. Henry, R. R., Gumbiner, B., Ditzler, T., et al. Intensive conventional insulin therapy for type II diabetes: metabolic effects during a 6-mo outpatient trial. *Diabetes Care* 1993; 16(1): 21–31. doi: 10.2337/diacare.16.1.21
3. Genuth, S. Insulin use in NIDDM. *Diabetes Care* 1990; 13(12): 1240–64. doi: 10.2337/diacare.13.12.1240
4. Holman, R. R., Thorne, K. I., Farmer, A. J., et al. Addition of biphasic, prandial, or basal insulin to oral therapy in type 2 diabetes. *New England Journal of Medicine* 2007; 357(17): 1716–30. doi: 10.1056/nejmoa075392
5. Kınık, M. F., Gönüllü, F. V., Vatansever, Z. & Karakaya, I. Diabulimia, a type I diabetes mellitus-specific eating disorder. *Türk Pediatri Arsivi* 2017; 52(1): 46–9. doi: 10.5152/turkpediatriars.2017.2366
6. Goebel-Fabbri, A. E., Fikkan, J., Franko, D. L. et al. Insulin restriction and associated morbidity and mortality in women with type 1 diabetes. *Diabetes Care* 2008; 31(3): 415–19. doi: 10.2337/dc07-2026
7. Kong, L. C., Wuillemin, P.-H., Bastard, J.-P., et al. Insulin resistance and inflammation predict kinetic body weight changes in response to dietary weight loss and maintenance in overweight and obese subjects by using a Bayesian network approach. *American Journal of Clinical Nutrition* 2013; 98(6): 1385–94. doi: 10.3945/ajcn.113.058099
8. Wright, C. E., Zborowski, J. V., Talbott, E. O., et al. Dietary intake, physical activity, and obesity in women with polycystic ovary syndrome. *International Journal of Obesity* 2004; 28(8): 1026–32. doi: 10.1038/sj.ijo.0802661
9. Lee, I., Cooney, L. G., Saini, S., et al. Increased risk of eating disorders in women with polycystic ovary syndrome. *Fertility and Sterility* 2016; 107(3): 796–802. doi: 10.1016/J.fertnstert.2016.12.014
10. Paganini, C., Peterson, G., Stavropoulos, V. & Krug, I. The overlap between binge eating behaviors and polycystic ovarian syndrome: an etiological integrative model. *Current Pharmaceutical Design* 2018; 24(9): 999–1006. doi: 10.2174/1381612824666171204151209
11. New Zealand Eating Disorders Clinic. Binge eating disorder. Online; accessed 3 July 2020. http://www.nzeatingdisordersclinic.co.nz/compulsive-overeating
12. Teede, H., Misso, M., Costello, M., et al. International evidence-based guideline for the assessment and management of polycystic ovary syndrome. Melbourne, VIC, Australia: Monash University, 2018.

Chapter 4

1. Teede, H., Misso, M., Costello, M., et al. International evidence-based guideline for the assessment and management of polycystic ovary syndrome. Melbourne, VIC, Australia: Monash University, 2018.
2. Legro, R. S., Barnhart, H. X., Schlaff, W. D. et al. Clomiphene, metformin, or both for infertility in the polycystic ovary syndrome. *Yearbook of Obstetrics, Gynecology and Women's Health* 2008; 153–5. doi: 10.1016/s1090-798x(08)79050-7

3. Palomba, S., Russo, T., Orio Jr, R. et al. Uterine effects of clomiphene citrate in women with polycystic ovary syndrome: a prospective controlled study. *Human Reproduction* 2006; 21(11): 2823–9. doi: 10.1093/humrep/del267

4. Morley, L. C., Tang, T., Yasmin, E., et al. Insulin-sensitising drugs (metformin, rosiglitazone, pioglitazone, d-chiro-inositol) for women with polycystic ovary syndrome, oligo-amenorrhoea and subfertility. *Cochrane Database of Systematic Reviews* 2017; 11(11): CD003053. doi: 10.1002/14651858.CD003053.pub6

5. Fujii, S., Akifumi, K., Kuki, A., et al. The effects of clomiphene citrate on normally ovulatory women. *Fertility and Sterility* 1997; 68(6): 997–9. doi: 10.1016/s0015-0282(97)00394-4

6. Gadalla, M.A., Huang, S. & Wang, R. Effect of clomiphene citrate on endometrial thickness, ovulation, pregnancy and live birth in anovulatory women: systematic review and meta-analysis. *Ultrasound Obstetrics and Gynacology* 2018; 51: 64–76

7. Liu, Q., Li, S., Quan, H. & Li, J. Vitamin B12 status in metformin treated patients: systematic review. *PloS One* 2014; 9(6): e100379. doi: 10.1371/journal.pone.0100379

8. Andrzejewski, S., Gravel, S.-P., Pollak, M. & St-Pierre, J. Metformin directly acts on mitochondria to alter cellular bioenergetics. *Cancer Metabolism* 2014; 2: 12. doi: 10.1186/2049-3002-2-12

9. Vanky, E., Zahlsen, K., Spigset, O. & Carlsen, S. M. Placental passage of metformin in women with polycystic ovary syndrome. *Fertility and Sterility* 2005; 83(5): 1575–8. doi: 10.1016/j.fertnstert.2004.11.051

10. Hu, S., Yu, S., Wang, Y., et al. Letrozole versus clomiphene citrate in polycystic ovary syndrome: a meta-analysis of randomized controlled trials. *Archives of Gynaecology & Obstetrics* 2018; 297(5): 1081–8. doi: 10.1007/s00404-018-4688-6

11. National Institutes of Health (NIH). News release: Progestin treatment for polycystic ovarian syndrome may reduce pregnancy chances. NIH, 24 May 2012. https://www.nih.gov/news-events/news-releases/progestin-treatment-polycystic-ovarian-syndrome-may-reduce-pregnancy-chances

12. Liu, M., Zhen, X., Song, H., et al. Low-dose lymphocyte immunotherapy rebalances the peripheral blood Th1/Th2/Treg paradigm in patients with unexplained recurrent miscarriage. *Reproductive Biology & Endocrinology* 2017; 15(1): 95. doi: 10.1186/S12958-017-0315-9

13. Ahmed, M. I., Duleba, A. J., El Shahat, O., et al. Naltrexone treatment in clomiphene resistant women with polycystic ovary syndrome. *Human Reproduction* 2008; 23(11): 2564–9. doi: 10.1093/humrep/den273

14. Sjaarda, L. A., Radin, R. G., Silver, R. M., et al. Preconception low-dose aspirin restores diminished pregnancy and live birth rates in women with low-grade inflammation: a secondary analysis of a randomized trial. *Journal of Clinical Endocrinology & Metabolism* 2017; 102(5): 1495–1504. doi: 10.1210/jc.2016-2917

15. Shamim, N., Usala, S. J., Biggs, W. C. & Mckenna, G. B. The elasticity of cervical-vaginal secretions is abnormal in polycystic ovary syndrome: case report of five PCOS women. *Indian Journal of Endocrinology & Metabolism* 2012; 16(6): 1019–21. doi: 10.4103/2230-8210.103030

16. Fordney-Settlage, D. A review of cervical mucus and sperm interactions in humans. *International Journal of Fertility* 1981; 26(3): 161–9

17. Shady Grove Fertility. Newsroom: Women with PCOS have higher intrauterine insemination (IUI) success rates compared to women with other causes of infertility. Shady Grove Fertility, 1 December 2016. https://www.shadygrovefertility.com/newsroom/pcos-women-have-high-iui-success-rates

18. Heijnen, E. M. E. W., Eijkemans, M. J. C., Hughes, E. G., et al. A meta-analysis of outcomes of conventional IVF in women with polycystic ovary syndrome. *Human Reproduction Update* 2006; 12(1): 13–21. doi: 10.1093/humupd/dmi036

19. Lebbi, I., Ben Temime, R., Fadhlaoui, A. & Feki, A. Ovarian drilling in PCOS: is it really useful? *Frontiers in Surgery* 2015; 2: 30. doi: 10.3389/fsurg.2015.00030

20. Campo, S. Ovulatory cycles, pregnancy outcome and complications after surgical treatment of polycystic ovary syndrome. *Obstetrical & Gynecological Survey* 1998; 53(5): 297–308. doi: 10.1097/00006254-199805000-00022

Chapter 5

1. Wilcox, A. J., Dunson, D. & Baird, D. D. The timing of the "fertile window" in the menstrual cycle: day specific estimates from a prospective study. *BMJ* 2000; 321:1259–62. doi: 10.1136/bmj.321.7271.1259

2. Hampton, K. D., Mazza, D. & Newton, J. M. Fertility-awareness knowledge, attitudes and practices of woman seeking fertility assistance. *Journal of Advanced Nursing* 2013; 69(5): 1076–84. doi: 10.1111/j.1365-2648.2012.06095.x

3. Righarts, A., Dickson, N. P., Parkin, L. & Gillett, W. R. Ovulation monitoring and fertility knowledge: their relationship to fertility experience in a cross-sectional study. *Australia and New Zealand Journal of Obstetrics & Gynaecology* 2017; 57(4): 412–19. doi: 10.1111/ajo.12606

4. Mahey, R., Gupta, M., Kandpal, S., et al. Fertility awareness and knowledge among Indian women attending a fertility clinic: a cross-sectional study. *BMC Women's Health* 2018; 18(1): 177. doi: 10.1186/s12905-018-0669-y

5. Diamant, Y. Z., Rimon, E. & Evron, S. High incidence of preeclamptic toxemia in patients with polycystic ovarian disease. *European Journal of Obstetrics, Gynecology & Reproductive Biology* 1982; 14(3): 199–204. doi: 10.1016/0028-2243(82)90097-1

6. Kousta, E., Cela, E., Lawrence, N., et al. The prevalence of polycystic ovaries in women with a history of gestational diabetes. *Clinical Endocrinology* 2000; 53(4) :501–7. doi: 10.1046/j.1365-2265.2000.01123.x

7. Dickey, R. P., Taylor, S. N., Curole, D. N., et al. Incidence of spontaneous abortion in clomiphene pregnancies. *Human Reproduction* 1996; 11(12): 2623–8. doi: 10.1093/oxfordjournals.humrep.a019182

8. Scialli, A. R. The reproductive toxicity of ovulation induction. *Fertility and Sterility* 1986; 45(3): 315–23. doi: 10.1016/s0015-0282(16)49209-5

9. Murafawa, H., Hasegawa, I., Kurabayashi, T. & Tanaka, K. Polycystic ovary syndrome. Insulin resistance and ovulatory responses to clomiphene citrate. *Journal of Reproductive Medicine* 1999; 44(1): 23–7

10. Centers for Disease Control and Prevention. National diabetes fact sheet: National estimates and general information on diabetes and prediabetes in the United States 2011. http://www.cdc.gov/diabetes/pubs/pdf/ndfs_2011.pdf

11. Baron-Cohen, S., Auyeung, B., Nørgaard-Pedersen, B., et al. Elevated fetal steroidogenic activity in autism. *Molecular Psychiatry* 2015; 20: 369–76. doi: 10.1038/mp.2014.48

12. Cherskov, A., Pohl, A., Allison, C., et al. Polycystic ovary syndrome and autism: a test of the prenatal sex steroid theory. *Translational Psychiatry* 2018; 8(1): 136. doi: 10.1038/s41398-018-0186-7

13. Kosidou, K., Dalman, C., Widman, L., et al. Maternal polycystic ovary syndrome and the risk of autism spectrum disorders in the offspring: a population-based nationwide study in Sweden.

Molecular Psychiatry 2016; 21(10): 1441–8. doi: 10.1038/mp.2015.183

14. Vanky, E., Zahlsen, K., Spigset, O. & Carlsen, S. Placental passage of metformin in women with polycystic ovary syndrome. *Fertility and Sterility* 2005; 83(5): 1575–8. doi: 10.1016/j.fertnstert.2004.11.05

15. Hanem, L. G. E., Stridsklev, S., Júlíusson, P. B., et al. Metformin use in PCOS pregnancies increases the risk of offspring overweight at 4 years of age: follow-up of two RCTs. *Journal of Clinical Endocrinology & Metabolism* 2008; 103(4): 1612–21. doi: 10.1210/jc.2017-02419

16. Jorquera G., Echiburú B., Crisosto N., et al. Metformin during pregnancy: effects on offspring development and metabolic function. *Front. Pharmacol.* 2020 https://doi.org/10.3389/fphar.2020.00653

17. Liu, Q., Li, S., Quan, H. & Li, J. Vitamin B12 status in metformin treated patients: systematic review. *PloS One* 2014; 9(6): e100379. doi: 10.1371/journal.pone.0100379

18. Reinstatler, L., Qi, Y. P., Williamson, R. S., et al. Association of biochemical B12 deficiency with metformin therapy and vitamin B12 supplements: the National Health and Nutrition Examination Survey, 1999–2006. *Diabetes Care* 2012; 35(2): 327–33. doi: 10.2337/dc11-1582

19. Kos, E., Liszek, M. J., Emanuele, M. A., et al. Effect of metformin therapy on vitamin D and vitamin B12 levels in patients with type 2 diabetes mellitus. *Endocrine Practice* 2012; 18(2): 179–84. doi: 10.4158/EP11009.OR

20. Molloy, A. M., Kirke, P. N., Troendle, J. F., et al. Maternal vitamin B12 status and risk of neural tube defects in a population with high neural tube defect prevalence and no folic acid fortification. *Pediatrics* 2009; 123(3): 917–23. doi: 10.1542/peds.2008–1173

21. Duggan, C., Srinivasan, K., Thomas, T., et al. Vitamin B-12 supplementation during pregnancy and early lactation increases maternal breast milk, and infant measures of vitamin B-12 status. *Journal of Nutrition* 2014; 144(5): 758–64. doi: 10.3945/jn.113.187278

22. Vighi, G., Marcucci, F., Sensi, L., et al. Allergy and the gastrointestinal system. *Clinical & Experimental Immunology* 2008; 153 (Suppl 1): 3–6. doi: 10.1111/j.1365-2249.2008.03713.x

23. Ismali, A. D., Alkhayl, F .F. A., Wilson, J., et al. The effect of short-duration resistance training on insulin sensitivity and muscle adaptation in overweight men. *Experimental Physiology* 2019; 104(4): 540–5. doi: 10.1113/EP087435

24. Konopka, A. R., Laurin, J. L., Schoenberg, H. M., et al. Metformin inhibits mitochondrial adaptations to aerobic exercise training in older adults. *Aging Cell* 2019; 18(1): e12880. doi: 10.1111/acel.12880

25. Walton, R. G., Dungan, C. M., Long, D. E., et al. Metformin blunts muscle hypertrophy in response to progressive resistance exercise training in older adults: a randomized, double-blind, placebo-controlled, multicenter trial: the MASTERS trial. *Aging Cell* 2019; 18(6): e13039. doi: 10.1111/acel.13039

26. Sharoff, C. G., Hagobian, T. A., Malin, S. K., et al. Combining short-term metformin treatment and one bout of exercise does not increase insulin action in insulin-resistant individuals. *American Journal of Physiology, Endocrinology & Metabolism* 2010; 298(4): E815–23. doi: 10.1152/ajpendo.00517.2009

27. Malin, S. K., Gerber, R., Chipkin, S. R. & Braun, B. Independent and combined effects of exercise training and metformin on insulin sensitivity in individuals with prediabetes. *Diabetes Care* 2012; 35(1): 131–6. doi: 10.2337/dc11-0925

28. Wycherley, T. P., Noakes, M., Clifton, P. M., et al. A high-protein diet with resistance exercise training improves weight loss and body composition in overweight and obese patients with type 2 diabetes. *Diabetes Care* 2010; 33(5): 969–76. doi: 10.2337/dc09-1974

29. Lee, Y. S., Kim, W. S., Kim, K. H., et al. Berberine, a natural plant product, activates AMP-activated protein kinase with beneficial metabolic effects in diabetic and insulin-resistant states. *Diabetes* 2006; 55(8): 2256–64. doi: 10.2337/db06-0006

30. Calderon-Margalit, R., Friedlander, Y., Yanetz, R., et al. Cancer risk after exposure to treatments for ovulation induction. *American Journal of Epidemiology* 2009; 169(3): 365–5. doi: 10.1093/aje/kwn318

31. Rizk, B. & Smitz, J. Ovarian hyperstimulation syndrome after superovulation using GnRH agonists for IVF and related procedures. *Human Reproduction* 1992; 7(3): 320–7. doi: 10.1093/oxfordjournals.humrep.a137642

32. Ratts, V. S., Pauls, R. N., Pinto, A. B., et al. Risk of multiple gestation after ovulation induction in polycystic ovary syndrome. *Journal of Reproductive Medicine* 2007; 52(10): 896–900.

33. American Society for Reproductive Medicine. Multiple pregnancy and birth: Twins, triplets, and high order multiples 2012.

34. Elster, N. Less is more: the risks of multiple births. The Institute for Science, Law, and Technology Working Group on Reproductive Technology. *Fertility and Sterility* 2000; 74(4): 617–23. doi: 10.1016/s0015-0282(00)00713-5

35. Klemetti, R., Sevón, T., Gissler, M. & Hemminki, E. Health of children born after ovulation induction. *Fertility and Sterility* 2010; 93(4): 1157–68. doi: 10.1016/j.fertnstert.2008.12.025

36. Sunderam, S., Kissin, D. M., Crawford, S. B., et al.; Centers for Disease Control and Prevention (CDC). Assisted reproductive technology surveillance— United States, 2011. *MMWR* 2014; 63: 1–28

37. RCOG Scientific Impact Paper. Multiple pregnancies following assisted conception. *BJOG* 2018; 125(5): e12–18. doi: 10.1111/1471-0528.14974

38. Pandey, S., Shetty, A., Hamilton, M., et al. Obstetric and perinatal outcomes in singleton pregnancies resulting from IVF/ICSI: a systematic review and meta-analysis. *Human Reproduction Update* 2012; 18(5): 485–503. doi: 10.1093/humupd/dms018

39. Hart, R. & Norman, R. J. The longer-term health outcomes for children born as a result of IVF treatment: Part I—General health outcomes. *Human Reproduction Update* 2013:19(3): 232–243. doi: https://doi.org/10.1093/humupd/dms062

40. Grand View Research. Press Room: IVF market size worth $37.7 billion by 2027. Grand View Research, February 2020. https://www.grandviewresearch.com/press-release/global-ivf-market

41. Kamphuis, E. I., Bhattacharya, S., van der Veen, F., et al. Are we overusing IVF? *BMJ* 2014; 348: g252. doi: 10.1136/bmj.g252

Chapter 6

1. Marshall, J. C. & Dunaif, A. Should all women with PCOS be treated for insulin resistance? *Fertility and Sterility* 2012; 97(1): 18–22. doi: 10.1016/J.fertnstert.2011.11.036

2. Stepto, N. K., Cassar, S., Joham, A. E., et al. Women with polycystic ovary syndrome have intrinsic insulin resistance on euglycaemic-hyperinsulaemic clamp. *Human Reproduction* 2013; 28(3): 777–84. doi:10.1093/humrep/des463

3. Guo, F., Moellering, D. R. & Garvey, W. T. Use of HbA1c for diagnoses of diabetes and prediabetes: comparison with diagnoses based on fasting and 2-hr glucose values and effects of gender, race, and age. *Metabolic Syndrome and Related Disorders* 2014; 12(5): 258–68. doi: 10.1089/met.2013.0128

4. Tirosh, A., Shai, I., Tekes-Manova, D., et al. Normal fasting plasma glucose levels and type 2 diabetes in young men. *New England Journal of Medicine* 2005; 353(14): 1454–62

doi: 10.1056/nejmoa050080

5. Kraft, J. R. Detection of diabetes mellitus *in situ* (occult diabetes). *Laboratory Medicine* 1975; 6(2): 10–22. doi: 10.1093/labmed/6.2.10

6. DiNicolantonio, J. J., Bhutani, J., OKeefe, J. H. & Crofts, C. Postprandial insulin assay as the earliest biomarker for diagnosing pre-diabetes, type 2 diabetes and increased cardiovascular risk. *Open Heart* 2017; 4(2): e000656. doi: 10.1136/openhrt-2017-000656

7. Teede, H., Misso, M., Costello, M., et al. *International evidence-based guideline for the assessment and management of polycystic ovary syndrome*. Melbourne, VIC, Australia: Monash University, 2018.

8. Altuntas, Y., Bilir, M., Ucak, S. & Gundogdu, S. Reactive hypoglycemia in lean young women with PCOS and correlations with insulin sensitivity and with beta cell function. *European Journal of Obstetrics & Gynecology & Reproductive Biology* 2005; 119(2):198–205. doi:10.1016/j.ejogrb.2004.07.038

9. Mastorakos, G., Koliopoulos, C., Deligeoroglou, E., et al. Effects of two forms of combined oral contraceptives on carbohydrate metabolism in adolescents with polycystic ovary syndrome. *Fertility and Sterility* 2006; 85(2): 420–7. doi: 10.1016/j.fertnstert.2005.07.1306

10. Wynn, V., Adams, P. W., Godsland, I., et al. Comparison of effects of different combined oral-contraceptive formulations on carbohydrate and lipid metabolism. *Lancet* 1979; 1(8125): 1045–9. doi: 10.1016/s0140-6736(79)92949-0

11. Dunaif, A. Insulin resistance and the polycystic ovary syndrome: mechanism and implications for pathogenesis. *Endocrine Reviews* 1997; 18(6): 774–800. doi: 10.1210/edrv.18.6.0318

12. Deng, Y., Zhang, Y., Li, S., et al. Steroid hormone profiling in obese and nonobese women with polycystic ovary syndrome. *Scientific Reports* 2017; 7(1): 14156. doi: 10.1038/s41598-017-14534-2

13. Nakamura, Y., Hornsby, P. J., Casson, P., et al. Type 5 17beta-hydroxysteroid dehydrogenase (AKR1C3) contributes to testosterone production in the adrenal reticularis. *Journal of Clinical Endocrinology & Metabolism* 2009; 94(6): 2192–8. doi: 10.1210/jc.2008-2374

14. Goodarzi, M. O., Carmina, E. & Azziz, R. DHEA, DHEA-S and PCOS. *Journal of Steroid Biochemistry & Molecular Biology* 2015; 145: 213–25. doi: 10.1016/j.jsbmb.2014.06.003

15. Harlow, S. D. & Matanoski, G. M. The association between weight, physical activity, and stress and variation in the length of the menstrual cycle. *American Journal of Epidemiology* 1991; 133(1): 38–49. doi: 10.1093/oxfordjournals.aje.a115800

16. Hendrickson-Jack, L. *The Fifth Vital Sign: master your cycles & optimize your fertility*. Fertility Friday Publishing Inc., 2019.

17. Sinha, U., Sinharay, K., Saha, S., et al. Thyroid disorders in polycystic ovarian syndrome subjects: a tertiary hospital based cross-sectional study from Eastern India. *Indian Journal of Endocrinology & Metabolism* 2013; 17(2): 304–9. doi: 10.4103/2230-8210.109714

18. Jokar, T. O., Fourman, L. T., Lee, H., et al. Higher TSH levels within the normal range are associated with unexplained infertility. *Journal of Clinical Endocrinology & Metabolism* 2018; 103(2): 632–9. doi: 10.1210/jc.2017-02120

19. Negro, R., Formoso, G., Mangieri, T., et al. Levothyroxine treatment in euthyroid pregnant women with autoimmune thyroid disease: effects on obstetrical complications. *Journal of Clinical Endocrinology & Metabolism* 2006; 91(7): 2587–91. doi: 10.1210/jc.2005-1603

20. Glinoer, D. Iodine nutrition requirements during pregnancy. *Thyroid* 2006; 16(10): 947–8. doi: 10.1089/thy.2006.16.947

21. Zimmermann, M. B., Burgi, H. & Hurrell, R. F. Iron deficiency predicts poor maternal thyroid

status during pregnancy. *Journal of Clinical Endocrinology & Metabolism* 2007; 92(9): 3436–40. doi: 10.1210/jc.2007-1082

22. Pop, V. J., Kuijpens, J. L., van Baar, A. L., et al. Low maternal free thyroxine concentrations during early pregnancy are associated with impaired psychomotor development in infancy. *Clinical Endocrinology (Oxford)* 1999; 50(2): 149–55. doi: 10.1046/j.1365-2265.1999.00639.x

23. Mueller, A., Schöfl, C., Dittrich, R., et al. Thyroid-stimulating hormone is associated with insulin resistance independently of body mass index and age in women with polycystic ovary syndrome. *Human Reproduction* 2009; 24(11): 2924–30. doi: 10.1093/humrep/dep285

24. Maratou, E., Hadjidakis, D. J., Kollias, A., et al. Studies of insulin resistance in patients with clinical and subclinical hypothyroidism. *European Journal of Endocrinology* 2009: 160(5); 785–90

25. Deyneli, O., Akpınar, İ. N. & Meriçliler, Ö. S. Effects of levothyroxine treatment on insulin sensitivity, endothelial function and risk factors of atherosclerosis in hypothyroid women. *Annales d'Endocrinologie* 2014: 75(4): 220–6

26. Demers, L. M. & Spencer, C. A. Laboratory medicine practice guidelines: laboratory support for the diagnosis and monitoring of thyroid disease. *Clinical Endocrinology (Oxford)* 2003; 58(2): 138–40. doi: 10.1046/j.1365-2265.2003.01681.x

27. Yoshioka, W., Amino, N., Ide, A., et al. Thyroxine treatment may be useful for subclinical hypothyroidism in patients with female infertility. *Endocrine Journal* 2015; 62(1): 87–92. doi: 10.1507/endocrj.ej14-0300

28. Kumar, N. & Singh, A. K. Trends of male factor infertility, an important cause of infertility: a review of literature. *Journal of Human Reproductive Sciences* 2015; 8(4): 191–6. doi: 10.4103/0974-1208.170370

29. Levine, H., Jørgensen, N., Martino-Andrade, A., et al. Temporal trends in sperm count: a systematic review and meta-regression analysis. *Human Reproduction Update* 2017; 23(6): 646–59. doi: 10.1093/humupd/dmx022

30. Cooper, T. G., Noonan, E., Eckardstein, S. V., et al. World Health Organization reference values for human semen characteristics. *Human Reproduction Update* 2010; 16(3): 231–45. doi: 10.1093/humupd/dmp048

31. Guzick, D. S., Overstreet, J. W., Factor-Litvak, P., et al. Sperm morphology, motility, and concentration in fertile and infertile men. *New England Journal of Medicine* 2001; 345(19): 1388–93. doi: 10.1056/NEJMoa003005

32. Künzle, R., Mueller, M. D., Hänggi, W., et al. Semen quality of male smokers and nonsmokers in infertile couples. *Fertility and Sterility* 2003; 79(2): 287–91. doi: 10.1016/s0015-0282(02)04664-2

33. Budin, S. B., Kho, J. H., Lee, J. H., et al. Low-dose nicotine exposure induced the oxidative damage of reproductive organs and altered the sperm characteristics of adolescent male rats. *Malaysian Journal of Medical Sciences* 2017; 24(6): 50–7. doi: 10.21315/mjms2017.24.6.6

34. Gundersen, T. D., Jørgensen, N., Andersson, A.-M., et al. Association between use of marijuana and male reproductive hormones and semen quality: a study among 1,215 healthy young men. *American Journal of Epidemiology* 2015; 182(6): 473–81. doi: 10.1093/aje/kwv135

35. Hembree III, W. C., Nahas, G. G., Zeidenberg, P. & Huang, H. F. Changes in human spermatozoa associated with high dose marihuana smoking. *Advances in the Biosciences* 1978; 22–23: 429–39. doi: 10.1016/b978-0-08-023759-6.50038-x

36. Durairajanayagam, D., Agarwal, A. & Ong, C. Causes, effects and molecular mechanisms of testicular heat stress. *Reproductive Biomedicine Online* 2015; 30(1): 14–27. doi: 10.1016/j.rbmo.2014.09.018

37. Jensen, T. K., Gottschau, M., Madsen, J. O. B., et al. Habitual alcohol consumption associated with reduced semen quality and changes in reproductive hormones; a cross-sectional study among 1221 young Danish men. *BMJ Open* 2014; 4(9): e005462. doi: 10.1136/bmjopen-2014-005462

38. Giahi, L., Mohammadmoradi, S., Javidan, A. & Sadeghi, M. R. Nutritional modifications in male infertility: a systematic review covering 2 decades. *Nutrition Reviews* 2016; 74(2): 118–30. doi: 10.1093/nutrit/nuv059

39. Environmental Working Group (EWG). Dirty Dozen™. Online; accessed 21 July 2020. https://www.ewg.org/foodnews/dirty-dozen.php

40. Safarinejad, M. R., Azma, K. & Kolahi, A. A. The effects of intense, long-term treadmill running on reproductive hormones, hypothalamus-pituitary-testis axis, and semen quality: a randomized controlled study. *Journal of Endocrinology* 2009; 200(3): 259–71. doi: 10.1677/JOE-08-0477

41. Tremellen, K. Oxidative stress and male infertility—a clinical perspective. *Human Reproduction Update* 2008; 14(3): 243–58. doi: 10.1093/humupd/dmn004

42. Aitken, R. J. & De Iuliis, G. N. Origins and consequences of DNA damage in male germ cells. *Reproductive Biomedicine Online* 2007; 14(6): 727–33. doi: 10.1016/s1472-6483(10)60676-1

43. Moslemi, M. K. & Tavanbakhsh, S. Selenium–vitamin E supplementation in infertile men: effects on semen parameters and pregnancy rate. *International Journal of General Medicine* 2011; 4: 99–104. doi: 10.2147/IJGM.S16275

44. Wong, W. Y., Merkus, H. M. W. M., Thomas, C. M. G., et al. Effects of folic acid and zinc sulfate on male factor subfertility: a double-blind, randomized, placebo-controlled trial. *Fertility and Sterility* 2002; 77(3): 491–8. doi: 10.1016/s0015-0282(01)03229-0

45. Safarinejad, M. R. The effect of coenzyme Q10 supplementation on partner pregnancy rate in infertile men with idiopathic oligoasthenoteratozoospermia: an open-label prospective study. *International Urology and Nephrology* 2012; 44(3): 689–700. doi: 10.1007/s11255-011-0081-0

46. Safarinejad, M. R. & Safarinejad, S. Efficacy of selenium and/or N-acetyl-cysteine for improving semen parameters in infertile men: a double-blind, placebo controlled, randomized study. *Journal of Urology* 2009; 181(2): 741–51. doi: 10.1016/j.juro.2008.10.015

47. Pazirandeh, S. & Burns, D. L. Overview of vitamin D. *Uptodate*. Online; updated 14 October 2019. https://www.uptodate.com/contents/overview-of-vitamin-d

48. Nguyen, H. C. T. Vitamin D3 25-hydroxyvitamin D. *Medscape*. Online; updated 20 November 2019. https://emedicine.medscape.com/article/2088694-overview#showall

49. de Angelis, C., Galdiero, M., Pivonello, C. et al. The role of vitamin D in male fertility: a focus on the testis. *Reviews in Endocrine & Metabolic Disorders* 2017; 18(3): 285–305. doi: 10.1007/S11154-017-9425-0

50. Amory, J. K., Ostrowski, K. A., Gannon, J. R., et al. Isotretinoin administration improves sperm production in men with infertility from oligoasthenozoospermia: a pilot study. *Andrology* 2017; 5(6): 1115–23. doi: 10.1111/andr.12420

51. Opotowsky, A. R. & Bilezikian, J. P. Serum vitamin A concentration and the risk of hip fracture among women 50 to 74 years old in the United States: a prospective analysis of the NHANES I follow-up study. *American Journal of Medicine* 2004; 117(3): 169–74. doi: 10.1016/j.amjmed.2004.02.045

52. Myhre, A. M., Carlsen, M. H., Bøhn, S. K., et al. Water-miscible, emulsified, and solid forms of retinol supplements are more toxic than oil-based preparations. *American Journal of Clinical Nutrition* 2003; 78(6): 1152–9. doi: 10.1093/ajcn/78.6.1152

53. Office of Dietary Supplements (ODS). Vitamin D: fact sheet for health professionals. USA: ODS, National Institutes of Health. Online; updated 24 March 2020. https://ods.od.nih.gov/factsheets/VitaminD-HealthProfessional

54. Stukenborg, J.-B., Kjartansdóttir, K. R., Reda, A., et al. Male germ cell development in humans. *Hormone Research in Paediatrics* 2014; 81(1): 2–12. doi: 10.1159/000355599

Chapter 7

1. Luddi, A., Capaldo A., Focarelli, R., et al. Antioxidants reduce oxidative stress in follicular fluid of aged women undergoing IVF. *Reproductive Biology & Endocrinology* 2016; 14(1): 57. doi: 10.1186/s12958-016-0184-7

2. Shamasbi, S. G., Dehgan, P., Charandabi, S. M.-A., et al. The effect of resistant dextrin as a prebiotic on metabolic parameters and androgen level in women with polycystic ovarian syndrome: a randomized, triple-blind, controlled, clinical trial. *European Journal of Nutrition* 2019: 58(2): 629–40. doi: 10.1007/s00394-018-1648-7

3. Clemens, R., Kranz, S., Mobley, A. R., et al. Filling America's fiber intake gap: summary of a roundtable to probe realistic solutions with a focus on grain-based foods. *Journal of Nutrition* 2012; 142(7): 1390S–401S. doi: 10.3945/jn.112.160176

4. Hamer, M. & Chida, Y. Intake of fruit, vegetables, and antioxidants and risk of type 2 diabetes: systematic review and meta-analysis. *Journal of Hypertension* 2007; 25(12): 2361–9. doi: 10.1097/hjh.0b013e3282efc214

5. Aune, D., Giovannucci, E., Boffetta, P., et al. Fruit and vegetable intake and the risk of cardiovascular disease, total cancer and all-cause mortality—a systematic review and dose–response meta-analysis of prospective studies. *International Journal of Epidemiology* 2017; 46(3): 1029–56. doi: 10.1093/ije/dyw319

6. Torres, P. J., Siakowska, M., Banaszewska, B., et al. Gut microbial diversity in women with polycystic ovary syndrome correlates with hyperandrogenism. *Journal of Clinical Endocrinology & Metabolism* 2018; 103(4): 1502–11. doi:10.1210/jc.2017-02153

7. Cornell, R. P. Endogenous gut-derived bacterial endotoxin tonically primes pancreatic secretion of insulin in normal rats. *Diabetes* 1985; 34(12): 1253–9. doi: 10.2337/diab.34.12.1253

8. Duleba, A. J. & Dokras, A. Is PCOS an inflammatory process? *Fertility and Sterility* 2012; 97(1): 7–12. doi: 10.1016/j.fertnstert.2011.11.023

9. Lee-Kwan, S. H., Moore, L. V., Blanck, H. M., et al. Disparities in state-specific adult fruit and vegetable consumption— United States, 2015. *MMWR Morbidity and Mortality Weekly Report* 2017; 66: 1241–7. doi: 10.15585/mmwr.mm6645a1

10. Nichols, L. *Real food for pregnancy: the science and wisdom of optimal prenatal nutrition.* United States: Lily Nichols, 2018.

11. Duggan, C., Srinivasan, K., Thomas, T., et al. Vitamin B-12 supplementation during pregnancy and early lactation increases maternal, breast milk, and infant measures of vitamin B-12 status. *Journal of Nutrition* 2014; 144(5): 758–64. doi: 10.3945/jn.113.187278

12. Leung, W. C., Hessel, S., Méplan, C., et al. Two common single nucleotide polymorphisms in the gene encoding beta-carotene 15,15'-monoxygenase alter beta-carotene metabolism in female volunteers. *FASEB Journal* 2009; 23(4): 1041–53. doi: 10.1096/fj.08-121962

13. Beck, K. L., Conlon, C. A., Kruger, R. & Coad, J. Dietary determinants of and possible solutions to iron deficiency for young women living in industrialized countries: a review. *Nutrients* 2014: 6(9): 3747–76. doi: 10.3390/nu6093747

14. Blanco-Rojo, R., Baeza-Richer, C., López-Parra, A. M. et al. Four variants in transferrin and *HFE*

genes as potential markers of iron deficiency anaemia risk: an association study in menstruating women. *Nutrition & Metabolism* 2011; 8: 69. doi: 10.1186/1743-7075-8-69

15. Weathersbee, P. & Lodge, J. A review of ethanol's effects on the reproductive process. *Journal of Reproductive Medicine* 1978; 21: 63–78.

16. Abel, E. L. *Marijuana, tobacco, alcohol, and reproduction.* Boca Raton, FL: CRC Press, 1983.

17. Becker, U. The influence of ethanol and liver disease on sex hormones and hepatic oestrogen receptors in women. *Danish Medical Bulletin* 1993; 40(4): 447–50.

18. Klonoff-Cohen, H., Lam-Kruglick, P. & Gonzalez, C. Effects of maternal and paternal alcohol consumption on the success rates of in vitro fertilization and gamete intrafallopian transfer. *Fertility and Sterility* 2003; 79(2): 330–9. doi: 10.1016/s0015-0282(02)04582-x

19. DiNicolantonio, J. J., Bhutani, J., OKeefe, J. H. & Crofts, C. Postprandial insulin assay as the earliest biomarker for diagnosing pre-diabetes, type 2 diabetes and increased cardiovascular risk. *Open Heart* 2017; 4(2): e000656. doi: 10.1136/openhrt-2017-000656

20. Altuntas, Y., Bilir, M., Ucak, S. & Gundogdu, S. Reactive hypoglycemia in lean young women with PCOS and correlations with insulin sensitivity and with beta cell function. *European Journal of Obstetrics, Gynecology & Reproductive Biology* 2005; 119(2): 198–205. doi: 10.1016/j.ejogrb.2004.07.038

21. Bell, K. J., Gray, R., Munns, D., et al. Estimating insulin demand for protein-containing foods using the Food Insulin Index. *European Journal of Clinical Nutrition* 2014; 68: 1055–9. doi: 10.1038/ejcn.2014.126

22. Holt, S. H., Miller, J. C. & Petocz, P. An insulin index of foods: the insulin demand generated by 1000-kJ portions of common foods. *American Journal of Clinical Nutrition* 1997; 66(5): 1264–76. doi: 10.1093/ajcn/66.5.1264

23. Rahman, S. A., Grant, L. K., Gooley, J. J., et al. Endogenous circadian regulation of female reproductive hormones. *Journal of Clinical Endocrinology & Metabolism* 2019; 104(12): 6049–59. doi: 10.1210/jc.2019-00803

24. Jakubowicz, D., Barnea, M., Wainstein, J. & Froy, O. Effects of caloric intake timing on insulin resistance and hyperandrogenism in lean women with polycystic ovary syndrome. *Clinical Science (London)* 2013; 125(9): 423–32. doi: 10.1042/cs20130071

25. Zumoff, B., Freeman, R., Coupey, S., et al. A chronobiologic abnormality in luteinizing hormone secretion in teenage girls with the polycystic-ovary syndrome. *New England Journal of Medicine* 1983; 309(20): 1206–9. doi: 10.1056/NEJM198311173092002

26. Prelević, G. M., Würzburger, M. I. & Balint-Perić, L. 24-hour serum cortisol profiles in women with polycystic ovary syndrome. *Gynecology & Endocrinology* 1993; 7(3): 179–84.

27. Loucks, A. B. & Verdun, M. Slow restoration of LH pulsatility by refeeding in energetically disrupted women. *American Journal of Physiology* 1998; 275(4): R1218–26. doi: 10.1152/ajpregu.1998.275.4.R1218

28. Ruge, T., Hodson, L., Cheeseman, J., et al. Fasted to fed trafficking of fatty acids in human adipose tissue reveals a novel regulatory step for enhanced fat storage. *Journal of Clinical Endocrinology & Metabolism* 2009; 94(5): 1781–8. doi: 10.1210/jc.2008-2090

29. Morgan, L. M., Shi, J. W., Hampton, S. M. & Frost, G. Effect of meal timing and glycaemic index on glucose control and insulin secretion in healthy volunteers. *British Journal of Nutrition* 2012; 108(7): 1286–91. doi: 10.1017/S0007114511006507

30. Nestler, J. E. & Jakubowicz, D. J. Decreases in ovarian cytochrome P450c17 alpha activity and serum free testosterone after reduction of insulin secretion in polycystic ovary syndrome. *New England Journal of Medicine* 1996; 335(9): 617–23. doi: 10.1056/NEJM199608293350902

31. Leidy, H. J., Bossingham, M. J., Mattes, R. D. & Campbell, W. W. Increased dietary protein consumed at breakfast leads to an initial and sustained feeling of fullness during energy restriction compared to other meal times. *British Journal of Nutrition* 2009; 101(6): 798–803. doi: 10.1017/s0007114508051532

32. Veldhorst, M., Smeets, A., Soenen, S., et al. Protein-induced satiety: effects and mechanisms of different proteins. *Physiology and Behaviour* 2008: 94(2); 300–7. doi: 10.1016/j.physbeh.2008.01.003

33. Leidy, H. J. & Racki, E. M. The addition of a protein-rich breakfast and its effects on acute appetite control and food intake in "breakfast-skipping" adolescents. *International Journal of Obesity* 2010: 34(7): 1125–33. doi: 10.1038/ijo.2010.3

34. Kerchner, A., Lester, W., Stuart, S. P. & Dokras, A. Risk of depression and other mental health disorders in women with polycystic ovary syndrome: a longitudinal study. *Fertility and Sterility* 2009; 91(1): 201–12. doi: 10.1016/j.fertnstert.2007.11.022

35. Bell, K. J., Gray, R., Munns, D., et al. Clinical application of the Food Insulin Index for mealtime insulin dosing in adults with type 1 diabetes: a randomized controlled trial. *Diabetes Technology & Therapeutics* 2016; 18(4): 218–25. doi: 10.1089/dia.2015.0254

36. Bell, K. Clinical application of the food insulin index to diabetes mellitus [Dissertation]. University of Sydney: School of Molecular and Microbial Bioscience, University of Sydney; 2014.

37. Diabetes UK. Healthy swaps: snacks. Online; accessed 21 July 2020. https://www.diabetes.org.uk/Guide-To-Diabetes/Enjoy-Food/Eating-With-Diabetes/Healthy-Swaps/Healthy-Swaps-Snacks

38. Suez, J., Korem, T., Zilberman-Schapira, G., et al. Non-caloric artificial sweeteners and the microbiome: findings and challenges. *Gut Microbes* 2015; 6(2): 149–155. doi:10.1080/19490976.2015.1017700

39. Hoffmann, B. R., Ronan, G. & Haspula, D. The influence of sugar and artificial sweeteners on vascular health during the onset and progression of diabetes. FASEB Journal. 2018; 32(1): 603.20.

40. Katta, R. & Desai, S. P. Diet and dermatology: the role of dietary intervention in skin disease. *Journal of Clinical & Aesthetic Dermatology* 2014; 7(7): 46–51.

41. Greer, S. M., Goldstein, A. N. & Walker, M. P. The impact of sleep deprivation on food desire in the human brain. *Nature Communications* 2013; 4: 2259. doi: 10.1038/ncomms3259

42. Kahleova, H., Belinova, L., Malinska, H., et al. Eating two larger meals a day (breakfast and lunch) is more effective than six smaller meals in a reduced-energy regimen for patients with type 2 diabetes: a randomised crossover study. *Diabetologia* 2014; 57(8): 1552–60. doi: 10.1007/s00125-014-3253-5 [Published correction appears in *Diabetologia* 2014; 58(1): 205.]

43. Dumesic, D. A., Padmanabhan, V. & Abbott, D. H. Polycystic ovary syndrome and oocyte developmental competence. *Obstetrical & Gynecological Survey* 2008; 63(1): 39–48. doi: 10.1097/OGX.0b013e31815e85fc

44. Loucks, A. B. & Thuma, J. R. Luteinizing hormone pulsatility is disrupted at a threshold of energy availability in regularly menstruating women. *Journal of Clinical Endocrinology & Metabolism* 2003; 88(1): 297–311. doi: 10.1210/jc.2002-020369

45. Sollid, L. M. & Jabri, B. Triggers and drivers of autoimmunity: lessons from coeliac disease. *Nature Reviews Immunology* 2013; 13(4): 294–302. doi: 10.1038/nri3407

46. Roy, A., Laszkowska, M., Sundström, J., et al. Prevalence of celiac disease in patients with autoimmune thyroid disease: a meta-analysis. *Thyroid*. 2016; 26(7): 880–90. doi: 10.1089/

thy.2016.0108

47. Liontiris, M. I. & Mazokopakis, E. E. A concise review of Hashimoto thyroiditis (HT) and the importance of iodine, selenium, vitamin D and gluten on the autoimmunity and dietary management of HT patients. Points that need more investigation. *Hellenic Journal of Nuclear Medicine* 2017; 20(1): 51–6. doi: 10.1967/s002449910507

48. Sapone, A., Lammers, K. M., Mazzarella, G., et al. Differential mucosal IL-17 expression in two gliadin-induced disorders: gluten sensitivity and the autoimmune enteropathy celiac disease. *International Archives of Allergy and Immunology* 2010; 152(1): 75–80. doi:10.1159/000260087

49. Di Sabatino, A., Volta, U., Salvatore, C., et al. Small amounts of gluten in subjects with suspected nonceliac gluten sensitivity: a randomized, double-blind, placebo-controlled, cross-over trial. *Clinical Gastroenterology & Hepatology* 2015; 13(9): 1604–12. doi: 10.1016/j.cgh.2015.01.029

50. Carroccio, A., Mansueto, P., Iacono G., et al. Non-celiac wheat sensitivity diagnosed by double-blind placebo-controlled challenge: exploring a new clinical entity. *American Journal of Gastroenterology* 2012; 107(12): 1898–906. doi: 10.1038/ajg.2012.236

51. Carroccio, A., D'Alcamo, A., Cavataio, F., et al. High proportions of people with nonceliac wheat sensitivity have autoimmune disease or antinuclear antibodies. *Gastroenterology* 2015; 149(3): 596–603. doi: 10.1053/j.gastro.2015.05.040

52. Jianqin, S., Leiming, X., Lu, X., et al. Effects of milk containing only A2 beta casein versus milk containing both A1 and A2 beta casein proteins on gastrointestinal physiology, symptoms of discomfort, and cognitive behavior of people with self-reported intolerance to traditional cows' milk. *Nutrition Journal* 2016; 15: 35. doi: 10.1186/s12937-016-0147-z [Published correction appears in *Nutrition Journal* 2016; 15: 45.]

53. Brooke-Taylor, S., Dwyer, K., Woodford, K. & Kost, N. Systematic review of the gastrointestinal effects of A1 compared with A2 b-casein. *Advanced Nutrition* 2017; 8(5): 739–48. doi: 10.3945/an.116.013953

54. Marziali, M., Venza, M., Lazzaro, S., et al. Gluten-free diet: a new strategy for management of painful endometriosis related symptoms? *Minerva Chirurgica* 2012; 67(6): 499–504.

Chapter 8

1. Hatch, M. C., Figa-Talamanca, I. & Salerno, S. Work stress and menstrual patterns among American and Italian nurses. *Scandinavian Journal of Work, Environment & Health* 1999; 25(2): 144–50. doi: 10.5271/sjweh.417

2. Fenster, L., Waller, K., Chen, J., et al. Psychological stress in the workplace and menstrual function. *American Journal of Epidemiology* 1999; 149(2): 127–34. doi: 10.1093/oxfordjournals. aje.a009777

3. An, Y., Sun, Z., Li, L., et al. Relationship between psychological stress and reproductive outcome in women undergoing in vitro fertilization treatment: psychological and neurohormonal assessment. *Journal of Assisted Reproduction & Genetics* 2013; 30(1): 35–41. doi: 10.1007/s10815-012-9904-x

4. Carmina, E. & Lobo, R. A. Pituitary–adrenal responses to ovine corticotropin-releasing factor in polycystic ovary syndrome and in other hyperandrogenic patients. *Gynecological Endocrinology* 1990; 4(4): 225–32. doi: 10.3109/09513599009024976

5. Leproult, R., Copinschi, G., Buxton, O. & Van Cauter, E. Sleep loss results in an elevation of cortisol levels the next evening. *Sleep* 1997; 20(10): 865–70.

6. Buxton, O. M., Pavlova, M., Reid, E. W., et al. Sleep restriction for 1 week reduces insulin sensitivity in healthy men. *Diabetes* 2010; 59(9): 2126–33. doi: 10.2337/db09-0699

7. Meier-Ewert, H., Ridker, P. M., Rifai, N., et al. Effect of sleep loss on C-reactive protein, an inflammatory marker of cardiovascular risk. *Journal of the American College of Cardiology* 2004; 43(4): 678–83. doi: 10.1016/j.jacc.2003.07.050

8. West, K. E., Jablonski, M. R., Warfield, B., et al. Blue light from light-emitting diodes elicits a dose-dependent suppression of melatonin in humans. *Journal of Applied Physiology* 2011; 110(3): 619–26. doi: 10.1152/japplphysiol.01413.2009

9. National Coffee Association USA. Infographic: American coffee consumption 2020. Online; accessed 22 July 2020. https://www.ncausa.org/Industry-Resources/Market-Research/NCDT/NCDT-Infographic

10. Patz, M. D., Day, H. E. W., Burow, A. & Campeau, S. Modulation of the hypothalamo–pituitary–adrenocortical axis by caffeine. *Psychoneuroendocrinology* 2006; 31(4): 493–500. doi: 10.1016/j.psyneuen.2005.11.008

11. Nehlig, A. Is caffeine a cognitive enhancer? *Journal of Alzheimer's Disease* 2010; 20(Suppl 1): S85–94. doi: 10.3233/JAD-2010-091315

12. Cornelis, M. C., Byrne, E. M., Esko, T., et al.; Coffee and Caffeine Genetics Consortium. Genome-wide meta-analysis identifies six novel loci associated with habitual coffee consumption. *Molecular Psychiatry* 2015; 20(5): 647–56. doi: 10.1038/mp.2014.107

13. Palatini, P., Benetti, E., Mos, L., et al. Association of coffee consumption and CYP1A2 polymorphism with risk of impaired fasting glucose in hypertensive patients. *European Journal of Epidemiology* 2015; 30(3): 209–17. doi: 10.1007/s10654-015-9990-z

14. El-Sohemy, A., Cornelis, M. C., Kabagambe, E. K. & Campos, H. Coffee, CYP1A2 genotype and risk of myocardial infarction. *Genes & Nutrition* 2007; 2(1): 155–6. doi: 10.1007/s12263-007-0043-4

15. Palatini, P., Ceolotto, G., Ragazzo, F., et al. CYP1A2 genotype modifies the association between coffee intake and the risk of hypertension. *Journal of Hypertension* 2009; 27(8): 1594–601. doi: 10.1097/HJH.0b013e32832ba850

16. Patwardhan, R. V., Desmond, P. V., Johnson, R. F. & Schenker, S. Impaired elimination of caffeine by oral contraceptive steroids. *Journal of Laboratory & Clinical Medicine* 1980; 95(4): 603–8.

17. Hill, E. E., Zack, E., Battaglini, C., et al. Exercise and circulating cortisol levels: the intensity threshold effect. *Journal of Endocrinological Investigation* 2008; (31): 587–91. doi: 10.1007/BF03345606

18. Duclos, M., Corcuff, J. B., Rashedi, M., et al. Trained versus untrained men: different immediate post-exercise responses of pituitary adrenal axis. A preliminary study. *European Journal of Applied Physiology & Occupational Physiology* 1997; 75(4): 343–50. doi: 10.1007/s004210050170

19. Freeman, R., Pollack, R. & Rosenbloom, E. Assessing impaired glucose tolerance and insulin resistance in polycystic ovarian syndrome with a muffin test: an alternative to the glucose tolerance test. *Endocrine Practice* 2010; 16(5): 810–17. doi: 10.4158/EP09330.OR

20. Shaw, K., Gennat, H., O'Rourke, P. & Del Mar, C. Exercise for overweight or obesity. *Cochrane Database of Systematic Reviews* 2006; 18(4): CD003817. doi: 10.1002/14651858.CD003817.pub3

21. Finlayson, G., Bryant, E., Blundell, J. & King, N. Acute compensatory eating following exercise is associated with implicit hedonic wanting for food. *Physiology & Behavior* 2009; 97(1): 62–7. doi: 10.1016/j.physbeh.2009.02.002

22. Teede, H., Misso, M., Costello, M., et al. *International evidence-based guideline for the assessment and management of polycystic ovary syndrome.* Melbourne, VIC, Australia: Monash University, 2018.

23. Adams, O. P. The impact of brief high-intensity exercise on blood glucose levels. *Diabetes, Metabolic Syndrome and Obesity* 2013; 6: 113–22. doi: 10.2147/DMSO.S29222

24. Trapp, E. G., Chisholm, D. J., Freund, J. & Boutcher, S. H. The effects of high-intensity intermittent exercise training on fat loss and fasting insulin levels of young women. *International Journal of Obesity* 2008: 32(4): 684–91. doi: 10.1038/sj.ijo.0803781

25. Pelly, J. *Want to reduce your mental load? Stop delegating and start specializing.* Parent Co. Online; published 4 December 2017. https://www.parent.com/want-reduce-mental-load-stop-delegating-start-specializing/

26. Moore, A., Gruber, T., Derose, J. & Malinowski, P. Regular, brief mindfulness meditation practice improves electrophysiological markers of attentional control. *Frontiers in Human Neuroscience* 2012; 6: 18. doi: 10.3389/fnhum.2012.00018

27. Zeidan, F., Matucci, K. T., Kraft R. A., et al. Neural correlates of mindfulness meditation-related anxiety relief. *Social Cognitive and Affective Neuroscience* 2014; 9(6): 751–9. doi: 10.1093/scan/nst041

Chapter 9

1. Hampton, K. D., Mazza, D. & Newton, J. M. Fertility-awareness knowledge, attitudes, and practices of women seeking fertility assistance. *Journal of Advanced Nursing* 2013; 69(5): 1076–84. doi: 10.1111/j.1365-2648.2012.06095.x

2. Mahey, R., Gupta, M., Kandpal, S., et al. Fertility awareness and knowledge among Indian women attending an infertility clinic: a cross-sectional study. *BMC Women's Health* 2018; 18(1): 177. doi: 10.1186/s12905-018-0669-y

3. Righarts, A., Dickson, N. P., Parkin, L. & Gillett, W. R. Ovulation monitoring and fertility knowledge: their relationship to fertility experience in a cross-sectional study. *Australian and New Zealand Journal of Obstetrics & Gynaecology* 2017; 57(4): 412–19. doi: 10.1111/ajo.12606

4. Mu, Q. & Fehring, R. J. Efficacy of achieving pregnancy with fertility-focused intercourse. *MCN American Journal of Maternal Child Nursing* 2014; 39(1): 35–40. doi: 10.1097/nmc.0b013e3182a76b88

5. Frank-Herrmann, P., Jacobs, C., Jenetzky, E., et al. Natural conception rates in subfertile couples following fertility awareness training. *Archives of Gynecology and Obstetrics* 2017; 295(4): 1015–24. doi: 10.1007/s00404-017-4294-z

6. Fehring, R. J. Accuracy of the peak day of cervical mucus as a biological marker of fertility. *Contraception* 2002; 66(4): 231–5. doi: 10.1016/s0010-7824(02)00355-4

7. Colombo, B. & Masarotto, G. Daily fecundability: first results from a new data base. *Demographic Research* 2000: 3: 39

8. Pallone, S. R. & Bergus, G. R. Fertility awareness-based methods: another option for family planning. *Journal of the American Board of Family Medicine* 2009; 22(2): 147–57. doi: 10.3122/jabfm.2009.02.080038

9. Wilcox, A. J., Weinberg, C. R. & Baird, D. D. Timing of sexual intercourse in relation to ovulation. Effects on the probability of conception, survival of the pregnancy, and sex of the baby. *New England Journal of Medicine* 1995; 333(23): 1517–21. doi: 10.1056/NEJM199512073332301

10. Dunson, D. B., Baird, D. D., Wilcox, A. J. & Weinberg, C. R. Day-specific probabilities of clinical pregnancy based on two studies with imperfect measures of ovulation. *Human Reproduction* 1999; 14(7): 1835–9. doi: 10.1093/humrep/14.7.1835

11. Treloar, A. E., Boynton, R. E., Behn, B. G. & Brown, B. W. Variation of the human menstrual

cycle through reproductive life. *International Journal of Fertility* 1967; 12(1 Pt 2): 77–126. doi: 10.1097/00006254-196801000-00019

12. Prior, J. C., Naess, M., Langhammer, A. & Forsmo, S. Ovulation prevalence in women with spontaneous normal-length menstrual cycles—a population-based cohort from HUNT3, Norway. *PloS One* 2015; 10(8): e0134473. doi: 10.1371/journal.pone.0134473

13. Freis, A., Freundl-Schütt, T., Wallwiener, L.-M., et al. Plausibility of menstrual cycle apps claiming to support conception. *Frontiers in Public Health* 2018; 6: 98. doi: 10.3389/fpubh.2018.00098

14. Robinson, S., Rodin, D. A., Deacon, A., et al. Which hormone tests for the diagnosis of polycystic ovary syndrome? *British Journal of Obstetrics & Gynaecology* 1992; 99(3): 232–8. doi: 10.1111/j.1471-0528.1992.tb14505.x

15. Clearblue. Clearblue fertility monitor. Online; updated 5 November 2019. https://uk.clearblue.com/ovulation-tests/fertility-monitor

16. Prior, J. C., Vigna, Y. M., Schechter, M. T. & Burgess, A. E. Spinal bone loss and ovulatory disturbances. *New England Journal of Medicine* 1990; 323(18): 1221–7. doi:10.1056/nejm199011013231801

17. Meenakumari, K. J., Agarwal, S., Krishna, A. & Pandey, L. K. Effects of metformin treatment on luteal phase progesterone concentration in polycystic ovary syndrome. *Brazilian Journal of Medical & Biological Research* 2004; 37(11): 1637–44. doi: 10.1590/S0100-879x2004001100007

18. Fauser, B. C. J. M. & Devroey, P. Reproductive biology and IVF: ovarian stimulation and luteal phase consequences. *Trends in Endocrinology & Metabolism* 2003; 14(5): 236–42. doi: 10.1016/s1043-2760(03)00075-4

Chapter 10

1. Yin, J., Xing, H. & Ye, J. (2008). Efficacy of berberine in patients with type 2 diabetes mellitus. *Metabolism* 2008; 57(5): 712–17. doi: 10.1016/j.metabol.2008.01.013

2. Banszewska, B., Wrotyńska-Barczyńska, J., Spaczynski, R. Z., et al. Effects of resveratrol on polycystic ovary syndrome: a double-blind, randomized, placebo-controlled trial. *Journal of Clinical Endocrinology & Metabolism* 2016; 101(11): 4322–8. doi: 10.1210/jc.2016-1858

3. Tremellen, K. Oxidative stress and male infertility—a clinical perspective. *Human Reproduction Update* 2008; 14(3): 243–58. doi:10.1093/humupd/dmn004

4. Fowke, J. H., Morrow, J. D., Motley, S., et al. Brassica vegetable consumption reduces urinary F2-isoprostane levels independent of micronutrient intake. *Carcinogenesis* 2006; 27(10): 2096–q02. doi: 10.1093/carcin/bgl065

5. Burton-Freeman, B. M. & Sesso, H. D. Whole food versus supplement: comparing the clinical evidence of tomato intake and lycopene supplementation on cardiovascular risk factors. *Advances in Nutrition* 2014; 5(5): 457–85. doi: 0.3945/an.114.005231

6. MacFarquhar, J. K., Broussard, D. L., Melstrom, P., et al. Acute selenium toxicity associated with a dietary supplement. *Archives of Internal Medicine* 2010; 170(3): 256–61. doi: 10.1001/archinternmed.2009.495

7. Davis, D. R., Epp, M. D. & Riordan, H. D. Changes in USDA food composition data for 43 garden crops, 1950 to 1999. *Journal of the American College of Nutrition* 2004; 23(6): 669–82. doi: 10.1080/07315724.2004.10719409

8. Larner, J. D-chiro-inositol—its functional role in insulin action and its deficit in insulin resistance. *International Journal of Experimental Diabetes Research* 2002; 3(1): 47–60

doi: 10.1080/15604280212528

9. Abdel Hamid, A. M. S., Ismail Madkour, W. A. & Borg, T. F. Inositol versus metformin administration in polycystic ovary syndrome patients. *Evidence-Based Women's Health* 2015; 5(3): 93–8. doi: 10.1097/01.EBX.0000466599.33293.cf

10. Benelli, E., Del Ghianda, S., Di Cosmo, C. & Tonacchera, M. A combined therapy with myo-inositol and D-chiro-inositol improves endocrine parameters and insulin resistance in PCOS young overweight women. *International Journal of Endocrinology* 2016; 2016: 3204083. doi: 10.1155/2016/3204083

11. Unfer, V., Nestler, J. E., Kamenov, Z. A., et al., Effects of inositol(s) in women with PCOS: a systematic review of randomized controlled trials. *International Journal of Endocrinology* 2016; 2016: 1849162. doi: 10.1155/2016/1849162

12. Nordio, M. & Proietti, E. The combined therapy with myo-inositol and D-chiro-inositol reduces the risk of metabolic disease in PCOS overweight patients compared to myo-inositol supplementation alone. *European Review for Medical & Pharmacological Sciences* 2012; 16(5): 575–81

13. Kaya, C., Cengiz, S. D. & Satiroğlu, H. Obesity and insulin resistance associated with lower plasma vitamin B12 in PCOS. *Reproductive Biomedicine Online* 2010; 19(5): 721–6. doi: 10.1016/j.rbmo.2009.06.005

14. Setola, E., Monti, L. D., Galluccio, E., et al. Insulin resistance and endothelial function are improved after folate and vitamin B12 therapy in patients with metabolic syndrome: relationship between homocysteine levels and hyperinsulinemia. *European Journal of Endocrinology* 2004; 151(4): 483–9. doi: 10.1530/eje.0.1510483

15. Larijani, B. *Journal of Diabetes and Metabolic Disorders*: launch editorial. *Journal of Diabetes and Metabolic Disorders* 2012; 11(1): 1. doi: 10.1186/2251-6581-11-1

16. Reinstatler, L., Qi, Y. P., Williamson, R. S., et al. Association of biochemical B12 deficiency with metformin therapy and vitamin B12 supplements: the National Health and Nutrition Examination Survey, 1999–2006. *Diabetes Care* 2012; 35(2): 327–33. doi: 10.2337/dc11-1582

17. Kos, E., Liszek, M. J., Emanuele, M. A., et al. Effect of metformin therapy on vitamin D and vitamin B12 levels in patients with type 2 diabetes mellitus. *Endocrine Practice* 2012; 18(2): 179–84. doi: 10.4158/EP11009.OR

18. Dharmarajan, T. S., Adiga, G. U. & Norkus, E. P. Vitamin B12 deficiency. Recognizing subtle symptoms in older adults. *Geriatrics* 2003; 58(3): 30–4, 37–8

19. Moini, A., Shirzad, N., Ahmadzadeh, M., et al. Comparison of 25-hydroxyvitamin D and calcium levels between polycystic ovarian syndrome and normal women. *International Journal of Fertility & Sterility* 2015; 9(1): 1–8. doi: 10.22074/ijfs.2015.4201

20. Alvarez, J. A. & Ashraf, A. Role of vitamin D in insulin secretion and insulin sensitivity for glucose homeostasis. *International Journal of Endocrinology* 2010; 2010: 351385. doi: 10.1155/2010/351385

21. Krul-Poel, Y. H., Snackey, C., Louwers, Y., et al. The role of vitamin D in metabolic disturbances in polycystic ovary syndrome: a systematic review. *European Journal of Endocrinology* 2013; 169(6): 853–65. doi: 10.1530/EJE-13-0617

22. Medscape. Vitamin D3 25-hydroxyvitamin D. Online; updated 20 November 2019. https://emedicine.medscape.com/article/2088694-overview#showall

23. Irani, M. & Merhi, Z. Role of vitamin D in ovarian physiology and its implication in reproduction: a systematic review. *Fertility and Sterility* 2014; 102(2): 460–8.e3. doi:10.1016/j.fertnstert.2014.04.046

24. Butts, S. F., Seifer, D. B., Koelper, N., et al. Vitamin D deficiency is associated with poor ovarian stimulation outcome in PCOS but not unexplained infertility. *Journal of Clinical Endocrinology & Metabolism* 2019; 104(2): 369–78. doi: 10.1210/jc.2018-00750

25. Maio, C.-Y., Fang, X.-J., Chen, Y. & Zhang, Q. Effect of vitamin D supplementation on polycystic ovary syndrome: a meta-analysis. *Experimental and Therapeutic Medicine* 2020; 19(4): 2641–9. doi: 10.3892/etm.2020.8525

26. Fang, F., Ni., K., Cai, Y., et al. Effect of vitamin D supplementation on polycystic ovary syndrome: a systematic review and meta-analysis of randomized controlled trials. *Complementary Therapies in Clinical Practice* 2017; 26: 53–60. doi: 10.1016/j.ctcp.2016.11.008

27. Bischoff-Ferrari, H. A., Giovannucci, E., Willett W. C., et al. Estimation of optimal serum concentrations of 25-hydroxyvitamin D for multiple health outcomes. *American Journal of Clinical Nutrition* 2006; 84(1): 18–28. doi: 10.1093/ajcn/84.1.18

28. Lee, Y. S., Kim, W. S., Kim, K. H., et al. Berberine, a natural plant product, activates AMP-activated protein kinase with beneficial metabolic effects in diabetic and insulin-resistant states. *Diabetes* 2006; 55(8): 2256–64. doi: 10.2337/db06-0006

29. Thakker, D., Raval, A., Patel, I. & Walia, R. *N*-acetylcysteine for polycystic ovary syndrome: a systematic review and meta-analysis of randomized controlled clinical trials. *Obstetrics & Gynecology International* 2015; 2015: 817849. doi: 10.1155/2015/817849

30. Oner, G. & Muderris, I. I. Clinical, endocrine and metabolic effects of metformin vs *N*-acetyl-cysteine in women with polycystic ovary syndrome. *European Journal of Obstetrics, Gynecology & Reproductive Biology* 2011; 159(1): 127–31. doi: 10.1016/j.ejogrb.2011.07.005

31. Amooee, S., Parsanezhad, M. E., Ravanbod Shirazi, M., et al. Metformin versus chromium picolinate in clomiphene citrate-resistant patients with PCOS: a double-blind randomized clinical trial. *Iranian Journal of Reproductive Medicine* 2013; 11(8): 611–18.

32. Fazelian, S., Rouhani, M. H., Bank, S. S. & Amani, R. Chromium supplementation and polycystic ovary syndrome: a systematic review and meta-analysis. *Journal of Trace Elements in Medicine & Biology* 2017; 42: 92–6. doi: 10.1016/j.jtemb.2017.04.008

33. Anon. A scientific review: the role of chromium in insulin resistance. *Diabetes Education* 2004; Suppl: 2–14.

34. de Baaij, J. H. F., Hoenderop, J. G. & Bindels, R. J. M. Magnesium in man: implications for health and disease. *Physiological Reviews* 2015; 95(1): 1–46. doi: 10.1152/physrev.00012.2014

35. Krostov, K. Effects of magnesium deficiency on mechanisms of insulin resistance in type 2 diabetes: focusing on the processes of insulin secretion and signaling. *International Journal of Molecular Sciences* 2019; 20(6): 1351. doi: 10.3390/ijms20061351

36. Barbagallo, M. & Dominguez, L. J. Magnesium and type 2 diabetes. *World Journal of Diabetes* 2015; 6(10): 1152–7. doi: 10.4239/wjd.v6.i10.1152

37. Veronese, N., Watutantrige-Fernando, S., Luchini, C., et al. Effect of magnesium supplementation on glucose metabolism in people with or at risk of diabetes: a systematic review and meta-analysis of double-blind randomized controlled trials. *European Journal of Clinical Nutrition* 2016; 70(12): 1354–9. doi: 10.1038/ejcn.2016.154

38. Rodríguez-Morán, M. & Guerrero-Romero, F. Oral magnesium supplementation improves insulin sensitivity and metabolic control in type 2 diabetic subjects: a randomized double-blind controlled trial. *Diabetes Care* 2003; 26(4): 1147–52. doi: 10.2337/diacare.26.4.1147

39. Seo, J. W. & Park, T. J. Magnesium metabolism. *Electrolyte & Blood Pressure* 2008; 6(2): 86–95. doi: 10.5049/EBP.2008.6.2.86

40. Choi, Y.-H., Miller. J. M., Tucker, K. L., et al. Antioxidant vitamins and magnesium and the

risk of hearing loss in the US general population. *American Journal of Clinical Nutrition* 2014; 99(1):148–55. doi: 10.3945 /ajcn.113.068437

41. Vighi, G., Marcucci, F., Sensi, L., et al. Allergy and the gastrointestinal system. *Clinical & Experimental Immunology* 2008; 153(Suppl 1): 3–6. doi: 10.1111/j.1365-2249.2008.03713.x

42. Utzschneider, K. M., Kratz, M., Damman, C. J. & Hullar, M. Mechanisms linking the gut microbiome and glucose metabolism. *Journal of Clinical Endocrinology & Metabolism* 2016; 101(4): 1445–54. doi: 10.1210/jc.2015-4251

43. Larsen, N., Vogensen, F. K., van den Berg, F. W. J., et al. Gut microbiota in human adults with type 2 diabetes differs from non-diabetic adults. *PloS One* 2010; 5(2): e9085. doi: 10.1371/journal.pone.000908543

44. Qin, J., Li, Y., Cai, Z., et al. A metagenome-wide association study of gut microbiota in type 2 diabetes. *Nature* 2012; 490(7418): 55–60. doi: 10.1038/nature11450

45. Tabuchi, M., Ozaki, M., Tamura, A., et al. Antidiabetic effect of *Lactobacillus* GG in streptozotocin-induced diabetic rats. *Bioscience, Biotechnology, & Biochemistry* 2003; 67(6): 1421–4. doi: 10.1271/bbb.67.1421

46. Cropley, M., Banks, A. P. & Boyle, J. The effects of *Rhodiola rosea L.* extract on anxiety, stress, cognition and other mood symptoms. *Phytotherapy Research* 2015; 29(12): 1934–9. doi: 10.1002/ptr.5486

47. Edwards, D., Heufelder, A. & Zimmermann, A. Therapeutic effects and safety of *Rhodiola rosea* extract WS° 1375 in subjects with life-stress symptoms—results of an open-label study. *Phytotherapy Research* 2012; 26(8): 1220–5. doi: 10.1002/ptr.3712

48. Xia, N., Li, J., Wang, H., et al. *Schisandra chinensis* and *Rhodiola rosea* exert an anti-stress effect on the HPA axis and reduce hypothalamic c-Fos expression in rats subjected to repeated stress. *Experimental & Therapeutic Medicine* 2016; 11(1): 353–9. doi: 10.3892/etm.2015.2882

49. Seelig, M. S. Consequences of magnesium deficiency on the enhancement of stress reactions; preventive and therapeutic implications (a review). *Journal of the American College of Nutrition* 1994; 13(5): 429–46. doi: 10.1080/07315724.1994.10718432

50. Boyle, N. B., Lawton, C. & Dye, L. The effects of magnesium supplementation on subjective anxiety and stress—a systematic review. *Nutrients* 2017; 9(5): 429. doi: 10.3390/nu9050429

51. Thesing, C. S., Bot, M., Milaneschi, Y., et al. Omega-3 polyunsaturated fatty acid levels and dysregulations in biological stress systems. *Psychoneuroendocrinology* 2018; 97: 206–15. doi: 10.1016/j.psyneuen.2018.07.002

52. Delaru, J., Matzinger, O. Binnert, C. et al. Fish oil prevents the adrenal activation elicited by mental stress in healthy men. *Diabetes and Metabolism* 2003; 29(3): 289–95. doi: 10.1016/s1262-3636(07)70039-3

53. Tarasov, I. A., Sheibak, V. M. & Moïseenok, A. G. Adrenal cortex functional activity in pantothenate deficiency and the administration of the vitamin or its derivatives [in Russian]. *Voprosy Pitaniia* 1985; (4): 51–4.

54. Kelly, G. S. Nutritional and botanical interventions to assist with the adaptation to stress. *Alternative Medicine Review* 1999; 4(4): 249–65.

55. Mocelin, R., Marcon, M., D'Ambros, S., et al. *N*-Acetylcysteine reverses anxiety and oxidative damage induced by unpredictable chronic stress in zebrafish. *Molecular Neurobiology* 2019; 56(2): 1188–95. doi: 10.1007/s12035-018-1165-y

56. Bedaiwy, M. A., Al Inany, A., Rezk, H. & Falcone, T. *N*-acetyl cystein improves pregnancy rate in long standing unexplained infertility: a novel mechanism of ovulation induction. *Fertility and Sterility* 2004; 82(Suppl 2): S228. doi: 10.1016/j.fertnstert.2004.07.604

57. Nielsen, F. H. Effects of magnesium depletion on inflammation in chronic disease. *Current Opinion in Clinical Nutrition & Metabolic Care* 2014; 17(6): 525–30. doi: 10.1097/MCO.0000000000000093

58. Afshar Ebrahimi, F., Foroozanfard, F., Aghadavod, E., et al. The effects of magnesium and zinc co-supplementation on biomarkers of inflammation and oxidative stress, and gene expression related to inflammation in polycystic ovary syndrome: a randomized controlled clinical trial. *Biological Trace Element Research* 2018; 184(2): 300–7. doi: 10.1007/s12011-017-1198-5

59. Rosanoff, A., Weaver, C. M. & Rude, R. K. Suboptimal magnesium status in the United States: are the health consequences underestimated? *Nutrition Reviews* 2012; 70(3): 153–64. doi: 10.1111/j.1753-4887.2011.00465.x

60. Morris, G., Anderson, G., Dean, O., et al. The glutathione system: a new drug target in neuroimmune disorders. *Molecular Neurobiology* 2014; 50(3): 1059–84. doi: 10.1007/s12035-014-8705-x

61. Estany, S., Palacio, J. R., Barnadas, R., et al. Antioxidant activity of *N*-acetylcysteine, flavonoids and alpha-tocopherol on endometrial cells in culture. *Journal of Reproductive Immunology* 2007; 75(1): 1–10. doi: 10.1016/j.jri.2007.01.007

62. Luddi, A., Capaldo, A., Focarelli, R., et al. Antioxidants reduce oxidative stress in follicular fluid of aged women undergoing IVF. *Reproductive & Biological Endocrinology* 2016; 14(1): 57. doi: 10.1186/s12958-016-0184-7

63. Mohammadi, S., Karimzadeh Bardei, L., Hojati, V., et al. Anti-inflammatory effects of curcumin on insulin resistance index, levels of interleukin-6, C-reactive protein, and liver histology in polycystic ovary syndrome-induced rats. *Cell Journal* 2017; 19(3): 425–33. doi:10.22074/cellj.2017.4415

64. Sahebkar, A. Are curcuminoids effective C-reactive protein-lowering agents in clinical practice? Evidence from a meta-analysis. *Phytotherapy Research* 2014; 28(5): 633–42. doi: 10.1002/ptr.5045

65. ScienceDaily. Vitamin D deficiency related to increased inflammation in healthy women. Online; published 14 April 2009; sourced from University of Missouri-Columbia. https://www.sciencedaily.com/releases/2009/04/090408140208.htm

66. Lu, X., Farmer, P., Rubin, J. & Nanes, M. S. Integration of the NfkappaB p65 subunit into the vitamin D receptor transcriptional complex: identification of p65 domains that inhibit 1,25-dihydroxyvitamin D3-stimulated transcription. *Journal of Cell Biochemistry* 2004; 92(4): 833–48. doi: 10.1002/jcb.20143

67. Strieder, T. G. A., Prummel, M. F., Tijssen, J. G. P., et al. Risk factors for and prevalence of thyroid disorders in a cross-sectional study among healthy female relatives of patients with autoimmune thyroid disease. *Clinical Endocrinology* 2003; 59(3): 396–401. doi: 10.1046/j.1365-2265.2003.01862.x

68. Mengheri, E. Health, probiotics and inflammation. *Journal of Clinical Gastroenterology* 2008; 42(Suppl 3 Pt 2): S1777–8. doi: 10.1097/MCG.0b013e31817eedc4

69. Gärtner, R., Gasnier, B. C. H., Dietrich, J. W., et al. Selenium supplementation in patients with autoimmune thyroiditis decreases thyroid peroxidase antibodies concentrations. *Journal of Clinical Endocrinology & Metabolism* 2002; 87(4): 1687–91. doi: 10.1210/jcem.87.4.8421

70. Medsafe Editorial Team. Selenium. *Prescriber Update* 2000; 20: 39–42. Online; published July 2000. http://www.medsafe.govt.nz/profs/puarticles/sel.htm

71. Chung, H. R. Iodine and thyroid function. *Annals of Pediatric Endocrinology & Metabolism* 2014; 19(1): 8–12. doi: 10.6065/apem.2014.19.1.8

72. Zimmermann, M. B., Burgi, H. & Hurrell, R. F. Iron deficiency predicts poor maternal thyroid status during pregnancy. *Journal of Clinical Endocrinology & Metabolism* 2007; 92(9): 3436–40. doi: 10.1210/jc.2007-1082

73. Hurrell, R. & Egli, I., Iron bioavailability and dietary reference values. *American Journal of Clinical Nutrition* 2010; 91(5): 1461–7. doi: 10.3945/ajcn.2010.28674F

74. Hyder, S. M., Persson, L. A., Chowdhury, A. M., et al. Do side-effects reduce compliance to iron supplementation? A study of daily- and weekly-dose regimens in pregnancy. *Journal of Health, Population, and Nutrition* 2002; 20(2): 175–9.

75. Thurber, C., Dugas, L. R., Ocobock, C., et al. Extreme events reveal an alimentary limit on sustained maximal human energy expenditure. *Science Advances* 2019; 5(6): eaaw0341. doi: 10.1126/sciadv.aaw0341

76. Ladipo, O. A. Nutrition in pregnancy: mineral and vitamin supplements. *American Journal of Clinical Nutrition* 2000; 72(1 Suppl): 280S–290S. doi: 10.1093/Ajcn/72.1.280S

77. Plumptre, L., Masih, S. P., Sohn, K.-J., et al. Suboptimal maternal and cord plasma pyridoxal 5′ phosphate concentrations are uncommon in a cohort of Canadian pregnant women and newborn infants. *Maternal & Child Nutrition* 2018; 14(1): e12467. doi: 10.1111/mcn.12467

78. Kocyłowski, R., Lewicka, I., Grzesiak, M., et al. Assessment of dietary intake and mineral status in pregnant women. *Archives of Gynecology and Obstetrics* 2018: 297(6): 1433–40. doi: 10.1007/s00404-018-4744-2

79. Giddens, J. B., Krug, S. K., Tsang, R. C., et al. Pregnant adolescent and adult women have similarly low intakes of selected nutrients. *Journal of the American Dietetic Association* 2000; 100(11): 1334–40. doi: 10.1016/S0002-8223(00)00377-1

80. Nefic, H., Mackic-Djurovic, M. & Eminovic, I. The frequency of the 677C>T and 1298A>C polymorphisms in the methylenetetrahydrofolate reductase (MTHFR) gene in the population. *Medical Archives* 2018; 72(3): 164–9. doi: 10.5455/medarh.2018.72.164-169

81. Obeid, R., Holzgreve, A. & Pietrzik, K. Is 5-methyltetrahydrofolate an alternative to folic acid for the prevention of neural tube defects? *Journal of Perinatal Medicine* 2013; 41(5): 469–83. doi: 10.1515/jpm-2012-0256

82. Lamers, Y., Prinz-Langenohl, R., Brämswig, S. & Pietrzik, K. Red blood cell folate concentrations increase more after supplementation with [6 S]-5-methyltetrahydrofolate than with folic acid in women of childbearing age. *American Journal of Clinical Nutrition* 2006; 84(1): 156–61. doi: 10.1093/ajcn/84.1.156

83. Wallace, T. C. & Fulgoni III, V. L. Assessment of total choline intakes in the United States. *Journal of the American College of Nutrition* 2016; 35(2): 108–12. doi: 10.1080/07315724.2015.1080127

84. Caudill, M. A., Strupp, B. J., Muscalu, L., et al. Maternal choline supplementation during the third trimester of pregnancy improves infant information processing speed: a randomized, double-blind, controlled feeding study. *FASEB J* 2018; 32(4): 2172–80. doi: 10.1096/fj.201700692RR

85. Bae, S., West, A. A., Yan, J. et al. Vitamin B-12 status differs among pregnant, lactating, and control women with equivalent nutrient intakes. *Journal of Nutrition* 2015; 145(7): 1507–14. doi: 10.3945/jn.115.210757

86. Weiler, H., Fitzpatrick-Wong, S., Veitch, R., et al. Vitamin D deficiency and whole-body and femur bone mass relative to weight in healthy newborns. *Canadian Medical Association Journal* 2005; 172(6): 757–61. doi: 10.1503/cmaj.1040508

87. Javaid, M. K., Crozier, S. R., Harvey, N. C., et al. Princess Anne Hospital Study Group.

Maternal vitamin D status during pregnancy and childhood bone mass at age 9 years: longitudinal study. *Lancet* 2006; 367(9504): 36–43. doi: 10.1016/S0140-6736(06)67922-1

88. Hollis, B. W., Johnson, D., Hulsey, T. C., et al. Vitamin D supplementation during pregnancy: double-blind, randomized clinical trial of safety and effectiveness. *Journal of Bone and Mineral Research* 2011; 26(10): 2341–57. doi: 10.1002/jbmr.463

89. Mulligan, M. L., Felton, S. K., Reik, A. E., et al. Implications of vitamin D deficiency in pregnancy and lactation. *American Journal of Obstetrics & Gynaecology* 2010; 202(5): 429.e1–9. doi: 10.1016/j.ajog.2009.09.002

90. Shirahata, A., Nakamura, T. & Ariyoshi, N. Vitamin K1 and K2 contents in blood, stool, and liver tissues of neonates and young infants. In: S. Suzuki, W. E. Hathaway, J. Bonnar & A. H. Sutor (Eds), *Perinatal thrombosis and hemostasis*. Tokyo, Japan: Springer, 1991, pp. 213–23.

91. Skeaff, S. A. Iodine deficiency in pregnancy: the effect on neurodevelopment in the child. *Nutrients* 2011; 3(2): 265–3. doi: 10.3390/nu3020265

92. Knight, B. A., Shields, B. M., He, X., et al. Iodine deficiency amongst pregnant women in South-West England. *Clinical Endocrinology (Oxford)* 2017; 86(3): 451–5. doi: 10.1111/cen.13268

93. Leung, A. M., Pearce, E. N. & Braverman, L. E. Iodine content of prenatal multivitamins in the United States. *New England Journal of Medicine* 2009; 360(9): 939–40. doi: 10.1056/NEJMc0807851

94. Mioto, V. C. B., Monteiro, A. C. C. N. G., de Camargo, R. Y. A., et al. High prevalence of iodine deficiency in pregnant women living in adequate iodine area. *Endocrine Connections* 2018; 7(5): 762–7. doi: 10.1530/EC-18-0131

95. Institute of Medicine. *Dietary reference intakes for vitamin A, vitamin K, arsenic, boron, chromium, copper, iodine, iron, manganese, molybdenum, nickel, silicon, vanadium, and zinc.* Washington, DC: National Academies Press, 2001. doi: 10.17226/10026

96. Beaton, G. H. Iron needs during pregnancy: do we need to rethink our targets? *American Journal of Clinical Nutrition* 2000; 72(1 Suppl): 265S–271S. doi: 10.1093/ajcn/72.1.265S

97. Unfer, V., Casini, M. L., Costabile, L., et al. High dose of phytoestrogens can reverse the antiestrogenic effects of clomiphene citrate on the endometrium in patients undergoing intrauterine insemination: a randomized trial. *Journal of the Society for Gynecologic Investigation* 2004; 11(5): 323–8. doi: 10.1016/j.jsgi.2003.12.007

98. Unfer, V., Casini, M. L., Gerli, S., et al. Phytoestrogens may improve the pregnancy rate in in vitro fertilization–embryo transfer cycles: a prospective, controlled, randomized trial. *Fertility and Sterility* 2004; 82(6): 1509–13. doi: 10.1016/j.fertnstert.2004.07.934

99. Shahin, A. Y. & Mohammed, S. A. Adding the phytoestrogen *Cimicifugae racemosae* to clomiphene induction cycles with timed intercourse in polycystic ovary syndrome improves cycle outcomes and pregnancy rates—a randomized trial. *Gynecological Endocrinology* 2014; 30(7): 505–10. doi: 10.3109/09513590.2014.895983

100. Rachoń, D., Vortherms, T., Seidlová-Wuttke, D. & Wuttke, W. Effects of black cohosh extract on body weight gain, intra-abdominal fat accumulation, plasma lipids and glucose tolerance in ovariectomized Sprague–Dawley rats. *Maturitas* 2008; 60(3): 209–15. doi: 10.1016/j.maturitas.2008.06.001

101. Kamel, H. H. Role of phyto-oestrogens in ovulation induction in women with polycystic ovarian syndrome. *European Journal of Obstetric, Gynecology & Reproductive Biology* 2013; 168(1): 60–3. doi: 10.1016/j.ejogrb.2012.12.025

102. Shahin, A. Y., Ismail, A. M. & Shaaban, O. M. Supplementation of clomiphene citrate cycles with *Cimicifuga racemosa* or ethinyl oestradiol—a randomized trial. *Reproductive Biomed Online*

2009; 19(4): 501–7. doi: 10.1016/j.rbmo.2009.06.007

103. Shahin, A. Y., Ismail, A. M., Zahran, K. M. & Makhlouf, A. M. Adding phytoestrogens to clomiphene induction in unexplained infertility—a randomized trial. *Reproductive Biomed Online* 2008; 16(4): 580–8. doi: 10.1016/s1472-6483(10)60465-8

104. Akdogan, M., Ozguner, M., Kocak, A., et al. Effects of peppermint teas on plasma testosterone, follicle-stimulating hormone, and luteinizing hormone levels and testicular tissue in rats. *Urology* 2004; 64(2): 394–8. doi: 10.1016/j.urology.2004.03.046

105. Grant, P. Spearmint herbal tea has significant anti-androgen effects in polycystic ovarian syndrome. A randomized controlled trial. *Phytotherapy Research* 2010; 24(2): 186–8. doi:10.1002/ptr.2900

106. Armanini, D., Mattarello, M. J., Fiore, C., et al. Licorice reduces serum testosterone in healthy women. *Steroids* 2004; 69(11–12): 763–6. doi: 10.1016/j.steroids.2004.09.005

107. Takahashi, K. & Kitao, M. Effect of TJ-68 (shakuyaku-kanzo-to) on polycystic ovarian disease. *International Journal of Fertility and Menopausal Studies* 1994; 39(2): 69–76.

Chapter 11

1. Diamond, M. P., Christianson, C., Daniell, J. F. & Wentz, A. C. Pregnancy following use of the cervical cup for home artificial insemination utilizing homologous semen. *Fertility and Sterility* 1983; 39(4): 480–4. doi: 10.1016/S0015-0282(16)46936-0

2. Corson, S. L., Batzer, F. R., Otis, C. & Fee, D. The cervical cap for home artificial insemination. *Journal of Reproductive Medicine* 1986; 31(5): 349–52.

3. Centers for Disease Control and Prevention (CDC). STDs & infertility. Online; page reviewed 30 October 2013. https://www.cdc.gov/std/infertility/default.htm

4. Castrillón-Duque, E. X., Puerta Suárez, J., Cardona Maya, W. D. Yeast and fertility: effects of *in vitro* activity of *Candida* spp. on sperm quality. *Journal of Reproduction & Infertility* 2018; 19(1): 49–55.

5. Haahr, T., Jensen, J. S., Thomsen, L., et al. Abnormal vaginal microbiota may be associated with poor reproductive outcomes: a prospective study in IVF patients. *Human Reproduction* 2016; 31(4): 795–803. doi: 10.1093/humrep/dew026

6. Behzadi, P., Behzadi, E. & Ranjbar, R. Urinary tract infections and *Candida albicans*. *Central European Journal of Urology* 2015; 68(1): 96–101. doi: 10.5173/ceju.2015.01.474

7. Rodrigues, C. F., Rodrigues, M. E. & Henriques, M. *Candida* sp. infections in patients with diabetes mellitus. *Journal of Clinical Medicine* 2019; 8(1): 76. doi: 10.3390/jcm8010076

8. Guo, Y., Qi, Y., Yang, X., et al. Association between polycystic ovary syndrome and gut microbiota. *PloS One* 2016; 11(4): e0153196. doi: 10.1371/journal.pone.0153196

9. Burrello, N., Salmeri, M., Perdichizzi, A., et al. *Candida albicans* experimental infection: effects on human sperm motility, mitochondrial membrane potential and apoptosis. *Reproductive Biomedicine Online* 2009; 18(4): 496–501. doi: 10.1016/S1472-6483(10); 60125–3

10. Eskenazi, B. & Warner, M. L. Epidemiology of endometriosis. *Obstetrics & Gynecology Clinics of North America* 1997; 24: 235–58. doi: 10.1016/S0889-8545(05)70302-8

11. Editor. World's first blood test for endometriosis can detect up to 9 out of 10 cases. *Lifescience Industry* news, 5 April 2019. https://www.lifescienceindustrynews.com/clinical-need/worlds-first-blood-test-for-endometriosis-can-detect-up-to-9-out-of-10-cases

12. Khan, K. N., Kitajima, M., Inoue, T., et al. 17β-Estradiol and lipopolysaccharide additively promote pelvic inflammation and growth of endometriosis. *Reproductive Sciences* 2015; 22(5): 585–94. doi: 10.1177/1933719114556487

13. Carmina, E., Dewailly, D., Escobar-Morreale, H. F., et al. Non-classic congenital adrenal hyperplasia due to 21-hydroxylase deficiency revisited: an update with a special focus on adolescent and adult women. *Human Reproduction Update* 2017; 23(5): 580–99. doi: 10.1093/humupd/dmx014

14. Speiser, P. W., Serrat, J., New, M. I. & Gertner, J. M. Insulin insensitivity in adrenal hyperplasia due to nonclassical steroid 21-hydroxylase deficiency. *Journal of Clinical Endocrinology & Metabolism* 1992; 75(6): 1421–4. doi: 10.1210/jcem.75.6.1464643

15. Azziz, R., Sanchez, L. A., Knochenhauer, E. S., et al. Androgen excess in women: experience with over 1000 consecutive patients. *Journal of Clinical Endocrinology & Metabolism* 2004; 89(2): 453–62. doi: 10.1210/jc.2003-031122

16. Bradbury, R. A., Lee, P. & Smith, H. C. Elevated anti-Müllerian hormone in lean women may not indicate polycystic ovarian syndrome. *Australian and New Zealand Journal of Obstetrics & Gynaecology* 2017; 57(5): 552–7. doi: 10.1111/ajo.12647

17. McCulloch, F. Natural treatments for autoimmune infertility concerns. *American College for Advancement in Medicine (ACAM) Integrative Medicine Blog*, 7 February 2013; updated 29 January 2014. https://www.acam.org/blogpost/1092863/179527/Natural-Treatments-for-Autoimmune-Infertility-Concerns

18. Yasin, Anas L., Yasin, Ahmad L. & Basha, W. S. The epidemiology of anti-sperm antibodies among couples with unexplained infertility in North West Bank, Palestine. *Journal of Clinical & Diagnostic Research* 2016; 10(3): QC01–3. doi: 10.7860/jcdr/2016/15788.7380

19. Botto, L. D. & Yang, Q. 5,10-Methylenetetrahydrofolate reductase gene variants and congenital anomalies: a HuGE review. *American Journal of Epidemiology* 2000; 151(9): 862–77. doi: 10.1093/oxfordjournals.aje.a010290

20. Cotter, A. M., Molloy, A. M., Scott, J. M. & Daly, S. F. Elevated plasma homocysteine in early pregnancy: a risk factor for the development of severe preeclampsia. *American Journal of Obstetrics & Gynecology* 2001; 185(4): 781–5. doi: 10.1067/mob.2001.117304

21. Guéant, J. L., Anello, G., Bosco, P., et al. Homocysteine and related genetic polymorphisms in Down's syndrome IQ. *Journal of Neurology, Neurosurgery & Psychiatry* 2005; 76(5): 706–9. doi: 10.1136/jnnp.2004.039875

22. Genetic and Rare Diseases Information Center (GARD), National Center for Advancing Translational Sciences, National Institutes of Health. MTHFR gene variant: not a rare disease; summary. Online; updated 25 January 2018. https://rarediseases.info.nih.gov/diseases/10953/mthfr-gene-mutation

Chapter 12

1. Thurber, C., Dugas, L. R., Ocobock, C., et al. Extreme events reveal an alimentary limit on sustained maximal human energy expenditure. *Science Advances* 2019; 5(6): eaaw0341. doi: 10.1126/sciadv.aaw0341

2. Sonagra, A. D., Biradar, S. M., Dattatreya, K., et al. Normal pregnancy—a state of insulin resistance. *Journal of Clinical & Diagnostic Research* 2014; 8(11): CC01–3. doi: 10.7860/jcdr/2014/10068.5081

3. Buchanan, T. A., Xiang, A., Kjos, S. L., et al. What is gestational diabetes? *Diabetes Care* 2007; 30(Suppl 2): S105–11. doi: 10.2337/dc07-s201

4. Wrighton, K. (original writer). News article: Babies of mothers with gestational diabetes have more body fat, scans reveal. *ScienceDaily*, 12 May 2016. https://www.sciencedaily.com/releases/2016/05/160512102612.htm

5. Mayor, S. More babies born to mothers with gestational diabetes have adverse outcomes, study shows. *BMJ* 2017; 356: j846. doi: 10.1136/bmj.j846

6. Mitanchez, D., Yzydorczyk, C. & Simeoni, U. What neonatal complications should the pediatrician be aware of in case of maternal gestational diabetes? *World Journal of Diabetes* 2015; 6(5): 734–43. doi: 10.4239/wjd.v6.i5.734

7. D'Anna, R., Di Benedetto, V., Rizzo, P., et al. Myo-inositol may prevent gestational diabetes in PCOS women. *Gynecological Endocrinology* 2012; 28(6): 440–2. doi: 10.3109/09513590.2011.633665

8. Mikola, M., Hiilesmaa, V., Halttunen, M., et al. Obstetric outcome in women with polycystic ovarian syndrome. *Human Reproduction* 2001; 16(2): 226–9. doi: 10.1093/humrep/16.2.226

9. Tuso, P. Prediabetes and lifestyle modification: time to prevent a preventable disease. *Permanente Journal* 2014; 18(3): 88–93. doi: 10.7812/tpp/14-002

10. Glueck, C. J., Wang, P., Kobayashi, S., et al. Metformin therapy throughout pregnancy reduces the development of gestational diabetes in women with polycystic ovary syndrome. *Fertility and Sterility* 2002; 77(3): 520–5. doi:10.1016/s0015-0282(01)03202-2

11. Joham, A. E., Boyle, J. A., Ranasinha, S. et al. Contraception use and pregnancy outcomes in women with polycystic ovary syndrome: data from the Australian Longitudinal Study On Women's Health. *Human Reproduction* 2014; 29(4): 802–8. doi: 10.1093/humrep/deu020

12. Jakubowicz, D. J., Iuorno, M. J., Jakubowicz, S., et al. Effects of metformin on early pregnancy loss in the polycystic ovary syndrome. *Journal of Clinical Endocrinology & Metabolism.* 2002; 87(2): 524–9. doi: 10.1210/jcem.87.2.8207

13. Chason, R. J., Richter, K. S., Widra, E. A. & Segars, J. H. A diagnosis of polycystic ovary syndrome (PCOS) is associated with an increased likelihood of pregnancy loss with assisted reproduction. *Fertility and Sterility* 2010; 94(4 Suppl): S25. doi: 10.1016/j.fertnstert.2010.07.094

14. Magnus, M. C., Wilcox, A. J., Morken, N.-H., et al. Role of maternal age and pregnancy history in risk of miscarriage: prospective register based study. *BMJ* 2019; 364: l869. doi: 10.1136/bmj.l869

15. Fedorcsák, P., Storeng, R., Dale, P. O., et al. Obesity is a risk factor for early pregnancy loss after IVF or ICSI. *Acta Obstetricia et Gynecologica Scandinavica* 2000; 79(1): 43–8. doi: 10.1034/j.1600-0412.2000.079001043.x

16. Meenakumari, K. J., Agarwal, S., Krishna, A. & Pandey, L. K. Effects of metformin treatment on luteal phase progesterone concentration in polycystic ovary syndrome. *Brazilian Journal of Medical and Biological Research* 2004; 37(11):1637–44. doi: 10.1590/s0100-879x2004001100007

17. Gabbe, S. G., Niebyl, J. R., Galan, H. L., et al. *Obstetrics: normal and problem pregnancies*, 6th edn, Ch 17, pp. 592–3. Saint Louis, Mo. USA: Saunders, 2012.

18. Society for Endocrinology web-based project. You and your hormones. Progesterone. Online; last reviewed February 2018. https://www.yourhormones.info/hormones/progesterone

19. Csapo, A. I., Pulkkinen, M. O., Ruttner, B., et al. The significance of the human corpus luteum in pregnancy maintenance. I. Preliminary studies. *American Journal of Obstetrics & Gynecology* 1972; 112(8): 1061–7. doi: 10.1016/0002-9378(72)90181-0

20. Ikoma, D. M., Hulteen, L. & Holden, J. Threshold progesterone level of 25 ng/ml to sustain pregnancy in first trimester in women with history of infertility or miscarriage. *Clinical Obstetrics, Gynecology & Reproductive Medicine* 2017; 4. doi: 10.15761/cogrm.1000205

21. Homburg, R., Armar, N. A., Eshel, A., et al. Influence of serum luteinising hormone

concentrations on ovulation, conception, and early pregnancy loss in polycystic ovary syndrome. *BMJ* 1988; 297(6655): 1024–6. doi: 10.1136/bmj.297.6655.1024

22. Zhang, Y., Wang, H., Pan, X., et al. Patients with subclinical hypothyroidism before 20 weeks of pregnancy have a higher risk of miscarriage: a systematic review and meta-analysis. *PLoS One* 2017: 12(4): e0175708. doi: 10.1371/journal.pone.0175708

23. Brown, R. S. Minireview: developmental regulation of thyrotropin receptor gene expression in the fetal and newborn thyroid. *Endocrinology* 2004; 145(9): 4058–61. doi: 10.1210/en.2004-0458

24. Khandelwal, D. & Tandon, N. Overt and subclinical hypothyroidism: who to treat and how. *Drugs* 2012; 72(1): 17–33. doi: 10.2165/11598070-000000000-00000

25. Abalovich, M., Gutierrez, S., Alcaraz, G., et al. Overt and subclinical hypothyroidism complicating pregnancy. *Thyroid* 2002; 12(1): 63–8. doi: 10.1089/105072502753451986

26. Stagnaro-Green, A., Abalovich, M., Alexander, E., et al.; The American Thyroid Association Taskforce on Thyroid Disease During Pregnancy and Postpartum. Guidelines of the American Thyroid Association for the diagnosis and management of thyroid disease during pregnancy and postpartum. *Thyroid* 2011; 21(10): 1081–125. doi: 10.1089/thy.2011.0087

27. Stagnaro-Green, A. Thyroid antibodies and miscarriage: where are we at a generation later? *Journal of Thyroid Research* 2011: 2011: 841949. doi: 10.4061/2011/841949

28. Janssen, O. E., Mehlmauer, N., Hahn, S., et al. High prevalence of autoimmune thyroiditis in patients with polycystic ovary syndrome. *European Journal of Endocrinology* 2004; 150(3): 363–9. doi: 10.1530/eje.0.1500363

29. Mincer, D. L. & Jialal, I. *Hashimoto thyroiditis*. In: Statpearls [Internet]. Treasure Island, FL: Statpearls Publishing, 2020.

30. Thangaratinam, S., Tan, A., Knox, E., et al. Association between thyroid autoantibodies and miscarriage and preterm birth: meta-analysis of evidence. *BMJ* 2011; 342: d2616. doi: 10.1136/bmj.d2616

31. Ghafoor, F., Mansoor, M., Malik, T., et al. Role of thyroid peroxidase antibodies in the outcome of pregnancy. *Journal of the College of Physicians and Surgeons—Pakistan* 2006; 16(7): 468–71. doi: 7.2006/jcpsp.468471

32. Negro, R., Formoso, G., Mangieri, T., et al. Levothyroxine treatment in euthyroid pregnant women with autoimmune thyroid disease: effects on obstetrical complications. *Journal of Clinical Endocrinology & Metabolism* 2006; 91(7): 2587–91. doi: 10.1210/jc.2005-1603

33. Ozdemir, O., Yenicesu, G. I., Silan, F., et al. Recurrent pregnancy loss and its relation to combined parental thrombophilic gene mutations. *Genetic Testing and Molecular Biomarkers* 2011; 16(4): 279–86. doi: 10.1089/gtmb.2011.0191

34. Nelen, W. L., Steegers, E. A., Eskes, T. K. & Blom, H. J. Genetic risk factor for unexplained recurrent early pregnancy loss. *Lancet* 1997; 350(9081): 861. doi: 10.1016/S0140-6736(97)24038-9

35. Zetterberg, H. Methylenetetrahydrofolate reductase and transcobalamin genetic polymorphisms in human spontaneous abortion: biological and clinical implications. *Reproductive Biology &Endocrinology* 2004; 2: 7. doi: 10.1186/1477-7827-2-7

36. Tara, S.-S., Ghaemimanesh, F., Zarie, S., et al. Methylenetetrahydrofolate reductase C677T and A1298C polymorphisms in male partners of recurrent miscarriage couples. *Journal of Reproductive Infertility* 2015; 16(4): 193–8.

37. Raziel, A., Kornberg, Y., Friedler, S., et al. Hypercoagulable thrombophilic defects and hyperhomocysteinemia in patients with recurrent pregnancy loss. *American Journal of*

Reproductive Immunology 2001; 45(2): 65–71. doi: https://doi.org/10.1111/j.8755-8920.2001.450201.x

38. Dong, Y. & Yu, J.-L. An overview of morbidity, mortality and long-term outcome of late preterm birth. *World Journal of Pediatrics* 2011; 7(3): 199–204. doi: 10.1007/s12519-011-0290-8

39. Yu, H.-F., Chen, H.-S., Rao, D.-P. & Gong, J. Association between polycystic ovary syndrome and the risk of pregnancy complications: a PRISMA-compliant systematic review and meta-analysis. *Medicine (Baltimore)* 2016; 95(51): e4863. doi: 10.1097/MD.0000000000004863

40. Naver, K. V., Grinsted, J., Larsen, S. O., et al. Increased risk of preterm delivery and pre-eclampsia in women with polycystic ovary syndrome and hyperandrogenaemia. *BJOG* 2014; 121(5): 575–81. doi: 10.1111/1471-0528.12558

Chapter 13

1. Gnoth, C., Frank-Herrmann, P., Schmoll, A., et al. Cycle characteristics after discontinuation of oral contraceptives. *Gynecological Endocrinology* 2002; 16(4): 307–17.

2. Steele, S. J., Mason, B. & Brett, A. Amenorrhoea after discontinuing combined oestrogen–progestogen oral contraceptives. *British Medical Journal* 1973; 4(5888): 343–5. doi: 10.1136/bmj.4.5888.343

3. Kumar, N. & Singh, A. Trends of male factor infertility, an important cause of infertility: a review of literature. *Journal of Human Reproductive Science* 2015; 8(4): 191–6. doi: 10.4103/0974-1208.170370

4. Ullmann, G., & Hammerstein, J. Inhibition of sperm motility in vitro by copper wire. *Contraception* 1972: 6(1): 71–6. doi: 10.1016/S0010-7824(72)80007-6

5. Belhadj, H., Sivin, I., Diaz, S., et al. Recovery of fertility after use of the levonorgestrel 20 mcg/d or Copper T 380 Ag intrauterine device. *Contraception* 1986; 34(3): 261–7. doi: 10.1016/0010-7824(86)90007-7

6. Committee on Adolescent Health Care Long-Acting Reversible Contraception Working Group, The American College of Obstetricians and Gynecologists. Committee opinion no. 539: adolescents and long-acting reversible contraception: implants and intrauterine devices. *Obstetrics & Gynecology* 2012; 120(4): 983–8. doi: 10.1097/AOG.0b013e3182723b7d

7. Trussell, J., Aiken, A. R. A., Micks, E. & Guthrie, K. A. Efficacy, safety, and personal considerations. In: R. A. Hatcher (Ed.), *Contraceptive technology*, 21st edn. New York, NY: Ayer Company Publishers, 2018.

8. Grimes, D. A. Intrauterine devices (IUDs). In: R. A. Hatcher, J. Trussell, A. L. Nelson et al., *Contraceptive technology,* 19th edn, pp. 117–43. New York, NY: Ardent Media, 2009.

9. Russo, A. J. Decreased zinc and increased copper in individuals with anxiety. *Nutrition and Metabolic Insights* 2001: 4; 1–5. doi: 10.4137/NMI.S6349

10. Islam, M. R. Ahmed, M. U., Mitu, S. A., et al. Comparative analysis of serum zinc, copper, manganese, iron, calcium, and magnesium level and complexity of interelement relations in generalized anxiety disorder patients. *Biological Trace Element Research* 2013; 154(1): 21–7. doi: 10.1007/s12011-013-9723-7

11. Imani, S., Moghaddam-Banaem, L., Roudbar- Mohammed, S. Changes in copper and zinc serum levels in women wearing a copper TCu-380A intrauterine device. *European Journal of Contraception and Reproductive Health Care* 2014; 19(1): 45–50. doi: 10.3109/13625187.2013.856404

12. CooperSurgical Inc. Paragard safety information. Online; accessed 15 July 2020. https://www.paragard.com/safety-information

13. Frank-Herrmann, P., Heil, J., Gnoth, C., et al. The effectiveness of a fertility awareness-based method to avoid pregnancy in relation to a couple's sexual behaviour during the fertile time: a prospective longitudinal study. *Human Reproduction* 2007; 22(5): 1310–19. doi: 10.1093/humrep/dem003

14. Pallone, S. R. & Bergus, G. R. Fertility awareness-based methods: another option for family planning. *Journal of The American Board of Family Medicine* 2009; 22(2): 147–57. doi: 10.3122/jabfm.2009.02.080038

15. Hatcher, R. A., Trussell, J., Stewart, F., et al. *Contraceptive technology*, 18th rev. edn. New York, NY: Ardent Media, 2004.

Final word

1. Joham, A.E, Boyle, J.A, Ranasinha, S., et al. Contraception use and pregnancy outcome in women with polycystic ovary syndrome: data from the Australian Longitudinal Study on Women's Health. *Human Reproduction* 2014; 29(4): 802–8.

2. Hudecova, M., Holte, J., Olovsson, M. & Sundström Poromaa, I. Long-term follow-up of patients with polycystic ovary syndrome: reproductive outcome and ovarian reserve. *Human Reproduction* 2009; 24(5): 1176–83. doi: 10.1093/humrep/den482

Glossary

ACTH	adrenocorticotropic hormone
AMH	anti-Müllerian hormone
ATA	American Thyroid Association
BBT	basal body temperature
BCAA	branched-chain amino acid
BMI	body mass index
CF	cervical fluid
CFS	chronic fatigue syndrome
CRP	c-reactive protein
DFI	DNA fragmentation index
DHEA-S	dehydroepiandrosterone sulfate
DHT	dihydrotestosterone
FAM	fertility awareness method
FSH	follicle-stimulating hormone
GI	glycemic index
HA	hypothalamic amenorrhea
Hb1Ac	glycolated hemoglobin, a measure of blood sugar levels over time
HBC	hormonal birth control
hCG	human chorionic gonadotropin
HIIT	high-intensity interval training
HSG	hysterosalpingogram
IBS	irritable bowel syndrome
IGF-1	insulin-growth factor
IUD	intrauterine device
IUI	intrauterine insemination
IVF	in-vitro fertilization
kcal	(kilo)calories

LH	luteinizing hormone
LPS	lipopolysaccharide
MTHFR	methyltetrahydrofolate reductase (enzyme)
NAC	N-acetylcysteine
NCAH	non-congenital adrenal hyperplasia
NCGS	non-celiac wheat/gluten sensitivity
OD	ovarian drilling
OHSS	ovarian hyperstimulation syndrome
PCOS	polycystic ovary syndrome
PID	pelvic inflammatory disease
PMS	premenstrual tension syndrome
RCT	randomized controlled trial, the "gold standard" for research studies
RDA	recommended dietary allowance
rT_3	reverse T_3
SHBG	sex-hormone-binding globulin
STI	sexually transmitted infection
T_3	triiodothyronine, the active form of T_4
T_4	thyroxine, a thyroid hormone
TCM	traditional Chinese medicine
TPO	thyroid peroxidase
TSH	thyroid-stimulating hormone
UTI	urinary tract infection

Resources

Downloads/links from www.thepcosnutritionist.com

Root cause identifier workshop: https://thepcosnutritionist.com/rootcause

PDF printout for BBT: https://thepcosnutritionist.com/chart

List of prenatal formulas: https://thepcosnutritionist.com/prenatals

Downloads from other websites

2018 PCOS guidelines: https://www.monash.edu/__data/assets/pdf_file/0004/1412644/PCOS_Evidence-Based-Guidelines_20181009.pdf

Dr. Jerrilyn Prior and the Centre for Menstrual Cycle and Ovulation Research, PDF handout on cyclical progesterone therapy (micronized progesterone): https://www.cemcor.ubc.ca/resources/cyclic-progesterone-therapy

Video of how The Stork works: https://www.youtube.com/watch?v=qBN9FyTrQ6s

Endometriosis UK PDF download: https://www.endometriosis-uk.org/sites/default/files/files/Information/consultation_questionnaire.pdf

Cyrex Laboratories Array 4 gluten-sensitivity test: https://www.cyrexlabs.com/CyrexTestsArrays (you'll need a practitioner to order this for you)

Podcasts

Chantelle's podcast: https://thepcosnutritionist.com/e21

Ciara's podcast: https://thepcosnutritionist.com/e27

Danah's podcast: https://thepcosnutritionist.com/e2

Destynne's podcast: https://thepcosnutritionist.com/e30

Dimity's podcast: https://thepcosnutritionist.com/e6

Sara's podcast: https://thepcosnutritionist.com/e9

Kellie-Anne's podcast: https://thepcosnutritionist.com/e32

Apps

Blue light f.lux for Mac laptop: https://justgetflux.com/

Blue light blocker for Android: https://play.google.com/store/apps/

details?id=com.eyefilter.nightmode.bluelightfilter&hl=en_NZ

1 Giant Mind free meditation app: https://www.1giantmind.com

Meditation Minis podcasts: http://meditationminis.com

Books

Briden, Laura, *Period Repair Manual: Every woman's guide to better periods*, MacMillan, 2018

Hendrickson Jacks, Lisa, *The Fifth Vital Sign: Master your cycles & optimize your fertility*, Fertility Friday Publishing Inc., 2019

Nichols, Lily, *Real Food for Gestational Diabetes*, https://realfoodforgd.com/book/

Nichols, Lily, *Real Food for Pregnancy: The science and wisdom of optimal pre-natal nutrition*, https://realfoodforpregnancy.com/book/

Weschler, Toni, *Taking Charge of Your Fertility*, https://www.tcoyf.com/taking-charge-of-your-fertility/

Acknowledgments

To all the wonderful women I've worked with as clients, who have generously shared their stories on the podcast and allowed me to include them in this book, especially Danah, Ciara, Chantelle, Destynne, Dimity, Francesca, Sarah and Kellie-Anne. Your stories are what bring these concepts to life and help other women see that there is hope for them. Thank you so much.

Thanks to my team, who make it possible to do such wonderful work, for having as much passion for our women with PCOS as I do. Special thanks to Sophia and Rodge for your help with the writing process, for your book cover ideas and opinions, and for giving me the space to get on with another round of book updates while you held down the fort.

Thanks to everyone in the Point Publishing team who helped me so much. To have an idea for a book and a draft is very different from having a book that's actually going to be helpful and engaging, so thank you for getting me here. Special thanks to my publishing manager, the wonderful Debra, for patiently allowing me to update references right until the last moment(!), and for bringing your incredible publishing experience to help me make this book a valuable resource for women with PCOS. It is really appreciated.

And, finally, to my wonderful family, friends and Scott for your unwavering support and patience hearing about 'the book' for 18 long months!

Index

164, 249
embryo transfer 78–79, 91–92
endometriosis 79, 94, 110, 168, 171–72,
    269–71
    causes 272
    diagnosis 271
    links to PCOS and infertility 76, 271–72
    symptoms 272
endometrium *see* uterine lining (uterine bed)
environment factors 33, 34–35, 40, 41–42,
    120
Environmental Working Group, "Dirty
    Dozen" 122
epigenetics 120
erythritol 152
estrogen 27–28, 53, 67, 68, 73, 75, 140, 214,
    215, 260
estrogen breakthrough bleeding 215
estrogen mimickers 123
European Society of Human Reproduction
    and Embryology 92
exercise 13, 15, 37, 41, 45, 58, 66, 82, 164,
    166, 186, 188, 189, 190
    best types for PCOS 202–03
    effect of too much exercise 43, 122, 187,
        198–200
    endurance exercise 10, 31, 44, 109, 167,
        199, 200, 202, 203
    exercising to lose weight is wrong
        approach 10–11, 200–01, 209
    high-intensity exercise 11, 167, 199, 200,
        201, 202–03
    how much to do 201–02
    low-intensity exercise 72, 203
    resistance exercise 89–90
expectations 84, 204

F
facial hair 24, 25, 26, 39, 49, 243, 260, 273,
    274, 275
families 35, 44
fatigue 15, 23, 72, 73, 75, 87, 100, 102, 108,
    113, 150, 169, 212, 245, 270, 297
fats, dietary 134, 137, 144, 148, 161, 167,
    246–47
FatSecret 165, 167
Femara (letrozole) 74–75, 76, 82
FemCap 267
fertile window 82–83, 140–41, 208–11,
    213–14, 216, 226, 266, 267
fertility assistance 81–86, 93–94

see also fertility medications; intrauterine
    insemination (IUI); in-vitro fertilization
    (IVF); surgery
fertility awareness method (FAM) 211–17,
    267, 294, 298–99, 300
fertility decision tree 264
fertility medications 32, 66–77
    risks 87–91
fertility process and ingredients 16–17,
    26–27, 39–40, 42–43, 45, 58, 85, 210
    see also infertility
    improving by increasing vegetable
        intake 131–33
fight-or-flight hormone (adrenaline) 42, 105,
    188
folate 88, 124–25, 235, 254–55, 277–78,
    279
follicle-stimulating hormone (FSH) 28, 67,
    68, 75, 104, 106, 259, 260, 276
    in PCOS 29–30, 40, 48, 217
follicles *see* "cysts" in PCOS; eggs; ovulation
fruit in the diet 129

G
gastric bypass or sleeve 79–80
genes 33–34, 35, 36, 40–41
genetic mutation 278
gestational diabetes 85, 91, 281–82
ghrelin 146
Glucophage *see* metformin
glucose 11, 38, 50, 74, 92, 99, 199–200
    fasting blood glucose 72, 101, 102, 142,
        197
    impact of stress 99, 109, 111
    insulin and blood sugar
        rollercoaster 143–44, 154–55, 163–64
    oral glucose challenge 101, 102
glutathione 125–26, 236, 247, 248
gluten 168–70, 171–72
glycemic index (GI) 147, 155
gonadotropins 75–76, 78, 90
    see also human chorionic gonadotropin
        (hCG)
Gram-negative bacteria 272
gut health 42, 49, 53, 89, 129, 132–33, 153,
    169, 244–45, 250, 268–69

H
hair growth 23, 24, 42, 45, 48, 150, 203, 243,
    260, 273
hair loss 23, 24, 26, 39, 42, 48, 113, 203, 274

Made in the USA
Las Vegas, NV
06 April 2021

20873688R00204